Critical Care Pearls

STEVEN A. SAHN, M.D.

Professor of Medicine
Director, Division of Pulmonary
  and Critical Care Medicine
Medical University of South Carolina
Codirector, Medical Intensive Care Unit
Medical University Hospital
Charleston, South Carolina

JOHN E. HEFFNER, M.D.

Associate Professor of Medicine
Division of Pulmonary
  and Critical Care Medicine
Medical University of South Carolina
Codirector, Medical Intensive Care Unit
Medical University Hospital
Charleston, South Carolina

HANLEY & BELFUS, INC.,/Philadelphia
THE C.V. MOSBY COMPANY/St. Louis • Toronto • London

Publisher: HANLEY & BELFUS, INC.
                210 S. 13th Street
                Philadelphia, PA 19107

North American and worldwide sales and distribution:

                THE C.V. MOSBY COMPANY
                11830 Westline Industrial Drive
                St. Louis, MO 63146

In Canada: THE C.V. MOSBY COMPANY
                120 Melford Drive
                Scarborough, Canada M1B 2X5

CRITICAL CARE PEARLS   ISBN 0-932883-24-9

Library of Congress catalog card number 89-84782

Last digit is the print number: 9 8 7 6 5 4 3 2 1

Dedication

To our wives,

Ellie Sahn
Ann Heffner

for their love, patience, and understanding,

And our parents,

Irwin and Mildred Sahn
Jack and Hazel Heffner

for their inspiration and support.

CONTENTS

CONTRIBUTORS

Robert J. Anderson, M.D.
Professor of Medicine, University of Colorado Health Sciences Center; Chief, Medical Service, Denver Veterans Administration Medical Center, Denver, Colorado

Blase A. Carabello, M.D.
Professor of Medicine, Medical University of South Carolina; Staff Cardiologist, Charleston Veterans Administration Medical Center, Charleston, South Carolina

Nelson S. Gwinn, M.D.
Fellow in Cardiology, Medical University of South Carolina, Charleston, South Carolina

Jan V. Hirschmann, M.D.
Associate Professor of Medicine, University of Washington School of Medicine; Medical Service, Seattle Veterans Administration Medical Center, Seattle, Washington

Randy L. Howard, M.D.
Fellow in Renal Diseases, University of Colorado Health Sciences Center, Denver, Colorado

Jerome E. Kurent, M.D.
Assistant Professor of Neurology, Medical University of South Carolina; Attending Neurologist, Medical University Hospital, Veterans Administration Hospital, and Charleston Memorial Hospital, Charleston, South Carolina

William M. Lee, M.D.
Professor of Medicine, and Director, Division of Gastroenterology, Medical University of South Carolina; Medical University Hospital, Charleston, South Carolina

Maurie Markman, M.D.
Vice Chairman, Department of Medicine, Memorial Sloan-Kettering Cancer Center, New York, New York

Thomas A. Raffin, M.D.
Associate Professor of Medicine; Acting Chief, Division of Respiratory Medicine; and Assistant Chief of Medicine, Stanford University School of Medicine, Stanford, California

Bruce W. Usher, M.D.
Professor of Medicine, Division of Cardiology, Medical University of South Carolina, Charleston, South Carolina

Gary P. Zaloga, M.D.
Associate Professor of Anesthesia (Critical Care) and Medicine (Endocrinology), Bowman Gray School of Medicine, Wake Forest University; Attending Physician, Critical Care, Baptist Hospital, Winston-Salem, North Carolina

FOREWORD

I have always believed that practicing medicine (or whatever line of "work" one has chosen) should be fun. Learning about medicine should be fun, too. However, reading about a disease in a standard text or dissecting a research study can also be tedious. *Critical Care Pearls* returns to a traditional method of teaching which is both very instructive and also "fun."

Traditionally, medicine is taught through study and discussion of actual patients and their problems (so-called "cases"). The individual patient becomes the framework on which to hang the information regarding a particular disease process or clinical problem. This framework allows the perpetual student of medicine to select the most salient aspects of such a discussion (and hopefully to be able to recall them at some later time). Not only are common features of the disease process that the patient illustrates easier to remember, but atypical aspects often prove useful as well. Atypical or unusual aspects allow one to more readily remember the usual presentation along with important exceptions and give the student an idea of the variability that commonly occurs when dealing with human disease.

I was delighted, then, by the appearance of both this book and its predecessor, *Pulmonary Pearls*. These volumes are extremely welcome at a time when case reports are disappearing from the literature or seem limited to bizarre and uncommon presentations or complications, and when the patient presentation is often eliminated from Grand Rounds. Steve Sahn and John Heffner have organized these critical care case reports, discussions, and clinical pearls around the problems commonly seen in intensive care units. The cases selected reflect the major categories of critical care which were covered in the first American Board of Internal Medicine Examination in Critical Care Medicine. I found the discussions very readable and educational. They obviously were written by physicians with practical experience in the management of such problems. The method of listing the clinical pearls at the end of the discussion is particularly useful in helping the reader to summarize the take-home messages.

I found reading these "critical care pearls" not only a painless method of learning but actually a very enjoyable way to learn or review important aspects of critical care medicine. In other words, it was fun and instructive too.

LEONARD D. HUDSON, M.D.
Professor of Medicine
Head, Division of Pulmonary
   and Critical Care Medicine
University of Washington
Harborview Medical Center
Seattle, Washington

PREFACE

Critical Care Medicine has come of age in the 1980s. Previously an offshoot of various medical and surgical specialties, the management of critically ill patients has matured into a unified discipline with broad-based educational requirements, specialized therapies, and singular ethical dilemmas. These unique qualities, in addition to an emphasis on technological innovations, physiologic monitoring, and interventional procedures, often foster the mistaken impression that critical care medicine is somehow different in principle and practice from more traditional branches of medicine. In reality, the management of critically ill patients requires the same basic physician skills common to all medical specialties: astute bedside observation, careful differential diagnosis, and analytical therapeutic decision-making.

Critical Care Pearls is dedicated to these fundamental skills. Expert contributors representing the major disciplines in critical care medicine present 100 patient cases written as brief clinical summaries. The reader is challenged to formulate a differential diagnosis, diagnostic approach, and therapeutic plan, much as the critical care specialist is challenged during actual clinical practice. In most instances, the case presentation is accompanied by an illustration. The diagnosis is discussed succinctly on the following pages with an emphasis on unifying basic principles and highlighting unique and interesting aspects of the patients' courses. The major topics achieving "pearl" status are listed at the end of the discussion for easily accessible future reference. The extensive informational content and comprehensive indexing allow *Critical Care Pearls* to serve as a reference resource.

We anticipate that *Critical Care Pearls* will be stimulating and enjoyable reading for a broad range of physicians from the house officer during his initial intensive care unit experience to the seasoned critical care specialist seeking to update and fortify his management skills. As proved true for this book's companion volume, *Pulmonary Pearls*, the case summary format will assist physicians in studying for critical care board certification examinations.

We and the contributing authors wish to acknowledge the help of our friends and colleagues in the completion of this book. Specifically, the tireless efforts of Terri Kelly, Louisa Cory, and Jeanne Jaeger were indispensable and extraordinary. The advice, guidance, and support of our exceptional publishers, Jack Hanley and Linda Belfus, were greatly valued and appreciated. And most importantly, we recognize our patients, whose trust and faith in our critical care skills inspire us to be our best.

STEVEN A. SAHN, M.D.
JOHN E. HEFFNER, M.D.

CHAPTER 1

Pulmonary Medicine

Steven A. Sahn, M.D.
John E. Heffner, M.D.

PATIENT 1

A 49-year-old man with fever, delirium, and myoclonic jerks

A 49-year-old man was transferred from a psychiatric hospital to the medical ICU because of fever, delirium, and uncontrollable myoclonic jerks. One week earlier he had required admission for depression with an episode of psychosis. He improved with imipramine hydrochloride, 150 mg, and haloperidol, 10 mg, but several days later noted muscle rigidity that prevented walking. He quickly progressed to diaphoresis, delirium, myoclonus, and severe tremors.

Physical Examination: Temperature 100.3°; pulse 120; respirations 32; blood pressure 178/102. Thin male with agitated delirium, severe tremors, and frequent myoclonic jerks. Chest: diffuse basilar rales. Heart and abdomen: unremarkable. Neurologic: diffuse muscular rigidity without focal signs.

Laboratory Findings: Hct 37%; WBC 15,300/μl; ABG (room air): pH 7.52, PCO_2 28 mm Hg, PO_2 56 mm Hg; SGOT 125 IU/L (normal 8 to 30 IU/L); CPK 4,265 IU/L (normal 0 to 155 IU/L). Chest radiograph: bilateral alveolar infiltrates predominantly in lower lung zones. ECG: sinus tachycardia.

What are the major diagnostic considerations and your approach to therapy?

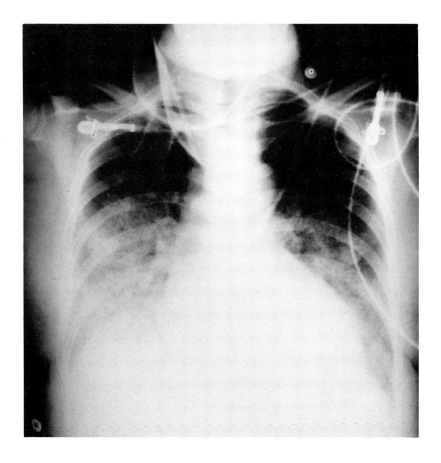

Diagnosis: Neuroleptic malignant syndrome with adult respiratory distress syndrome.

Discussion: Antipsychotic drugs (neuroleptics) are widely used for the control of agitation and psychosis because they combine the capacity to sedate, tranquilize, inhibit aggressive behavior, and control the bizarre thinking of psychosis while they preserve the higher intellectual functions. Unfortunately, adverse reactions are numerous. Anticholinergic effects are frequent, causing a wide range of extrapyramidal symptoms and dystonias. Tardive dyskinesia is a serious movement disorder that may be irreversible. Neuroleptic malignant syndrome is a rare yet potentially lethal complication that may present in a sudden and unpredictable fashion.

Neuroleptic malignant syndrome is characterized by muscular rigidity, hyperpyrexia, delirium, akinesia, and autonomic dysfunction manifested by tachycardia, labile hypertension, excessive sweating, sialorrhea, and cardiac arrhythmias. Fever may be as high as 106° and consciousness may alternate between coma and delirium with periods of alertness. Increased creatinine phosphokinase, liver function tests, and leukocytosis ranging from 15,000 to 30,000/μl are the major laboratory findings.

Drugs commonly associated with neuroleptic malignant syndrome include haloperidol, fluphenazine decanoate, chlorpromazine, thiothixene, and piperazine phenothiazine. The probability of developing neuroleptic malignant syndrome does not appear to be related to either the dose of the drug or the presence of drug interactions.

Young adult males are most commonly affected, and the presence of brain disorders, treatment with depot-injection preparations, physical exhaustion, heat stress, or dehydration appears to predispose to the condition. The overall mortality is 20 to 38% and the course is often complicated by cardiac arrhythmias, myocardial infarction, aspiration pneumonia, and thromboembolic disease. Rhabdomyolysis may be severe and precipitate myoglobinuria with renal failure. Occasional instances of the adult respiratory distress syndrome have been reported, as occurred in the present patient.

The etiology of neuroleptic malignant syndrome is unknown. A proposed mechanism suggests that neuroleptic agents impair dopaminergic function by blocking central dopaminergic receptor sites, thereby generating hyperpyrexia and muscle rigidity. It is also uncertain whether neuroleptic malignant syndrome is a specific entity or a variant of malignant hyperthermia, a condition characterized by skeletal muscle hypermetabolism and abnormal calcium transfer across the sarcoplasmic reticulum. Malignant hyperthermia is most commonly associated with administration of halogenated inhalational anesthetic agents and depolarizing muscle relaxants such as succinylcholine, and has a shorter duration compared with neuroleptic malignant syndrome (3 to 5 days versus 5 to 30 days).

There is no specific therapy for neuroleptic malignant syndrome. Supportive measures include cooling, correction of acid-base and electrolyte abnormalities, brisk diuresis to avoid myoglobinuric renal failure, and ventilatory assistance. Presynaptic dopamine agonists, such as amantadine hydrochloride, and anticholinergic agents, such as diphenhydramine hydrochloride, have been tried with only partial success. More encouraging results have been noted with dantrolene sodium, which inhibits calcium release from muscle storage sites in the sarcoplasmic reticulum, thereby reversing muscular rigidity. Dantrolene has proven especially beneficial for patients with malignant hyperthermia syndrome. Additional drugs that have been employed for neuroleptic malignant syndrome include bromocryptine mesylate, a postsynaptic dopamine agonist, and pancuronium, a curariform agent that prevents muscular rigidity and rhabdomyolysis through its paralyzing effects.

The present patient underwent supportive therapy that included intubation and mechanical ventilation. He improved only transiently with decreased muscular rigidity after receiving benztropine mesylate and diphenhydramine, but improved with dantrolene sodium. He did not develop myoglobinuric renal failure, and subsequently recovered with resolution of respiratory failure.

Clinical Pearls

1. Neuroleptic malignant syndrome occurs after the initiation of antipsychotic agents most commonly in young adult males, does not relate to drug dose, and presents with fever, muscular rigidity, tremors, and autonomic dysfunction.

2. Rhabdomyolysis with myoglobinuric renal failure is a major complication of the syndrome.

3. Dantrolene sodium can improve muscular rigidity by blocking calcium release from sarcoplasmic reticulum.

REFERENCES

1. Tollefson G: A case of neuroleptic malignant syndrome: In vitro muscle comparison with malignant hyperthermia. J Clin Psychopharmacol 2:266–270, 1982.
2. Sangal R, Dimitrijevic R: Neuroleptic malignant syndrome: Successful treatment with pancuronium. JAMA 254:2795–2796, 1985.

PATIENT 2

A 22-year-old man with chest pain and hemoptysis following an automobile accident

A 22-year-old man was involved in an automobile accident while driving to work. He was briefly unconscious at the scene but was alert during transport to the hospital. His major complaints were dyspnea, left anterior chest pain, and minimal hemoptysis.

Physical Examination: Temperature 98.9°; pulse 125; respirations 30; blood pressure 143/88. The patient periodically expectorated blood-streaked sputum. Bruises were apparent over the forehead and left pectoralis region. Chest: diffuse rales, increased resonance in left chest, and consolidative findings over left mid lung field posteriorly. Cardiac: normal. Neurologic: normal.

Laboratory Findings: CBC, electrolytes, and renal indices were normal. Chest radiograph after chest tube placement for a left pneumothorax: bilateral alveolar infiltrates without rib fractures. ECG: normal.

Hospital Course: The patient remained afebrile and had an uneventful course until the third hospital day when he expectorated brown sputum that was negative on Gram stain. Chest radiograph (below): left-sided alveolar infiltrates with multiple air-fluid levels (arrow).

The patient's course is compatible with which pulmonary disorder?

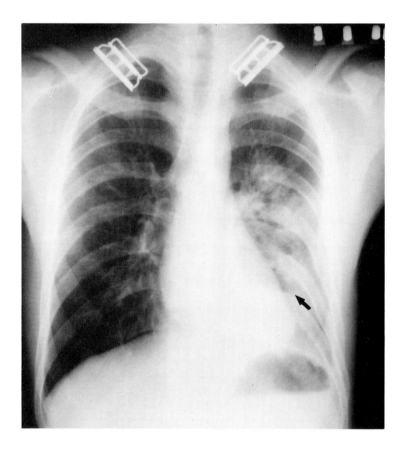

Diagnosis: Lung contusion and laceration with traumatic pneumatocele.

Discussion: Blunt chest trauma is associated with several disorders of the lung parenchyma. Pulmonary contusion is the most common, occurring in up to 70% of patients sustaining severe nonpenetrating chest trauma. The contusion consists of hemorrhage and edema formation in the alveoli and interstitium of the lung in the absence of parenchymal disruption. Shock waves and lung compression appear to disturb capillary permeability in local regions where the impact is most severely focused, thereby causing heightened membrane permeability.

The chest radiograph in pulmonary contusion typically ranges from patchy, ill-defined alveolar infiltrates to extensive regions of homogeneous consolidation. The infiltrate is most frequently located near the region of maximal chest trauma, but it can also develop at distant sites, including the contralateral lung, when a contrecoup effect occurs. Lung contusions are radiographically apparent in 70% of patients within 1 hour of trauma and invariably within 6 hours. A new pulmonary infiltrate occurring after this time period in a trauma victim suggests an alternate diagnosis. Most patients with contusions do well. Minimal hemoptysis occurs in 50% of patients and dyspnea with hypoxemia may occur if the contusion is extensive. Resolution of the infiltrate begins within 2 to 3 days but may require several weeks for complete resolution.

Pulmonary lacerations are rare complications of blunt chest trauma but can develop when the forces causing lung contusion are particularly severe or shearing. Traumatic airway closure contributes by promoting compression of alveolar gas that may result in an explosive regional injury. Lacerations may also result from penetrating injuries from the ends of broken ribs. Lung lacerations frequently extend through the pleural surface, presenting with a bronchopleural fistula and hemopneumothorax, and requiring thoracostomy tube drainage, although intrapulmonary lacerations without pleural manifestations also occur.

Hemorrhage within a laceration that is confined within the lung causes a localized pulmonary hematoma that appears radiologically as a spherical infiltrate with margins that are better defined than those of a pulmonary contusion. Hemoptysis occurs more frequently and to a greater degree than with contusion. The infiltrate related to a lung hematoma may require several weeks to clear and may present as a solitary pulmonary nodule months following the trauma.

Traumatic pneumatoceles may complicate pulmonary lacerations that are confined to the pulmonary parenchyma, although they are the least frequent pulmonary manifestation of blunt trauma. The intrinsically elastic lung contracts from the region of lung rupture and forms one or more cystic lesions from 2 to 14 cm in diameter and often contains air-fluid levels. Pneumatoceles may appear on admission chest radiographs immediately after trauma or present several hours or days later, as occurred in the present patient. Delayed presentation probably results for several reasons: (1) the pneumatoceles are initially thin-walled and may not contrast well on plain films; (2) coexisting contusion may obscure the cavities; and (3) the barotrauma of mechanical ventilation may promote progression of a simple laceration to a pneumatocele.

The radiographic appearance of traumatic pneumatoceles varies. One half of these lesions are cystic with or without air-fluid levels. If intracavitary hemorrhage occurred, they may appear solid with well-demarcated borders compatible with a pulmonary hematoma. Pneumatoceles usually have a benign course, although 4 to 6 months may be required for complete radiographic resolution. Occasionally superinfection occurs, progressing to a lung abscess. Antibiotics, however, should be withheld unless patients have clear signs of infection.

The present patient continued clinically well despite his impressive chest radiograph. A chest ultrasound excluded the possibility of pleural fluid. The radiographic abnormalities resolved after 7 months.

Clinical Pearls

1. Pulmonary lacerations contained within the lung present as pulmonary hematomas or traumatic pneumatoceles.

2. Pulmonary infiltrates from lung contusion develop within 6 hours of chest trauma and clear over the following few days. Later onset of infiltrates suggests alternate diagnoses.

3. Traumatic pneumatoceles may be single or multiple and often present several days after trauma.

REFERENCES

1. Shackford SR: Blunt chest trauma: The intensivist's perspective. J Intens Care Med 1:125–136, 1986.
2. Williams JR, Bonte FJ: Pulmonary damage in nonpenetrating chest injuries. Radiol Clin North Am 1:439–451, 1963.
3. Ganske JG, Dennis DL, Vanderveer JB: Traumatic lung cyst: Case report and literature review. J Trauma 21:493–496, 1981.

PATIENT 3

A 47-year-old woman with sudden cyanosis and coma after uterine dilatation and curettage

A 47-year-old woman underwent a uterine dilatation and curettage under epidural anesthesia for menorrhagia. After the brief procedure, she became suddenly agitated, diaphoretic, and cyanotic in the recovery room, lapsing into coma. She was promptly intubated and manually ventilated.

Physical Examination: Temperature 99.9°; pulse 44; respirations 22; blood pressure 82/64. Chest: scattered bibasilar rales. Cardiac: a "churning" murmur over left sternal border. Neurologic: unresponsive with midpoint pupils and left lateral gaze.

Laboratory Findings: ABG (100% O_2 Ambu bag): pH 7.32, PCO_2 28 mm Hg, PO_2 72 mm Hg. Chest radiograph after intubation: bilateral, diffuse alveolar infiltrates.

Consider the probable underlying diagnosis and your immediate course of action.

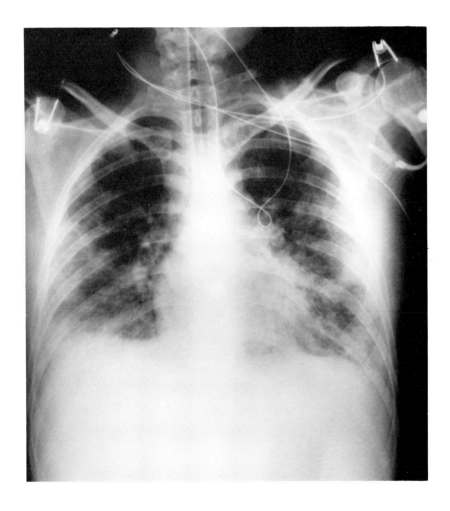

Diagnosis: Venous air embolism with paradoxical arterial embolization.

Discussion: The sudden occurrence of unexplained cardiopulmonary dysfunction with neurologic findings during or soon after a surgical procedure should suggest the possibility of venous air embolism. Introduction of small volumes of air into the venous circulation is a common event in surgical patients that is usually well tolerated. Whenever a surgical wound disrupts veins, creating a blood-air interface that lies above the level of the right atrium, there is a potential for negative intravascular pressure to create venous air emboli. Sensitive Doppler echocardiographic techniques demonstrate that 40% of patients undergoing cesarean section and 20 to 40% of craniotomy patients experience some degree of air embolization. Additional clinical situations associated with venous air emboli include epidural anesthesia (especially in pregnant women), cardiac pacemaker insertion, central line placement or manipulation, percutaneous needle aspiration of the lung, trauma, and positive pressure ventilation.

Patients remain asymptomatic during the progression of venous air emboli until sufficient air collects in the right ventricle and pulmonary arteries to cause pulmonary hypertension through a "vapor lock" effect that interferes with right ventricular outflow. Systemic hypotension and hypoxemia result, which are occasionally associated with noncardiogenic pulmonary edema, as occurred in the present patient. Paradoxical arterial air embolization may further complicate the course of these patients. The clinical impact of air in the arterial circulation is less dependent on the volume of air infused than on the particular organ to which air is embolized. Small volumes of air in the cerebral or coronary arteries are sufficient to cause major tissue infarction. Paradoxical emboli result from several mechanisms. As venous emboli increase right atrial pressure, a patent foramen ovale may open, thereby creating a right-to-left shunt through which air reaches the arterial circulation. Considering that 20 to 30% of the normal population have a potentially patent foramen ovale, this mechanism is a major cause of paradoxical arterial air emboli. As pulmonary hypertension progresses, precapillary pulmonary arteriovenous shunts are recruited, allowing an additional route of air emboli to the arterial circulation. Although the lung is considered an effective sieve for air bubbles, further increases in pulmonary artery pressure eventually force air emboli through the pulmonary microcirculation.

Diagnosis of venous air embolism requires awareness that the condition can occur after virtually any surgical procedure. Cardiac examination may demonstrate the classic "mill-wheel," murmur, as occurred in this patient. Chest radiographs may occasionally reveal lucencies in the pulmonary artery, and chest CT scans may demonstrate intracardiac air. The urgency of therapy, however, usually obviates the value of these examinations. Occasionally, aspiration of a central line catheter may return frothy blood or frank air. Doppler echocardiography may detect venous air bubbles as small as 0.25 ml, promoting the value of this technique for preventive intraoperative monitoring of surgical patients for the onset of air emboli.

Once venous air emboli are suspected, the patient should be quickly placed in the extreme left lateral decubitus position with the chest dependent so as to position intraventricular air away from the pulmonary outflow tract. Aspiration of a central line may allow removal of air. Transfer of the patient to a hyperbaric chamber may decrease the size of the intravascular bubbles, restoring tissue oxygenation and perfusion pending resorption of air. Patients sustaining intraoperative venous air emboli while undergoing nitrous oxide anesthesia should have the anesthetic immediately discontinued; nitrous oxide is 20 times more soluble than oxygen or nitrogen and diffuses rapidly into air bubbles, increasing their size.

The present patient was rapidly placed in a left-lateral tilt, head-down position by the critical care team. An internal jugular central line was placed and 200 ml of frothy blood was aspirated. Ventilation with 100% oxygen was continued, and the patient recovered within 30 minutes without neurologic sequelae.

Clinical Pearls

1. Patients are at risk for air emboli in any condition that disrupts veins, allowing a blood-air interface above the level of the right atrium.

2. Some degree of asymptomatic venous air emboli occurs in up to 40% of patients undergoing cesarean section or craniotomy in the upright position.

3. Paradoxical arterial air emboli result when venous air traverses a patent foramen ovale, precapillary pulmonary arteriovenous shunts, or the pulmonary microcirculation. The degree of arterial embolization correlates with the severity of pulmonary hypertension.

REFERENCES

1. Kizer KW, Goodman PC: Radiographic manifestations of venous air embolism. Radiology 144:35–39, 1982.
2. Gottdiener JS, Papademetriou V, Notargiacomo A, et al: Incidence and cardiac effects of systemic venous air embolism: Echocardiographic evidence of arterial embolization via noncardiac shunt. Arch Intern Med 148:795–800, 1988.

PATIENT 4

A 28-year-old man with dyspnea and hypotension 8 days after thoracic spine injury

A 28-year-old man was admitted to the trauma unit after sustaining a cerebral contusion and a thoracic spine injury in an automobile accident that left him paralyzed below the waist. After 3 days he was progressively more alert and began complaining of shortness of breath. Arterial blood gases and a chest radiograph were normal. Physicians reassured the patient after a lung scan (below left) was interpreted as "low probability" with matching subsegmental defects. He did well until 8 days after the accident when he became suddenly dyspneic, diaphoretic, and hypotensive.

Physical Examination: Temperature 100.9°; pulse 132; respirations 32; blood pressure 85/67. Chest: normal. Cardiac; second heart sound was widely split at the cardiac apex with an S_4 gallop. Lower extremities: paraplegic without edema.

Laboratory Findings: ABG (50% O_2 mask): pH 7.45, PCO_2 30 mm Hg, PO_2 62 mm Hg. Chest radiograph: bibasilar atelectasis; pulmonary angiogram (below right): pulmonary emboli.

How would you proceed with the management of this patient?

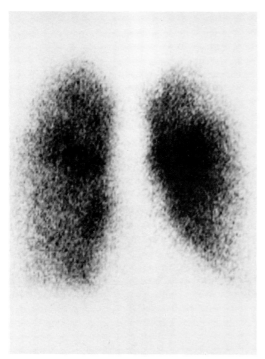 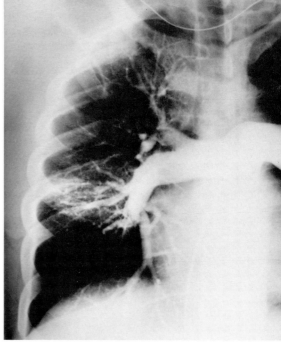

Diagnosis: Massive pulmonary thromboemboli with shock.

Discussion: Trauma patients are predisposed to deep venous thrombosis (DVT) and resultant pulmonary emboli (PE), with a 4 to 22% incidence of PE during initial hospitalization. Spinal injuries with head trauma are particularly associated with thromboembolic disease, with reported frequencies as high as 22%. Spinal cord disruption further increases risk: 90% of patients with complete paralysis develop DVT. The pathophysiology of DVT in trauma results from venous endothelial injury (which may occur in regions distant from the site of trauma), stasis in areas of trauma or due to immobilization, and the hypercoagulable state that develops in trauma. Stasis appears to be a particularly important factor, considering that the incidence of DVT increases with the duration of bedrest after injury: 19% after 4 days to 47% on day 7, and 90% in patients confined to bed for 28 days.

Diagnosis of PE is difficult in trauma patients because associated injuries may obscure clinical manifestations, and patients with altered mental status are unable to report symptoms. The high incidence of PE warrants its careful consideration in any trauma victim who manifests cardiopulmonary dysfunction. The initial evaluation in most patients is a lung scan, even though associated chest trauma may complicate interpretation. A normal lung scan excludes the diagnosis with equal sensitivity as a normal pulmonary angiogram. A high probability lung scan in a patient with clinical suspicion of PE is sufficient to initiate therapy unless the patient is at high risk for hemorrhagic complications of anticoagulation or if fibrinolytic therapy or inferior vena cava interruption is a consideration. In these circumstances, the diagnosis should be confirmed with pulmonary angiography. Low probability or intermediate probability lung scans, as occurred in the present patient, do not adequately diminish the possibility of PE to exclude the diagnosis. As many as 25 to 45% of patients with low probability scans actually have PE.

Diagnosis of PE in patients with nondiagnostic lung scans may be assisted by tests to detect lower extremity DVT, in that most emboli in trauma originate from the legs. Impedence plethysmography can detect 95% of fresh clots at the level of the popliteal veins or above and can be performed in the ICU. Unfortunately, injuries to the pelvis or legs may cause false-positive examinations or prevent placement of electrodes. Radiofibrinogen leg scanning, which identified 95% of DVT below mid thigh, is less applicable in acute thromboses because it requires serial examinations over 24 hours and may be falsely negative in patients receiving heparin. Doppler ultrasonic flow detectors are primarily limited to DVT below the knee. Contrast venography may assist diagnosis when noninvasive studies are inconclusive; this study requires transfer of trauma patients to the radiology department and may present difficulties in interpretation. Normal leg studies are found in 50% of patients with PE and do not exclude the diagnosis. Further investigation with pulmonary angiography is required.

The present patient underwent immediate pulmonary angiography because of the suspicion of massive PE that mandated confirmation of clot by angiography in anticipation of fibrinolytic therapy or inferior vena cava interruption. Massive PE is defined in hemodynamic terms as any anatomic degree of pulmonary vascular obstruction that results in circulatory insufficiency, particularly shock. Patients with previously normal cardiopulmonary function require obstruction of more than 50% of their pulmonary circulation before shock develops, whereas patients with comorbid conditions, such as congestive heart failure or emphysema, may incur circulatory collapse with smaller thromboembolic episodes.

The high mortality of patients with massive PE and shock, which is 33% (or 5 times the mortality of submassive PE), dictates urgent diagnosis and aggressive therapy. Although controversial, fibrinolytic agents are recommended for patients with PE and hemodynamic compromise because radiographic and hemodynamic evidence for clot resolution proceeds more rapidly than with heparin. No clear benefit in reducing mortality, however, has been demonstrated in any patient group, and therapy is contraindicated in many trauma patients because of hemorrhagic risk. Interruption of the inferior vena cava with a Greenfield filter can be performed with minimal morbidity and is indicated in trauma patients along with heparin in massive PE or without heparin in patients with contraindications to anticoagulation. Despite earlier impressions, these devices have good long-term patency rates and are usually not associated with the later development of collateral routes for PE, since embolic recurrences are probably less than 3%. The 50% mortality in massive PE attached to acute embolectomy, which is higher than that with heparin therapy, warrants avoiding this procedure unless shock is intractable to pressors and fluids during the first hour of therapy.

As often occurs in massive PE, the present patient stabilized during the first hour of therapy. Recent trauma contraindicated fibrinolytic therapy and the patient was managed with heparin and a Greenfield filter.

Clinical Pearls

1. Injury of the spinal cord is a major predisposition to thromboemboli, with 90% of paraplegic patients developing DVT.

2. The probability of PE with a low probability lung scan may be as high as 25 to 45%.

3. Development of shock from PE requires obstruction of 50% of the pulmonary circulation in patients with preexisting normal cardiopulmonary function.

REFERENCES

1. Shackford SR, Moser KM: Deep venous thrombosis and pulmonary embolism in trauma patients. J Intens Care Med 3:87–98, 1988.
2. Kanter B, Moser KM: The Greenfield vena cava filter. Chest 93:170–175, 1988.
3. Mohr DN, Ryu JH, Litin SC, Rosenow EC III: Recent advances in the management of venous thromboembolism. Mayo Clin Proc 63:281–290, 1988.

PATIENT 5

A 63-year-old woman with progressive dyspnea and stridor

A 63-year-old woman with a heavy smoking history was admitted because of a 2-week history of progressive dyspnea and stridor.

Physical Examination: Temperature 99°; pulse 125; respirations 35; blood pressure 150/90. The patient was diaphoretic and agitated with loud inspiratory stridor. She was able to speak short phrases with a normal voice between breaths. Chest: tubular breath sounds over the right upper lobe. Lymph nodes: abnormal nodes in both supraclavicular fossae.

Laboratory Findings: Hct 36%, WBC 8,600/μl. ABG (40% face mask): pH 7.31, PCO_2 69 mm Hg, PO_2 185 mm Hg. Chest radiograph: right upper lobe mass with widening of superior mediastinum.

What disorder is associated with inspiratory stridor and a preserved voice in a patient with a lung mass?

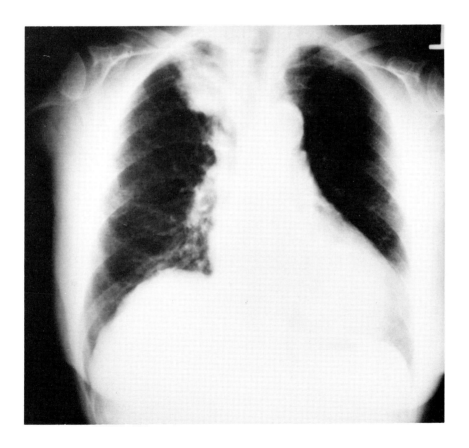

Diagnosis: Bilateral vocal cord paralysis resulting from lung cancer invading both recurrent laryngeal nerves.

Discussion: Unilateral vocal paralysis is a familiar mode of presentation for patients with lung cancer. Extension of tumor into the mediastinum disrupts the recurrent laryngeal nerve, causing denervation paralysis of the vocal cord. Patients develop hoarseness and occasionally symptoms related to aspiration, but upper airway obstruction is distinctively absent because the contralateral functioning vocal cord is able to abduct away from the midline during inspiration. The left vocal cord is more commonly involved because of the circuitous route of the left recurrent laryngeal nerve that enters the chest and circumnavigates the aortic arch. Various conditions, such as mediastinal tumor, left atrial or pulmonary outflow tract enlargement, and aortic aneurysms, are able to compress the nerve, thereby paralyzing the left vocal cord.

It is less well recognized that the right recurrent laryngeal nerve also traverses the thorax, placing it at jeopardy for injury from intrathoracic disorders. It enters from the neck and courses around the right subclavian artery at the level of the thoracic inlet. Right-sided Pancoast tumors or metastases to the right superior mediastinum may cause unilateral right vocal cord paralysis. It follows that extensive superior mediastinal cancer may disrupt both recurrent laryngeal nerves and cause bilateral vocal cord paralysis, as occurred in the present patient.

The functional consequences of bilateral and unilateral vocal cord paralysis differ significantly. In bilateral paralysis, both cords are adducted in the midline of the airway. During exhalation, the cords passively abduct, being pushed aside by positive airway pressure. Because of the neutral position of the cords in the midline, the voice may be relatively preserved. During inspiration, however, the flaccid cords abut, acting as one-way valves, thereby obstructing the airway. Varying degrees of stridor develop that may result in respiratory failure. Additional symptoms in less severely affected patients include nocturnal stridor, monotone voice, and conscious suppression of cough and laughter. Bilateral vocal cord paralysis may simulate aspirated foreign bodies or airway obstruction from laryngotracheal tumors, although these conditions typically have a component of expiratory stridor.

Visualization of the vocal cords can quickly confirm the presence of bilateral vocal cord paralysis. Severe instances of stridor and respiratory failure necessitating emergency intubation, however, may require timely consideration of the diagnosis so that cord function can be noted during placement of the airway. Although occasional patients may tolerate bilateral vocal cord paralysis, maintaining normal ventilation, most patients require intubation for management of airway obstruction. Patients can then be converted to a tracheotomy for long-term management, and a one-way valve can be attached to the tracheotomy tube to allow exhalation through the normal airway and preservation of speech. Rarely, radiation or chemotherapy directed at the mediastinal tumor may return function to one or both cords if the nerve was only compressed as opposed to disrupted by direct neoplastic invasion. More commonly, the vocal cord paralysis is permanent.

Several surgical procedures are available to allow removal of the tracheotomy tube. Surgical or laser arytenoidectomy with lateralization of a vocal cord removes sufficient glottic obstruction to allow ventilation, although patients may lose their voice. Newer surgical techniques involving reinnervation and arytenoidectomy without vocal cord displacement are considered in selected patients, since voice preservation is a potential benefit.

The present patient underwent translaryngeal intubation by fiberoptic bronchoscope. The trachea appeared normal but a right upper lobe tumor was biopsied, demonstrating small cell cancer. She did well with a tracheotomy, but vocal cord function did not improve after chemotherapy.

Clinical Pearls

1. Bilateral vocal cord paralysis results in inspiratory stridor that may progress to respiratory failure. Voice may be relatively preserved, because the paralyzed cords meet in the midline of the airway.

2. Although bilateral vocal cord paralysis may simulate aspirated foreign body or upper airway tumor, these latter conditions usually have a component of expiratory stridor.

3. The right recurrent laryngeal nerve enters the thoracic inlet and courses around the subclavian artery before returning to the larynx. This route places it at jeopardy for disruption by mediastinal tumors.

REFERENCES

1. Shaw GL: Airway obstruction due to bilateral vocal cord paralysis as a complication of stroke. South Med J 60:1432–1433, 1987.
2. Neel HB, Townsend GL, Devine KD: Bilateral vocal cord paralysis of undetermined etiology. Ann Otol 61:514–519, 1972.

PATIENT 6

A 59-year-old man with abdominal pain, diarrhea, and fever following corticosteroid and radiation therapy for adenocarcinoma

A 59-year-old Vietnam veteran was admitted with weight loss, dyspnea, and confusion. Bronchoscopy demonstrated an obstructing adenocarcinoma in the right upper lobe, and CT scanning detected two intracranial metastases with associated cerebral edema. The patient improved with dexamethasone and began radiation therapy to his head and mediastinum. Ten days later he experienced abdominal pain, low-grade fever, and diarrhea, which were followed 2 days later by the sudden onset of fever, confusion, dyspnea, and hypotension. He required intubation and transfer to the ICU.

Physical Examination: Temperature 103.2°; pulse 129; respirations 22; blood pressure 89/64 on pressors. Chest: diffuse rales over the lower lung fields. Abdomen: bowel sounds absent, moderate abdominal tenderness.

Laboratory Findings: Hct 36%; WBC 13,000/μl with 60% PMNs, 30% bands, and 10% lymphocytes. Chest radiograph: right paratracheal mass (smaller since admission) and bilateral alveolar infiltrates. Central line catheter and endotracheal tubes correctly positioned. Blood cultures were positive for *E. coli.*

What laboratory test should be urgently ordered?

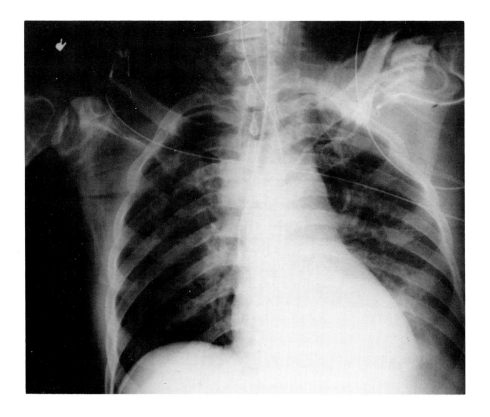

Answer: Stool examination for ova and parasites in consideration of *Strongyloides stercoralis* hyperinfection with associated gram-negative sepsis.

Discussion: Strongyloides stercoralis is a nematode that causes chronic infestation of the intestinal tract, producing varying degrees of abdominal pain, weight loss, and diarrhea. Because of the unique life cycle of Strongyloides which allows the organism to reproduce and mature entirely within the human host, immunocompromised patients can develop intense infection with a heavy intestinal burden of organism that is termed "hyperinfection." This condition produces a clinical picture of severe vomiting and diarrhea, abdominal pain, shock, respiratory failure, and gram-negative bacteremia, which may be a source of diagnostic confusion.

Strongyloides is present worldwide predominantly in tropical and subtropical zones. Initial infection results when filariform larvae contained in feces or contaminated soil penetrate the skin. The larvae then travel in venous blood to the lungs where they penetrate alveoli, gaining access to the tracheobronchial tree. They are then expectorated and swallowed, thereby entering the intestinal tract. In the proximal small bowel, adult worms develop and burrow into the intestinal wall where they lay eggs that hatch into rhabditiform larvae. These larvae may then be expelled in stool back into the soil where they metamorphose into filariform larvae, perpetuating the infectious form of the parasite and ensuring transmission to additional human hosts.

As eggs hatch, some rhabditiform larvae transform within the gut lumen into infective filariform larvae. These may then burrow directly into the gut wall or perianal skin and continue another life cycle migration through the lungs, establishing a new wave of adult worms in the small intestine. This process is termed "autoinfection" and allows Strongyloides to persist for as long as 30 years in patients without a subsequent reexposure to endemic regions. Additionally, factors that accelerate this autoinfection cycle, such as immunocompromise or prolonged intestinal transit times from ileus, can promote progressively more severe infections that lead to hyperinfection and disseminated disease.

Most patients maintain a tolerable burden of parasites by immunologic mechanisms that limit the degree of infection. Numerous conditions that result in compromised cell-mediated immunity, however, can attenuate these protective defenses and predispose patients to hyperinfection. Neoplastic disease, malnutrition, coexisting severe chronic infections, or immunosuppressive medications such as corticosteroids are responsible for most instances of hyperinfection.

A classic complication of hyperinfection strongyloidiasis is the development of bacterial sepsis. Repeated penetration of the intestinal wall by burrowing filariform larvae allows bowel flora either to seep into the bloodstream or be carried on or within the larvae. Subsequent bacteremia is distinctive in its constant nature, possibly because the larvae secrete bacteria into the blood, and may present with persistent sepsis syndrome, meningitis, or pneumonia.

Hyperinfection strongyloidiasis in the immunocompromised host may progress to disseminated disease when the migrating filariform larvae enter organs not normally a part of the worm's life cycle. Almost any organ can be involved, including liver, kidney, heart and brain, but the typical feature of disseminated infection is pulmonary infiltrates with pneumonitis. In these tissues the filariform larvae can mature into adult worms that may be present on biopsied specimens.

Diagnosis depends on considering the disorder in at-risk patients who develop persistent sepsis or pulmonary infiltrates in the setting of gastrointestinal symptoms. Because chronic disease can last decades, exposure histories should be carefully obtained. Eosinophilia is a common feature of chronic strongyloides, but is frequently absent in hyperinfection because of corticosteroid therapy or the effects of acute inflammation. Stools should be examined for rhabditiform larvae, and the presence of filariform larvae is strong evidence for hyperinfection. Because stool examinations are positive in only 20% of seriously ill patients with hyperinfection, duodenal aspirates should be performed, which are usually positive. In disseminated disease, sputum, transbronchial biopsy samples, or specimens from other infected organs may contain larvae or worms.

Because strongyloidiasis may be rapidly fatal, therapy should be initiated rapidly with thiabendazole. Immunosuppressive agents should be discontinued or tapered if clinically possible. Repeat stool examinations or duodenal aspirates should be monitored for parasites during therapy because thiabendazole is not universally effective and hyperinfection may recur after its discontinuation.

The present patient had a positive stool examination for both rhabditiform and filariform larvae. Endotracheal aspirates were also positive for parasites. Despite broad-spectrum antibiotics and the timely institution of thiabendazole, the patient died 48 hours later of unremitting sepsis.

Clinical Pearls

1. *Strongyloides stercoralis* is unique among human parasites for causing autoinfection that is associated with hyperinfection and disseminated disease.

2. Hyperinfection is associated with gram-negative sepsis that is often continuous in nature, possibly because larvae excrete bacteria into the bloodstream.

3. The presence of pulmonary infiltrates and persistent sepsis in the immunocompromised host with preexisting abdominal complaints should suggest strongyloidiasis.

REFERENCES

1. Scowden EB, Schaffner W, Stone WJ: Overwhelming strongyloidiasis. An unappreciated opportunistic infection. Medicine 57:527–544, 1978.
2. Barrett-Connor E: Parasitic pulmonary disease. Am Rev Respir Dis 126:558–563, 1982.

PATIENT 7

A 65-year-old man with congestive cardiomyopathy and transient pulmonary edema during weaning from mechanical ventilation

A 65-year-old man with severe congestive cardiomyopathy returned to the ICU after undergoing three-vessel coronary artery bypass graft surgery. He was initiated on assist-control mechanical ventilation (TV 800 ml, R 12/min, FiO_2 0.50, and PEEP 5 cm H_2O), resulting in excellent ABG values. The next morning the patient's chest radiograph showed cardiomegaly with clear lung fields (below left). ABG on the above ventilator settings were pH 7.39, PCO_2 40 mm Hg, PO_2 125 mm Hg. He was placed on a "T-piece" with an FiO_2 of 0.50 and did well for 15 minutes when he became diaphoretic, hypotensive, and hypoxic with a PO_2 of 59 mm Hg. The chest radiograph (below right) now demonstrated pulmonary edema. He improved 20 minutes later after reinitiation of mechanical ventilation. A Swan-Ganz catheter was placed showing the following parameters: PCW 22 mm Hg and CI 1.5 l/min/m².

Physical Examination: Pulse 115; respirations 15; blood pressure 98/65. Alert. Chest: bibasilar rales. Cardiac: S_3 with diffuse precordial impulse.

Laboratory Findings: Spontaneous ventilatory parameters: V_T 350 ml, VC 950 ml, V_E 9.5 L/min, negative inspiratory force (NIF) –25 cm H_2O.

Why did the patient suddenly decompensate on the T-piece during spontaneous respiration yet improve so quickly on the ventilator?

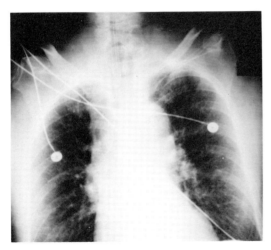 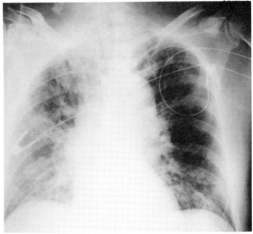

Answer: The patient developed cardiogenic pulmonary edema after the left ventricular unloading effects of positive airway pressure were removed.

Discussion: Positive pressure respiration with a mechanical ventilator or a mask that delivers continuous positive airway pressure (CPAP) is an effective means of improving arterial oxygenation in many patients with respiratory failure. The heart and lungs, however, work as a functional unit, and it is often difficult to predict the total physiologic benefit of therapy directed at the lungs without considering its cardiovascular impact. The hemodynamic effects of positive airway pressure are complex and multifactorial with clinical outcomes that depend on the adequacy of the patients' preexisting cardiac function and the status of their intravascular volume.

The principal determinants of cardiac stroke volume are ventricular preload, myocardial contractility, and ventricular afterload. Considering that the heart is contained within the thorax surrounded by the lungs, it is logical that variations of pleural pressure during respiration affect intracardiac pressures, thereby altering preload and afterload. Right ventricular preload, which is defined as end-diastolic intraventricular volume, is reduced because increased intrathoracic pressure decreases the venous gradient for right atrial filling. The resultant decreased right ventricular stroke volume may subsequently diminish left ventricular preload and cardiac output.

Increased intrathoracic pressure also raises pulmonary resistance which increases right ventricular afterload. The normal right ventricle compensates by increasing end-diastolic volume which maintains stroke volume. In certain circumstances, however, the compensatory increase in right ventricular volume bulges the interventricular septum leftward, encroaching on left ventricular volume and thereby reducing preload. This reduction in left ventricular diastolic compliance is further aggravated by high levels of PEEP that surround the intact pericardium, causing a pericardial constrictive effect. Cardiac function may be improved with the use of dopamine or dobutamine if reduction in intrathoracic pressure is not feasible. Dobutamine may have theoretical advantages since dopamine may increase wedge pressures by 50% in hypoxic respiratory failure.

Reduction of biventricular preload and increased right ventricular afterload in combination are usually considered to potentially reduce cardiac output in mechanically ventilated patients. In certain patients with poor left ventricular function and high left ventricular filling volumes, positive intrathoracic pressure may actually improve cardiac output by decreasing left ventricular afterload. Afterload is defined as the force or tension required in the ventricular wall during systole to maintain stroke volume. Since intrathoracic pressure is applied to the outside of the heart, it reduces the transmural ventricular pressure necessary to maintain any given cardiac output. In the setting of poor myocardial function and an increased pulmonary capillary wedge pressure, mechanical ventilation may not only reduce preload but also unload the left ventricle, thereby improving cardiac performance. Additionally, reflex decreases in heart rate in patients undergoing positive pressure ventilation may improve myocardial ischemia.

Augmentation of left ventricular function by positive airway pressure does not require mechanical ventilation. Spontaneously breathing patients with pulmonary edema have been noted to involuntarily "grunt" during exhalation, thereby raising airway pressure and improving cardiac output. Similarly, it appears that mean airway pressure may be more important than the pressure waveform in determining hemodynamic effects. CPAP masks, therefore, have been employed in cardiogenic pulmonary edema and found to improve cardiac output. Work of breathing may also be improved because of effects of positive pressure in improving functional residual capacity.

Despite fulfilling extubation criteria based on spontaneous ventilatory parameters and ABG values, patients with cardiomyopathy and high filling pressures should be suspected of having cardiotonic unloading effects from mechanical ventilation. Sudden extubation could result in pulmonary edema, as occurred in the present patient. Patients should receive maximal cardiac therapy and possibly undergo a transitional phase with CPAP before the complete withdrawal of ventilatory assistance if cardiac failure is still suspected.

The present patient improved with the reinstitution of positive pressure ventilation. After 24 hours of more vigorous diuresis, the wedge pressure decreased to 18 mm Hg, and the patient weaned without difficulty.

Clinical Pearls

1. Positive intrathoracic pressure may impair cardiac output through reduction of biventricular preload.

2. Patients with impaired left ventricular function and high filling pressures may experience improved cardiac output on positive pressure ventilation because of left ventricular unloading.

3. Consider weaning on positive pressure, such as with CPAP, in patients receiving benefit from left ventricular unloading effects of mechanical ventilation.

REFERENCES

1. Pinsky MR, Matuschak GM, Itzkoff JM: Respiratory augmentation of left ventricular function during spontaneous ventilation in severe left ventricular failure by grunting: An auto-EPAP effect. Chest 86:267–269, 1984.
2. Rasanen J, Nikki P, Heikkila J: Acute myocardial infarction complicated by respiratory failure: The effects of mechanical ventilation. Chest 85:21–28, 1984.

PATIENT 8

A 28-year-old man with shortness of breath and a flail chest following trauma

A 28-year-old male construction worker was admitted to the ICU after a one-story fall from scaffolding. He complained of severe sternal and left-sided thoracic pain that made breathing difficult.

Physical Examination: Pulse 111; respirations 25; blood pressure 125/85. Patient was alert but grimacing in pain during respiration. Chest: marked paradoxical movement of the sternum and left chest; breath sounds barely audible above the patient's groans.

Laboratory Findings: ABG (40% mask O_2): pH 7.34, PCO_2 42 mm Hg, PO_2 76 mm Hg. Chest radiograph: a left-sided pulmonary infiltrate, mediastinal and subcutaneous emphysema, and multiple rib fractures.

What criteria dictate whether the patient should be intubated and mechanically ventilated for management of his large flail chest?

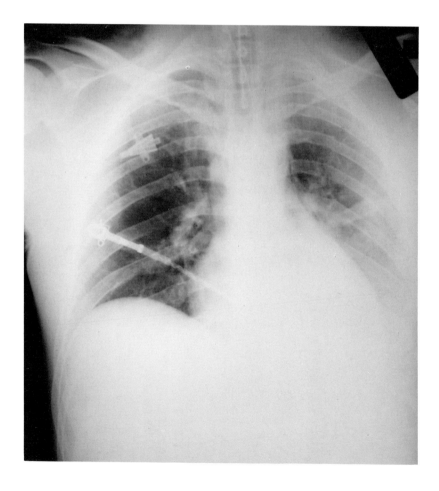

Answer: The decision to intubate a patient with a flail chest is determined by the presence of accompanying respiratory failure. Even a major flail chest is not by itself an indication for assisted ventilation if the patient maintains adequate respiration.

Discussion: Management techniques for flail chest injuries have evolved over the last two decades. Traditional concepts emphasized the pathophysiologic importance of paradoxical chest wall motion. In instances of severe unilateral flail chest, inspired gas was thought to flow from the lung affected by the flail into the normal hemithorax and back during expiration into the paradoxically moving flail lung. This pendulum-like gas flow *(pendulufft)* from one lung to the other was considered to increase dead space ventilation, thereby decreasing effective alveolar ventilation.

Based on these pathophysiologic concepts, therapeutic goals focused on stabilization of the thorax to prevent paradoxical chest wall motion. Sand bags with towel clips were employed in addition to surgical procedures with implants that repaired broken ribs and sternums. Later, intubation with mechanical ventilation provided the concept of "internal pressure splints" for chest wall stabilization. Because patients were considered to require several weeks to recover from flail chests, they received controlled ventilation with positive end-expiratory pressure (PEEP), undergoing early tracheotomy to prevent paradoxical chest wall motion. They were considered for extubation and spontaneous ventilation only after resolution of the flail chest.

Unfortunately, aggressive measures to stabilize flail chests did not improve mortality in blunt thoracic injuries. In fact, patients managed with prolonged mechanical ventilation developed nosocomial pneumonia that further complicated their course. Present therapeutic techniques are based on observations that the degree of respiratory compromise does not correlate with the severity of chest wall flail injury, and that respiratory failure most commonly occurs in patients with direct lung injuries, such as contusions, or with underlying pulmonary compromise, such as emphysema. Furthermore, the improved understanding that pendulufft respiration, although a logical concept, probably does not occur has deemphasized the importance of chest wall stabilization in flail chest.

The present approach requires that the physician evaluates how well the patient tolerates the flail chest injury. Spontaneously breathing patients who do not demonstrate respiratory compromise can be carefully observed. Bronchial hygiene is best managed with aggressive analgesia utilizing intercostal nerve blocks and epidural anesthesia, timing respiratory therapy and coughing exercises to periods of maximum pain control. The decision to intubate and ventilate is determined by the presence of respiratory failure with impaired gas exchange, which is defined by the same criteria as respiratory failure from any other cardiopulmonary disorder. Mechanical ventilation is directed at improving gas exchange rather than primarily stabilizing the unstable chest wall. Patients are aggressively weaned from the ventilator when they can support spontaneous respiration regardless of the status of paradoxical thoracic movement. Borderline patients with flail chest injuries not clearly in respiratory failure may be supported with continuous positive airway pressure (CPAP) masks for short periods until ventilation improves, thereby avoiding intubation.

The ideal mode of mechanical ventilation in flail chest is not yet defined. Surgical recommendations have emphasized the importance of intermittent mandatory ventilation (IMV) with PEEP, although no controlled studies have compared advantages of IMV to assist-control ventilation in flail chest. Cited studies are uncontrolled and compare IMV with older series employing prolonged controlled mechanical ventilation. It appears that assist-control and IMV would be equally successful as long as the physician recognizes the therapeutic principles of ventilating patients selectively who are in need of improved gas exchange and weaning patients aggressively as respiratory function allows.

The present patient sustained a flail chest with a left pulmonary contusion. Despite his discomfort, he ventilated adequately with acceptable ABG and did not require intubation. He became more comfortable with initiation of epidural analgesia, maintaining good pulmonary toilet and recovering with an uncomplicated course.

Clinical Pearls

1. Patients with flail chest injuries should be intubated and ventilated selectively as dictated by the presence of respiratory failure because the severity of the chest wall injury does not correlate with the degree of respiratory dysfunction.

2. Respiratory failure is more likely in flail chest if patients have accompanying lung injuries (contusion) or preexisting pulmonary conditions (emphysema).

3. Regardless of the status of paradoxical chest wall movement, wean patients from mechanical ventilation when recovery from respiratory insufficiency allows.

REFERENCES

1. Shackford SR, Virgilio RW, Peters RM: Selective use of ventilator therapy in flail chest injury. J Thorac Cardiovasc Surg 81:194–201, 1981.
2. Cullen P, Modell JH, Kirby RR, Klein EF Jr, Long W: Treatment of flail chest: Use of intermittent mandatory ventilation and positive end-expiratory pressure. Arch Surg 110:1099–1103, 1975.

PATIENT 9

A 23-year-old woman with massive hemoptysis following cocaine inhalation

A 23-year-old woman previously in good health was admitted with severe dyspnea and massive hemoptysis. She noted exertional dyspnea 3 weeks earlier accompanied by one episode of minimal hemoptysis that spontaneously resolved. The night before admission she had smoked a cigarette laced with free-base cocaine. The next morning she experienced the sudden onset of severe dyspnea and hemoptysis, which totaled "several" cups of blood.

Physical Examination: Temperature 102°; pulse 141; respirations 60; blood pressure 144/50. Chest: decreased breath sounds at the right lung base with coarse rales in both upper lung zones. Cardiac: normal. Neurologic: normal.

Laboratory Findings: Hct 15.2%; WBC 17,300/μl with 76% PMNs, 8% eosinophils; platelets 602,000/μl; prothrombin time 12 sec; partial thromboplastin time 29 sec. Peripheral blood smear: normal. Urinalysis: normal. ABG (room air): pH 7.32, PCO_2 25 mm Hg, PO_2 45 mm Hg. Chest radiograph: diffuse, bilateral alveolar infiltrates.

What is the most likely diagnosis, considering the patient's previously negative pulmonary history?

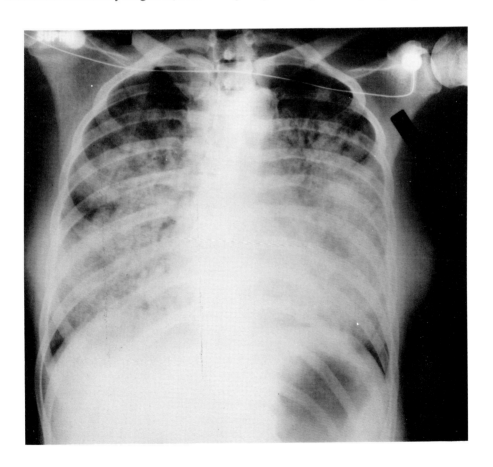

Diagnosis: Pulmonary hemorrhage and respiratory failure from inhalation of free-base cocaine.

Discussion: Cocaine addiction has reached epidemic proportions in the United States. Thirty million Americans have used the drug at least one time and an additional 5 million are habitual abusers. As cocaine has become more available, the purity of the street drug has risen, while the per gram cost is at an all-time low. Additionally, during the last 5 years, cocaine abuse has evolved from intranasal, recreational use to hardline addiction with the alkaloid form ("free-base" or "crack"). Free-base cocaine is obtained by extracting the drug from the solvent layer of a mixture of cocaine hydrochloride, an alkaline solution (baking soda), and a solvent (ether or alcohol), resulting in a nearly pure form of the drug. Injected intravenously or smoked in a water pipe or cigarette, free-base cocaine causes a rapid rise of extremely high cocaine levels in the bloodstream.

The massive widespread use of cocaine has been accompanied by the public misconception that it is a relatively innocuous drug unassociated with serious adverse complications. Increasing experience with cocaine abuse, however, clearly demonstrates that it has serious medical consequences. Neurologic and psychiatric disorders are the most apparent manifestations. Patients may develop seizures, focal neurologic deficits, headaches, and loss of consciousness. Seizures are typically generalized and self-limited, although status epilepticus has occurred, resulting in chronic encephalopathies. Focal neurologic events include visual, sensory, and motor disturbances. Also, intracranial hemorrhage from drug-induced hypertension and cerebral infarction related to the vasoconstrictive effects of cocaine have been observed. Transient loss of consciousness probably results from cardiac arrhythmias. Acute psychiatric disturbances include dysphoria, agitation, assaultiveness, paranoia, psychosis, and hallucinations, which probably result from cocaine effects on neurotransmitters. These conditions usually resolve after short-term psychiatric hospitalization but may provoke more serious injury when patients overdose on other drugs after the initial cocaine or fall from heights.

Recent reports have linked cocaine to almost every form of heart disease. Ischemic events with myocardial infarction are frequent manifestations, and an association appears to exist between cocaine use, contraction bands, and sudden arrhythmic death. Ventricular tachycardia and fibrillation have both been temporally related to cocaine abuse, and it appears clear that life-threatening cardiac complications are not limited to parenteral drug use but occur perhaps even more commonly after intranasal administration. Seizures or underlying heart disease are not prerequisites for serious cardiac complications. Cocaine may also precipitate myocarditis, cardiomyopathy, and valvular heart disease, although supporting evidence is less clear.

Rhabdomyolysis is a potentially life-threatening complication of cocaine use that is unrelated to muscle trauma. Up to one-third of patients with muscle injury develop renal failure that is often associated with disseminated intravascular coagulation, profound hypotension, hyperpyrexia, and markedly elevated creatinine phosphokinase levels of 28,000 IU/L or greater.

Pulmonary complications of cocaine abuse are being increasingly recognized. Up to 25% of free-base users have respiratory complaints of dyspnea, cough, hemoptysis, and nonspecific chest pain. Pneumomediastinum and rarely pneumothorax occur as a consequence of the Valsalva maneuver that is a part of the cocaine inhalation ritual. Varying degrees of noncardiogenic pulmonary edema, including the adult respiratory distress syndrome, result from cocaine use and are clinically similar to that observed after illicit use of heroin, propoxyphene, and ethchlorvynol. Pulmonary edema occurs a few to 24 hours after cocaine use typically in young patients, and may differ from other etiologies of noncardiogenic pulmonary edema only by the occasional presence of hypercapnia, which results from drug suppression of respiratory drive.

Other respiratory conditions include rare instances of hypersensitivity lung reactions accompanied by fever, pulmonary infiltrates, pruritus, increased serum IgE, and eosinophilia. Septic lung complications are similar to those that occur with other illicit drugs that predispose to bacteremia or to aspiration pneumonia during periods of suppressed consciousness. Cocaine has intense vasoconstrictive properties, and pathologic studies demonstrate that pulmonary artery hypertrophy and hyperplasia unassociated with foreign body reactions can develop with chronic use. Lung diffusion abnormalities with decreased $D_L CO$ measurements have been reported subsequent to chronic cocaine inhalation, but recent studies discount this relationship.

Pulmonary hemorrhage with hemoptysis has been reported in one previous patient who inhaled free-base cocaine. In that instance, respiratory failure was associated with diffuse pulmonary infiltrates and eosinophilia with negative serologic studies for collagen vascular disease. Open lung biopsy demonstrated acute alveolar hemorrhage and interstitial fibrosis without evidence of vasculitis or deposition of antibasement membrane antibodies. Other pathologic studies of patients dying from cocaine abuse demonstrate numerous hemosiderin-laden macrophages in lung tissue, suggesting that occult hemorrhage may occur more commonly than recognized in cocaine addiction.

The present patient required intubation and mechanical ventilation for respiratory failure and received corticosteroids for pulmonary hemorrhage. Other causes of pulmonary hemorrhage, such as Goodpasture's disease, collagen vascular diseases, and rapidly progressive glomerulonephritis, were eventually excluded by appropriate serum and urine studies. An open lung biopsy demonstrated numerous hemosiderin-laden macrophages and collagen deposition with increased presence of interstitial eosinophils. Because of the temporal relationship with cocaine use, idiopathic pulmonary hemosiderosis seemed an unlikely diagnosis, and the patient was counseled to discontinue cocaine use.

Clinical Pearls

1. Diffuse pulmonary hemorrhage with hemoptysis is a manifestation of cocaine abuse.

2. Young patients presenting with noncardiogenic pulmonary edema should be evaluated for cocaine ingestion, particularly if hypercapnia is present.

3. Peripheral eosinophilia may be a clinical clue to cocaine use in patients with diffuse pulmonary infiltrates.

REFERENCES

1. Murray RJ, Albin RJ, Mergner W, Criner GJ: Diffuse alveolar hemorrhage temporally related to cocaine smoking. Chest 93:427–429, 1988.
2. Cucco RJ, Yoo OH, Cregler L, Chang JC: Nonfatal pulmonary edema after "freebase" cocaine smoking. Am Rev Respir Dis 136:179–181, 1987.
3. Cregler LL, Mark H: Medical complications of cocaine abuse. N Engl J Med 315:1495–1500, 1986.

PATIENT 10

A 65-year-old woman with hypertension and tachycardia after receiving a muscle paralyzing drug for control of agitation during mechanical ventilation

A 65-year-old woman required intubation and mechanical ventilation for management of respiratory failure resulting from severe emphysema. She had not slept for several nights because of cough and dyspnea. Two months before admission her FEV_1 was 0.5 L and her ABGs on 2 L/min nasal cannula oxygen were pH 7.34, PCO_2 55 mm Hg, PO_2 65 mm Hg.

Physical Examination: Pulse 138; respirations 30 (triggering the ventilator); blood pressure 95/52. The patient was agitated attempting to sit up in bed and reach for his endotracheal tube. Chest: hyperresonant, decreased breath sounds.

Laboratory Findings: Hct 52%; electrolytes normal; BUN 42 mg/dl; creatinine 2.3 mg/dl; serum theophylline level 12 µg/ml; ABG (ventilator settings: V_T = 800 ml, FiO_2 = 0.5, assist-control rate = 12/min): pH 7.32, PCO_2 50 mm Hg, PO_2 92 mm Hg. Chest radiograph: hyperexpanded lungs with good position of the endotracheal tube.

Hospital Course: Because of the patient's uncontrolled agitation, pancuronium bromide (4 mg IV) was ordered. The patient relaxed as paralysis developed, but 5 minutes later her heart rate was 175 and blood pressure 245/130.

What was a possible cause of this patient's agitation? Why did she develop hypertension and tachycardia?

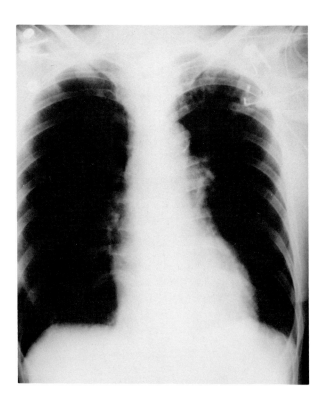

Answer: The agitation resulted from unrecognized intrinsic PEEP. The hypertensive episode was caused by a pancuronium-induced adrenergic response.

Discussion: Agitation is a frequent management problem in patients with underlying emphysema intubated for respiratory failure. Dyspnea from underlying lung disease, sleep deprivation, anxiety, confusion, underlying organic brain disorders, corticosteroids, and stress psychosis are all factors that contribute to patient excitability that may interfere with medical management. Agitation, however, may also be the presenting manifestation of medical complications of mechanical ventilation. Agitated patients, therefore, should be evaluated for pneumothorax, misplaced, occluded, or kinked endotracheal tubes, worsening pulmonary function with hypoxemia or hypercapnia, and ventilator malfunction or maladjustment.

Ventilated patients may develop agitation because of occult positive end-expiratory pressure ("auto-PEEP" or "intrinsic PEEP") that may not be measured by the ventilator airway pressure manometer. In these instances, insufficient time exists during expiration for alveolar pressure to return to zero (i.e., atmospheric pressure) before the next ventilator breath occurs. Subsequent "stacking" of breaths results in sufficiently raised alveolar pressures to cause lung hyperinflation and depressed cardiac output. This phenomenon occurs most commonly in patients with obstructive airway disease who have expiratory limitation of airflow. Intrinsic PEEP may be detected by occluding the expiratory ventilator port at end-expiration, allowing equilibration of pressures throughout the circuit and measurement of alveolar pressures on the ventilator manometer. Approaches to prevent intrinsic PEEP include keeping a low inspiratory/expiratory time ratio by increasing ventilator flow rates, decreasing tidal volumes, or attempting to decrease respiratory rate.

Frequently, patients remain agitated despite correction of aggravating medical conditions and require pharmacologic intervention to prevent self-injury. Several therapeutic options exist. Haloperidol is an especially appealing agent because it causes only minor effects on respiratory and hemodynamic function and seldom precipitates delirium in contrast to other agents such as diazepam. Its onset of action (10 to 20 min) is slower than diazepam, and increasing dosages may be required to produce the desired effect. Potential adverse reactions include extrapyramidal symptoms, which occur less commonly after the intravenous in contrast to oral route of drug administration.

Benzodiazepines are useful agents in intubated patients. Diazepam has a rapid onset of action after intravenous administration. Depression of blood pressure may be a consideration in patients with volume depletion, sepsis, or concomitant use of antihypertensive agents. It has a relatively long half-life (60 to 100 hours) and has an even longer acting metabolite, nordiazepam ($T_{1/2}$ = 100 to 200 hours) that can result in prolonged obtundation. Hepatic dysfunction further complicates its use by delaying drug metabolism. Lorazepam has advantages compared with other benzodiazepines, such as diazepam: negligible cardiopulmonary effects and a short half-life (15 hours) without any active metabolites. When combined with haloperidol, lorazepam is a particularly effective sedating agent.

Morphine is beneficial in managing agitated patients in pain because it produces sedation in addition to analgesia. However, morphine may adversely affect blood pressure, combine with other depressant drugs to cause oversedation, and aggravate delirium.

Nondepolarizing muscle relaxants are employed when sedating drugs are contraindicated or ineffective. These agents should be used reluctantly because undersedation produces a terrorizing experience and because complications (skin breakdown, deep venous thrombosis, and asphyxia during ventilator malfunction) are more likely. Pancuronium bromide is commonly used, although it is no longer the drug of choice in critically ill patients. Its muscarinic action and capacity to prevent neural reuptake of norepinephrine can generate increased heart rate and blood pressure, as occurred in the present patient. Newer agents, such as vecuronium bromide (Norcuron) and atracurium besylate (Tracrium) are devoid of any significant cardiovascular effects. Elimination of atracurium is not affected by hepatic or renal dysfunction since it breaks down spontaneously in the serum.

The present patient was administered metoprolol, a beta-blocker, intravenously and her heart rate and blood pressure stabilized. After recovery from muscle paralysis, she required sedation with low doses of lorazepam.

Clinical Pearls

1. Patients with emphysema undergoing mechanical ventilation may develop intrinsic PEEP with resulting lung hyperinflation that can manifest as agitation.

2. Pancuronium bromide prevents reuptake of norepinephrine, resulting in increased heart rate, blood pressure, and cardiac output. Vecuronium bromide and atracurium besylate are devoid of significant cardiovascular effects.

REFERENCES

1. Pepe PE, Marini JJ: Occult positive and end-expiratory pressure in mechanically ventilated patients with airflow obstruction: The auto-PEEP effect. Am Rev Respir Dis 126:166–170, 1982.
2. Griffiths RB, Hunter JM, Jones RS: Atracurium infusions in patients with renal failure on an ITU. Anaesthesia 41:375–381, 1986.
3. Tesar GE, Stern TA: Rapid tranquilization of the agitated intensive care unit patient. J Intens Care Med 3:195–201, 1988.

PATIENT 11

A 29-year-old woman with sickle C disease, back pain, fever, confusion, and respiratory distress

A 29-year-old black woman with sickle C disease was admitted with severe low back pain several days following a tracheobronchitis. The patient was gravida 3, AB 2 at 28 weeks' gestation. She was treated with analgesics and hydration.

Physical Examination: Temperature 98.9°; pulse 96; respirations 28. Alert patient in severe distress due to back pain. Splenomegaly.

Laboratory Findings: Hct 35%; WBC 15,000/μl with 80% PMNs, 15% lymphocytes. Peripheral smear: numerous target cells, a few nucleated RBCs and sickled forms. Chest radiograph: normal.

Hospital Course: Twenty-four hours following admission the patient developed a temperature to 102°, confusion, and respiratory distress. Physical examination demonstrated bronchial breathing bilaterally and conjunctival petechiae. A repeat chest radiograph is shown below.

What is the most likely diagnosis and what therapy should be instituted as soon as possible?

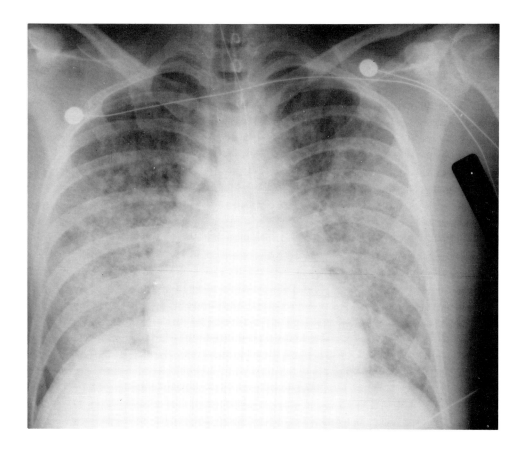

Diagnosis and Treatment: Massive fat embolism from bone marrow necrosis resulting from sickle C disease. Massive or exchange transfusion should be instituted.

Discussion: Almost all cases of the fat embolism syndrome (FES) are secondary to trauma, usually fractures of the bones of the lower extremities. Rarely, other conditions associated with FES include severe burns, diabetes mellitus, intraosseous venography, total hip replacement, seizures, corticosteroid therapy with and without fatty liver, acute osteomyelitis, pancreatitis, acute fatty liver of alcoholism, extracorporeal circulation, and bone marrow infarction with sickle cell crisis.

FES is a clinical diagnosis usually manifested by dyspnea, fever, altered mental status, and petechiae within an hour or up to 5 days following the injury; the most common time of onset is 24 to 72 hours following the event. Petechiae are most commonly found along the anterior axillary folds and in the conjunctiva and retina. The appearance of petechiae on the least dependent site is consistent with the skimming off of floating fat emboli in the blood and their selective distribution by branches arising from the top of the aortic arch. Petechiae are bilateral, appear in crops, and are visible for 6 to 24 hours. Fat may be detected in urine but is not diagnostic of FES and can be found in patients with trauma who do not develop the syndrome. Fat embolism following long bone fractures appears to be extremely common; however, only a small percentage of patients (probably less than 3%) develop the clinical syndrome.

The pathogenesis is thought to be related to bone marrow fat entering traumatically ruptured veins and circulating through the pulmonary vasculature as triglycerides. In the lung, triglycerides are converted to unsaturated fatty acids by lipase, leading to increased capillary permeability with intraalveolar hemorrhage. Catecholamine-induced lipolysis of tissue fat stores and intravascular coagulation may potentiate the syndrome.

Bone marrow necrosis in patients with sickle cell disease is a rare cause of FES and is usually fatal. The complication may be more common in SC than in SS disease and pregnancy may be an additional risk factor. Higher hematocrits and the relatively fatty marrow compared with SS disease may predispose patients with sickle C disease to bone marrow infarcts and fat embolism. The association with pregnancy may be explained by an enlarged uterus that compresses pelvic veins, elevated levels of coagulation factors, and induction of labor with posterior pituitary extract, resulting in decreased bone marrow blood flow.

Once a vasoocclusive phenomenon occurs, it may feed back in morbid fashion. Hypoxia-induced sickling leads to increased blood viscosity and capillary sludging; hypoxia from pulmonary fat emboli accelerates the cycle. Dual obstruction of pulmonary capillaries by fat and sickled cells results in a poor outcome in these patients.

Prophylactic corticosteroids may prevent FES in trauma patients with pelvic and long bone fractures: however, once FES occurs, treatment is basically supportive. The present patient developed ARDS from FES and was treated with mechanical ventilation and exchange transfusion but died within 48 hours of admission due to complications of tissue hypoxia.

Clinical Pearls

1. The fat embolism syndrome is diagnosed clinically when a known precipitating factor is followed within hours or up to 5 days by respiratory distress, altered mental status, and petechiae in nondependent regions of the upper torso.

2. The fat embolism syndrome is a rare manifestation of bone marrow necrosis in patients with sickle cell disease.

3. Patients with SC disease and near-term pregnancy appear to be at increased risk for the fat embolism syndrome.

REFERENCES
1. Shelley WM, Curtis EM: Bone marrow and fat embolism in sickle cell anemia and sickle cell-hemoglobin C disease. Bull Johns Hopkins Hosp 103:8–24, 1958.
2. Ober WB, Bruno MS, Simon RM, Weiner L: Hemoglobin S-C disease with fat embolism. Report of a patient dying in crisis: Autopsy findings. Am J Med 27:647–658, 1959.
3. Chmel H, Bertles KF: Hemoglobin S/C disease in a pregnant woman with crisis and fat embolization syndrome. Am J Med 58:563–566, 1975.
4. Shapiro MP, Hayes JA: Fat embolism in sickle cell disease. Arch Intern Med 144:181–182, 1984.

PATIENT 12

A 63-year-old woman with airway hemorrhage three weeks after placement of a tracheostomy

A 63-year-old woman was intubated for pneumonia with respiratory failure and converted to a tracheotomy after 10 days. At three weeks, while the patient was still ventilator-dependent, the nurses noted 5 to 10 ml of frank bleeding from her trachea during suctioning.

Physical Examination: Vital signs: normal. The patient was alert and cooperative. Tracheostomy stoma appeared free of infection and bleeding. Nasopharynx and oropharynx: normal except for a large-bore nasogastric feeding tube in the left nares. Chest: scattered rales.

Laboratory Findings: Hct 32%. Chest radiograph: diffuse infiltrates with a tracheotomy tube positioned 2 cm above the carina.

How would you evaluate the patient's minor degree of bleeding?

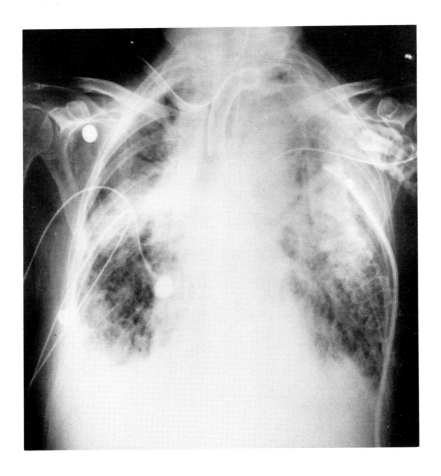

Answer: The tracheotomy tube should not be manipulated until a thoracic surgeon evaluates the patient in an operating room setting for the possibility of tracheoinnominate fistula.

Discussion: Modern tracheotomy techniques and tube design have markedly improved the management of patients who require prolonged mechanical ventilation for respiratory failure. Patients undergoing tracheotomy compared with continued translaryngeal intubation have improved comfort, enhanced ability to eat and mobilize, decreased risk of laryngeal injury, and greater opportunity to phonate and improve communication with family and medical staff. Unfortunately, tracheotomy, as with any surgical procedure performed in critically ill patients, has inherent complications that are aggravated by comorbid medical conditions and underlying debilitation.

Complications of tracheotomy occur either immediately or late in the postoperative period. Among immediate complications, inadvertent tracheal decannulation is the most serious because the stoma tract is not established for 3 to 5 days after surgery. Tube replacement attempts during this period may cause a false tract anterior to the trachea, thereby compressing and obstructing the airway. Patients experiencing earlier decannulation should be reintubated through the nose or mouth with an endotracheal tube whenever feasible. If the translaryngeal route is contraindicated or unavailable, an experienced surgeon familiar with the patient's anatomy should attempt tracheotomy tube replacement. Additional immediate complications that occur in 5% or less of patients include pneumothorax, pneumomediastinum, subcutaneous emphysema, aspiration, and incisional hemorrhage.

Delayed complications develop days to weeks after tracheotomy. Tracheal stenosis may be a source of major morbidity but occurs less frequently with high-volume, low-pressure cuffs. Nosocomial pneumonia is a concern because of the increased airway colonization incurred by patients undergoing tracheotomy compared with translaryngeal intubation.

Tracheoesophageal fistulae complicate the course of 1% of patients with tracheotomy and usually result from poorly fitted tracheotomy tubes or cuff overdistention. Malnutrition and concomitant presence of a large-bore nasogastric tube that impinges the tracheal and esophageal mucosa against the tracheotomy cuff predispose to this complication. Patients may present with obvious manifestations of aspiration or mild, nonspecific respiratory symptoms that can be misinterpreted as arising from their underlying pulmonary condition.

Tracheoinnominate fistula is the most feared late complication of tracheotomy because of its 75% mortality rate. Low placement of the tracheostomy allows the tube tip to erode into the innominate artery where it crosses the anterolateral surface of the trachea at the level of the upper sternum. Bleeding can result days or months after surgery; 50% of all tracheal bleeding longer than 48 hours after tracheotomy results from tracheoinnominate fistulae. Although the degree of bleeding may be initially minor, any tracheal blood may be the herald of sudden, massive hemoptysis. Patients with suspected tracheoinnominate fistulae should be moved to the operating room and examined by a thoracic surgeon before the tube or trachea is manipulated. If moderate to severe hemorrhage is already established, the tracheotomy cuff should be overinflated in an attempt to tamponade the artery. If unsuccessful, an endotracheal tube placed through the stoma with cuff placement adjacent to the fistula can be initiated while the patient is prepared for surgery. As a life-saving, temporizing procedure in severe hemorrhage, a finger inserted through a suprasternal notch incision can compress the artery against the sternum. Median sternotomy with resection of the necrotic section of artery is the definitive therapy. Tracheoinnominate artery fistulae can be prevented by avoiding low tracheotomies, using appropriate tube lengths that do not place the tip at the level of the innominate artery, and adequately securing the tracheotomy and ventilator hoses to avoid excessive tube movement.

The present patient was evaluated in the operating room and found to have a tracheoinnominate fistula with incipient major hemorrhage. She underwent emergency median sternotomy with successful resection of the necrotic arterial segment.

Clinical Pearls

1. Up to 50% of tracheal hemorrhages 48 hours or longer after tracheotomy result from tracheoinnominate fistulae.

2. Patients with suspected tracheoinnominate fistulae should be evaluated in the operating room because of the threat of sudden, massive hemorrhage after tube manipulation.

3. Symptoms from tracheoesophageal fistulae may be mild and nonspecific, simulating worsening of the underlying pulmonary condition.

REFERENCES

1. Heffner JE, Miller KS, Sahn SA: Tracheostomy in the intensive care unit. II. Complications. Chest 90:430–436, 1986.
2. Jones JW, Reynolds M, Hewitt RL, Drapanas T: Tracheoinnominate artery erosion: Successful surgical management of a devastating complication. Ann Surg 184:194–204, 1977.
3. Stauffer JL, Olson DE, Petty TL: Complications and consequences of endotracheal intubation and tracheostomy. Am J Med 70:65–76, 1981.

PATIENT 13

An 80-year-old man with disorientation

An 80-year-old widower was brought to the emergency room after being found by a neighbor in a disoriented state. He had been in relatively good health until he had a CVA 3 months earlier, which left him with residual hemiparesis.

Physical Examination: Temperature 89.7°; pulse 50; respirations 8; blood pressure 90/60. Chest: basilar rhonchi. Cardiac: heart sounds normal without gallops or murmurs. Neurologic: disoriented, dysarthric, sluggish pupillary responses, hyporeflexia.

Laboratory Findings: Hct 52%; WBC 5,000/μl, normal differential, platelets 120,000/μl; Na+ 132 mEq/L, K+ 5.0 mEq/L, glucose 150 mg/dl. ABG (room air): pH 7.32, PCO_2 45 mm Hg, PO_2 68 mm Hg. Chest radiograph: basilar atelectasis. ECG: shown below. Drug screen: negative.

What single diagnosis can explain the patient's presentation?

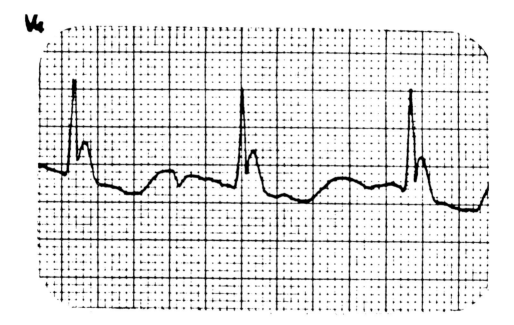

Diagnosis: Moderate (slowing) hypothermia.

Discussion: Hypothermia is defined as a core body temperature of < 95° F (35° C). Accidental hypothermia, an environmentally induced state with a high mortality, results from a spontaneous decrease in core temperature, generally in a cold environment. Most have an associated condition such as CNS disease or alcoholism. Hypothermia occurs most commonly in the elderly, the very young, and those immobilized, comatose, poisoned, or exercised to exhaustion in the cold. The elderly are susceptible to hypothermia because they have a decreased capacity to increase metabolic rate and augment heat production as needed to maintain normothermia, a limited peripheral vasoconstrictive response to cold, and decreased muscle mass. Additional predisposing factors include a high incidence of underlying disease (hypothyroidism), susceptibility to trauma, senility, and medications (phenothiazines) that impair self-protective behavior.

Emergency facilities should have a thermocouple rectal probe or specially designed thermometer capable of recording core body temperatures as low as 75° F so as to diagnose hypothermia. Clinical findings depend upon the degree of hypothermia and presence of associated conditions. Mild (responsive) hypothermia (90–95° F, 32–35° C) is characterized by increased metabolic rate, blood pressure, cardiac output, and respiratory rate. If otherwise normal, these patients can compensate physiologically for their hypothermia.

Moderate (slowing) hypothermia is defined by a body temperature < 90° F (32° C). This stage, as in the present patient, is characterized by impaired ability of the patient to generate heat. Hypoventilation and bradycardia occur, muscles stiffen, and shivering decreases. The ECG, as in the present patient, shows prolongation of the PR and QT intervals and J waves (Osborn's sign); J waves appear when the temperature is < 95° F. Cerebellar signs, cranial nerve deficits, decreased pupillary responses, and coma may develop. Tissue hypoxia leads to metabolic acidosis and, combined with the respiratory acidosis, displaces the oxygen-hemoglobin (O_2-Hgb) dissociation curve to the right, partially offsetting the left shift induced by the change in the P_{50} of Hgb. Hyperventilation or excessive bicarbonate during resuscitation can shift the O_2-Hgb dissociation curve further to the left and impair O_2 release to tissues and potentiate hypoxia. ABGs must be corrected for body temperature because gas solubilities change as a function of temperatures. As temperature decreases, the solubility of O_2 and CO_2 increases and, thus, the measured PO_2 and pH are higher than exists in the patient. For clinical purposes, however, temperature correction need to be done only for temperatures < 95° F.

Severe (poikilothermic) hypothermia is defined by core body temperatures < 86° F (30° C). The patient may be mistaken for a corpse and the differential diagnosis is death. Elderly patients have body temperatures that assume the prevailing ambient temperature.

Successful management requires early diagnosis and careful attention to rewarming. In moderate to severe hypothermia, blood volume is reduced, potentially inducing cardiac arrest with rewarming; 5% dextrose and normal saline should be given at 100–200 ml/hr with constant readjustment. Meticulous monitoring of temperature, intravascular volume, and ABGs must be done during rewarming. Passive external rewarming (PER) consists of placing the patient in a warm room and giving IV fluids at 98° F. Allowing the patient to warm at his own rate, using heat generated by the body, is preferred for the elderly and those with mild hypothermia. In severe hypothermia, PER may be too slow to prevent complications and metabolic consequences. Active external rewarming, accomplished by immersion in hot water or electric blankets, may cause a marked decreased in peripheral vascular resistance with hypotension, arrhythmias, and decreased coronary perfusion; it may be hazardous for the elderly with cardiovascular disease but may be more appropriate for the younger patient. Active core rewarming (ACR) for moderate to severe hypothermia uses inhalation of heated oxygen, peritoneal dialysis, colonic irrigation, or extracorporeal blood rewarming. Proponents of ACR claim preferential warming of the myocardium (decreasing cardiac irritability) and a more rapid return to normal core temperature. Patients should not be pronounced dead until their core temperature reaches normal following rewarming.

The present patient was placed in a warm room and given warm IV fluids with monitoring of ABGs and intravascular volume. He was discharged without new neurologic sequelae but a lower than normal body temperature.

Clinical Pearls

1. The elderly are susceptible to environmental hypothermia because they have decreased capacity to increase metabolic rate, limited muscle mass, decreased vasoconstrictive response, and a high incidence of underlying disease.

2. Therapy of hypothermia should be based on the degree of hypothermia, age of the patient, and underlying cardiovascular status.

3. Patients presenting with hypothermia should not be pronounced dead until core body temperature reaches normal with rewarming.

REFERENCES

1. Stoner HB, Frayn KN, Little RA, et al: Metabolic aspects of hypothermia in the elderly. Clin Sci 59:19–27, 1980.
2. Fitzgerald FT, Jessop C: Accidental hypothermia: A report of 22 cases and review of the literature. Adv Intern Med 27:127–150, 1982.
3. Lonning PE, Skulberg A, Abyholm F: Accidental hypothermia. Acta Anaesthesiol Scand 30:601–613, 1986.

PATIENT 14

A 59-year-old woman with Guillain-Barré syndrome, pulmonary embolism, and a discolored finger

A 59-year-old woman with Guillain-Barré syndrome of 1 week's duration was transferred to our hospital on a ventilator for plasmapheresis. Several hours after her second plasmapheresis she developed acute dyspnea, diaphoresis, and tachycardia. ABGs showed a widened A-a O_2 gradient. Ventilation/ perfusion lung scan revealed a high probability for pulmonary embolism with multiple mismatched segmental perfusion defects. The patient was given a bolus of heparin and begun on a continuous heparin infusion at 1000 U/hour. Clinical status improved. Five days later it was noted that the patient's right fifth finger was discolored but not cold. Radial and ulnar arteries were palpable, as were digital arteries of other digits.

Laboratory Findings: Hct 30%; WBC 12,500/μl with 87% PMNs, 10% lymphocytes; platelet count 130,000/μl; PT 13.4 sec, PTT 44.8 sec; BUN 8 mg/dl, Na+ 134 mEq/L, K+ 4.3 mEq/L, glucose 219 mg/dl. ABG (mechanical ventilator, FiO$_2$ 0.40): pH 7.46, PCO$_2$ 40 mm Hg, PO$_2$ 95 mm Hg. Chest radiograph (below): bilateral basal patchy infiltrates.

What diagnosis should be considered and what immediate action taken?

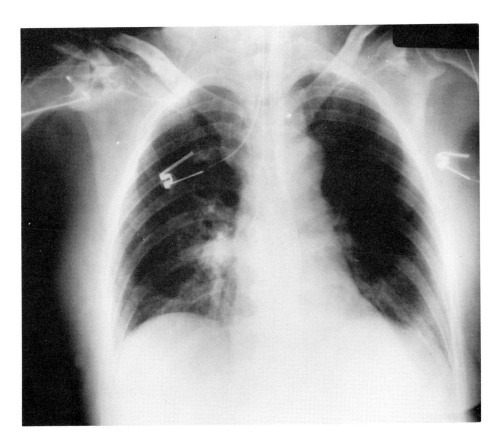

Diagnosis: Heparin-associated thrombocytopenia (HAT) with arterial thrombosis. Management should include discontinuation of heparin, placement of a Greenfield filter, and initiation of warfarin.

Discussion: Adverse effects of heparin therapy in the ICU include allergic reactions, hemorrhage, and HAT. HAT can be an asymptomatic laboratory abnormality or be associated with arterial and venous thrombosis (less common), causing marked morbidity and death. Approximately 20% of patients with HAT and thrombosis have required amputations and 30% have died. The incidence of HAT ranges widely between reports, with recent studies indicating rates of 1–5%. Severe thrombocytopenia, hemorrhage, and death have occurred in patients receiving mini-dose heparin. Bovine heparin appears to produce thrombocytopenia approximately three times more often than porcine heparin. HAT can develop on any day of treatment but most commonly occurs between days 5 and 12 of therapy; thrombocytopenia occurs earlier in patients previously exposed to heparin. The diagnosis of HAT is one of exclusion because no laboratory test is completely sensitive and specific. Alternate diagnoses causing thrombocytopenia in critically ill patients include sepsis, DIC, and other drug therapy. Furthermore, it should be certain that thrombocytopenia is a new rather than chronic event, and pseudothrombocytopenia is not present.

The pathogenesis of HAT has not been completely elucidated. The delay of onset of thrombocytopenia after initiation of heparin therapy is consistent with an immune mechanism. Most patients with HAT have increased platelet-associated IgG, and it has been suggested that heparin acts like a hapten and induces an immune response against heparin-platelet complexes. Recent studies support a reaction in some patients with HAT of antibodies with heparin-bound endothelial cells or with heparin sulfate synthesized by endothelial cells. These observations suggest that both the endothelial cell and platelet injury by immune mechanisms may be important in the development of thrombosis.

It is difficult to detect HAT in its earliest phase, because no predisposing factors identify the patient at risk. Because most patients with HAT and thrombosis develop thrombocytopenia and thrombosis simultaneously, serial platelet counts rarely provide a marker of impending thrombosis. However, it is prudent and probably cost-effective to perform a platelet count at the beginning and several days into heparin therapy so that a decreasing trend can be monitored. With mild thrombocytopenia, heparin may be continued with careful observation, since most patients will not develop thrombosis. Oral anticoagulants should be started at this time and heparin discontinued as soon as possible. At the documentation of thrombosis or severe thrombocytopenia, heparin should be discontinued immediately with institution of appropriate alternative forms of therapy such as vena cava filter, dextran, warfarin, or antiplatelet drugs. With occlusion of a large vessel, thrombosis may be remedial to surgical clot removal. Because HAT occurs most commonly after several days of heparin, 90% of instances of HAT can be avoided by starting warfarin concurrent with heparin to limit the duration of heparin therapy. Patients with HAT should never be rechallenged with heparin.

The present patient's heparin was discontinued, and she underwent a Greenfield filter insertion into the inferior vena cava and a warfarin anticoagulation. Thrombosis progressed in the fifth finger, requiring amputation, and also involved the third and fourth fingers. The platelet count reached a nadir of 29,000/μl 6 days after initiation of heparin and returned to $>$ 100,000/μl 5 days later.

Clinical Pearls

1. HAT with or without thrombosis has a peak incidence 5 to 12 days after initiation of heparin therapy. Occurrence is earlier in patients previously treated with heparin.

2. Arterial and venous thrombosis usually is associated with thrombocytopenia but, on occasion, can occur at near normal platelet counts.

3. Ninety percent (90%) of instances of HAT can be avoided by starting oral anticoagulation concurrent with heparin to limit the duration of heparin therapy.

REFERENCES
1. Weismann RE, Tobin RW: Arterial embolism occurring during systemic heparin therapy. Arch Surg 76:219–227, 1958.
2. Phelan BK: Heparin associated thrombosis without thrombocytopenia. Ann Intern Med 99:637–639, 1983.
3. King DJ, Kalton JG: Heparin associated thrombocytopenia. Ann Intern Med 100:535–540, 1984.

PATIENT 15

A 55-year-old man with pulmonary infiltrates following pneumonectomy

A 55-year-old man, treated for pulmonary tuberculosis 6 years prior, was admitted with massive hemoptysis. Chest radiograph revealed bilateral upper lobe disease, a large fungus ball in the right upper lobe, and alveolar infiltrates compatible with pulmonary hemorrhage. Pulmonary function studies 2 months prior showed an FEV_1 of 1.9 L. He continued to have large amounts of bleeding and was taken to the operating room. Rigid bronchoscopy documented hemorrhage from the left lung. Due to marked fibrosis, it was impossible to perform a left upper lobectomy; a pneumonectomy was accomplished. Intra- and post-operatively he received 3 units of packed RBCs and 4600 cc of crystalloid. Thirty hours after surgery, the patient became restless and felt that he "was not getting enough air."

Physical Examination: Temperature 100.6°; pulse 120; respirations 36 (on ventilator). Chest: diffuse rales on right.

Laboratory Findings: Hct 33%, WBC 12,500/μl with 83% PMNs, 11% lymphocytes. Gram stain (tracheal aspirate): moderate PMNs, gram-positive cocci, gram-negative bacilli. Chest radiograph (below): status post-pneumonectomy, alveolar-interstitial infiltrates on right. ABG (FiO_2 0.40): pH 7.47, PCO_2 38 mm Hg, PO_2 55 mm Hg. Peak pressure: 70 cm H_2O; static pressure: 60 cm H_2O. Pulmonary artery catheter: RA 11 mm Hg, PA (mean) 44 mm Hg, PCW 6 mm Hg, CI 4.1 L/min/m².

What is the most likely diagnosis?

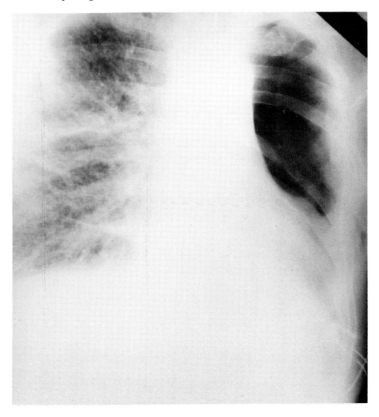

Diagnosis: Postpneumonectomy pulmonary edema (PPE).

Discussion: Pneumonectomy is associated with substantial morbidity and mortality that vary institutionally, depending on the patient's age, general state of health, and reason for pneumonectomy. The reported operative mortality ranges from < 5% up to 30%.

Improved surgical techniques and recognition of predisposing factors have decreased the incidence of many complications of pneumonectomy. Bronchopleural fistula, however, remains more common following pneumonectomy than with lesser resections. Empyema can occur with or without bronchopleural fistula with a reported incidence of 2 to 10%. Evidence for empyema can occur at any time after surgery but it is most often diagnosed in the early postoperative period. The pleural space may be contaminated at pneumonectomy, following bronchopleural fistula, or from bacteremia. Because postpneumonectomy empyema may be occult for months, diagnosis requires a high index of suspicion and should be considered in the postpneumonectomy patient with fever. Esophagopleural fistula is rare and usually follows right pneumonectomy for inflammatory disease. The diagnosis should be suspected in postoperative empyema without a bronchopleural fistula. Cardiac complications of pneumonectomy include atrial arrhythmias, which are common but rarely clinically important. Cardiac herniation is a rare, potentially life-threatening complication that occurs in the immediate postoperative period, presenting with shock and cardiac arrest. Vena caval obstruction results with right-sided herniation, and left ventricular compression follows left-sided herniation. Diagnosis is confirmed by chest radiograph and requires immediate thoracotomy to reduce the herniation. With intractable right heart failure, massive pulmonary embolism from a thrombus developing in the pulmonary arterial stump should be considered.

Pulmonary edema is a preventable complication of pneumonectomy that most commonly occurs with right pneumonectomy and iatrogenic perioperative fluid overload. As the right lung represents approximately 55% of lung mass and lymphatic capacity, following right pneumonectomy only 45% of the pulmonary vasculature and lymphatic system remains to transport blood volume and interstitial edema. Perioperative volume overload results in increased cardiac output and elevated pulmonary artery pressure. Because PCWP is normal in both man and animals in PPE, edema must result from increased capillary permeability. Following pneumonectomy, the mean pulmonary artery pressure increases and results in a greater difference between pressures in the arterial and venous ends of the capillary. Presumably, the higher upstream pressure results in the mean capillary pressure point moving toward the venous end of the capillary, resulting in a greater net filtration force and subsequent capillary leak. Excessive fluid administration with its effect on pulmonary artery pressure and cardiac output exacerbates this phenomenon. The lung lymphatics have tremendous reserve but cannot compensate for the increased filtration and, thus, pulmonary edema ensues.

PPE most often occurs between 24 and 48 hours postoperatively. Meticulous fluid balance is required during this period to maintain a normal cardiac index with careful replacement of blood and crystalloid. Pulmonary artery catheters benefit high-risk patients by monitoring vascular pressures and cardiac output. Postoperative preventive measures include positioning the patient with the remaining lung up and pain control to reduce catecholamine release and thus cardiac output and afterload. When PPE develops, diuresis should be instituted, monitoring cardiac output and pulmonary artery pressure.

The present patient received diuretic therapy, vascular pressure monitoring, and mechanical ventilation but died 7 days after surgery of nosocomial pneumonia.

Clinical Pearls

1. The major risk factor for PPE is excessive perioperative fluid administration.

2. Pulmonary edema results because excess fluid accumulation causes an increased cardiac output and elevated pulmonary artery pressure, resulting in increased fluid filtration that exceeds the limited lymphatic drainage of the remaining lung.

3. PPE is a preventable condition if fluid administration is judicious and cardiac output and pulmonary artery pressures are controlled.

REFERENCES

1. Gibbon JH Jr, Gibbon MH, Kraul CW: Experimental pulmonary edema following lobectomy and blood transfusion. J Thorac Surg 12:60–77, 1942.
2. Hutchin P, Terzi RG, Hollandsworth LA, et al: Pulmonary congestion following infusion of large fluid loads in thoracic surgical patients. Ann Thorac Surg 8:339–347, 1969.
3. Zeldin RA, Normandin D, Landtwing BS, Peters RM: Post-pneumonectomy pulmonary edema. J Thorac Cardiovasc Surg 87:359–365, 1984.

PATIENT 16

A 34-year-old man with dyspnea, chest tightness, and cough

A 34-year-old man with asthma for 15 years was seen in the emergency room because of severe dyspnea, chest tightness, and cough over the preceding 24 hours and gradual worsening of symptoms for the previous 2 weeks. He had recently moved to Charleston and had exhausted his medications 6 weeks prior. He had purchased an "over the counter" metered-dose inhaler and had been using up to 24 inhalations per day for the previous 2 days.

Physical Examination: Temperature 98.9°; pulse 120; respirations 32; blood pressure 130/80; pulsus paradoxus 15 mm Hg. Anxious with interrupted speech, use of accessory respiratory muscles, and positive Hoover's sign. Chest: poor airflow without wheezes.

Laboratory Findings: PEFR 100 L/min. ABG (4 L/min O_2): pH 7.31, PCO_2 51 mm Hg, PO_2 60 mm Hg. Chest radiograph (below): hyperinflation.

Hospital Course: The patient was given several doses of an inhaled beta-2 agonist and a loading dose of aminophylline over the next 30 minutes without improvement.

What are the diagnosis and immediate plan of management?

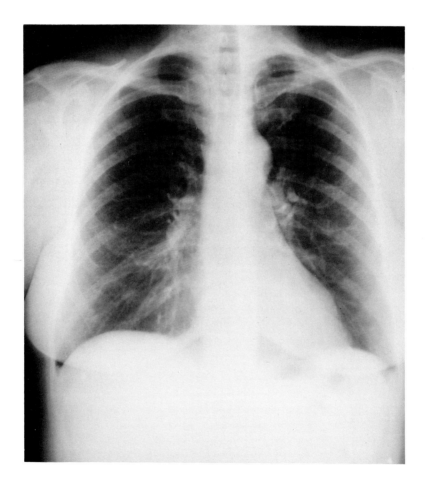

Diagnosis and Treatment: Status asthmaticus (SA) requiring aggressive pharmacologic therapy, including corticosteroids, in the ICU. ABGs should be monitored, sedation avoided, and intubation equipment readily available at the bedside.

Discussion: SA is a potentially fatal condition defined as acute, severe asthma refractory to beta-agonists and aminophylline after 30 minutes of therapy. Patients with SA do not respond to initial therapy because they have severe airway inflammation, edema, and mucus plugging in addition to bronchial hyperreactivity. These pathologic changes lead to expiratory airflow obstruction with air-trapping and hyperinflation. Enlarging lung volumes increase airway patency but place the respiratory muscles at a disadvantageous point on the length-tension curve, increasing the work of breathing and oxygen consumption of the respiratory muscles. Hypoxemia is universal and results from low V/Q units. If airway obstruction worsens, hypercapnia ensues, as hypoventilation from respiratory muscle fatigue compounds V/Q mismatching.

Early recognition with immediate and aggressive pharmacologic treatment can prevent most fatalities. Supplemental oxygen usually reverses hypoxemia. Inhaled beta-agonists should be given repeatedly or continuously until airway obstruction improves or the patient is markedly tremulous. The maintenance dose of IV aminophylline should be based on age, smoking history, and underlying disease. A continuous infusion of hydrocortisone (0.5 mg/kg/hr) after a 2 mg/kg bolus, or methylprednisolone 125 mg IV every 6 hours, has been shown to improve airflow obstruction significantly in the first 24 hours with the earliest improvement by 6 hours. When SA is diagnosed, IV corticosteroids should be given immediately, as procrastination will only delay their onset of action. Sedatives should be avoided because restlessness is a sign of respiratory distress in this setting.

The decision for mechanical ventilation in SA needs to be individualized and based on the constellation of clinical findings and not on a single ABG. Hypercapnia in acute asthma is rapidly reversible in most instances with aggressive therapy, and mechanical ventilation usually can be avoided. Indications for mechanical ventilation include impending or actual cardiorespiratory arrest, deteriorating mental status, and progressive hypercapnia. When a decision is made to intubate, an endotracheal tube ≥ 8 mm internal diameter should be placed by the oral route to decrease expiratory airway resistance and to allow for therapeutic bronchoscopy if indicated. Nasal endotracheal intubation should be avoided because of the required tube size and the high incidence of nasal polyps and sinusitis in these patients. The goals of mechanical ventilation are to assure adequate gas exchange and to rest the respiratory muscles until airway obstruction resolves with drug therapy. These goals need to be pursued while minimizing the risk of barotrauma, which is related to the peak airway pressure (PAP). PAP > 70 cm H_2O is associated with barotrauma in up to 50% of patients, PAP between 50 and 70 cm H_2O in $< 10\%$, and PAP < 50 cm H_2O rarely causes barotrauma. Barotrauma can be minimized by using low tidal volumes, low respiratory rates, and high I/E ratios. Controlled hypoventilation with low PAP and normalization of pH with bicarbonate infusion appear to be the best methods of minimizing barotrauma in SA.

Extubation usually can be accomplished successfully when PAP is < 50 cm H_2O with normal tidal volumes, FiO_2 is ≤ 0.40, minute ventilation is < 10 L/min, and maximum inspiratory pressure is < -25 cm H_2O.

The present patient remained alert, did not develop progressive hypercapnia, and began to reverse his airway obstruction by 6 hours; hypercapnia resolved following 12 hours of therapy.

Clinical Pearls

1. Patients with hypercapnia in SA generally have severe airflow obstruction and manifest a pulsus paradoxus > 10 mm Hg, use of accessory respiratory muscles, and a quiet chest on physical examination.

2. Hypercapnia per se is not an indication for mechanical ventilation; the decision for ventilatory support should be made after assessment of the total clinical presentation and serial ABGs.

3. Barotrauma in patients ventilated for SA occurs in close to 50% of patients if the PAP is greater than 70 cm H_2O; it is virtually nonexistent if the PAP is < 50 cm H_2O. PAP can be minimized by controlled hypoventilation and acidemia corrected with intravenous bicarbonate.

REFERENCES

1. Peterson GW, Baier H: Incidence of pulmonary barotrauma in a medical ICU. Crit Care Med 11:67–69, 1982.
2. Menitove SM, Golding RM: Combined ventilator and bicarbonate strategy in the management of status asthmaticus. Am J Med 74:898–901, 1983.
3. Mountain RD, Sahn SA: Clinical features and outcome in patients with acute asthma presenting with hypercapnia. Am Rev Respir Dis 138:535–539, 1988.

PATIENT 17

A 70-year-old man with confusion and tachypnea

A 70-year-old man was brought to the emergency room after his wife found him "confused and breathing rapidly." He had undergone a transurethral prostatectomy 2 months earlier.

Physical Examination: Temperature 101.5°; pulse 110; respirations 32, blood pressure 85/55. Chest: scattered rhonchi. Cardiac: grade II/VI ejection murmur. Abdomen: non-tender, no organomegaly. Neurologic: disoriented.

Laboratory Findings: Hct 39%, WBC 13,000/μl with 80% PMNs, 7% bands; BUN 36 mg/dl, creatinine 1.2 mg/dl; glucose 160 mg/dl. Urinalysis: many PMNs, gram-negative bacilli. Urine and blood cultures: *E. coli.*

Hospital Course: The patient received IV fluids and antibiotics for urosepsis with improvement in mental status, blood pressure, and urine output. On the third hospital day, however, he developed ARDS and required mechanical ventilation. Swan-Ganz catheter: PA (mean) 30 mm Hg, PCW 5 mm Hg, CI 5.24 L/min/m², SVR 440 dyn•cm. Ten days after admission, respiratory status improved with maintenance of negative fluid balance. Laboratory findings: bilirubin 3.5 mg/dl, glucose 180 mg/dl, BUN 52 mg/dl, creatinine 2.6 mg/dl. Tracheal aspirate: *P. aeruginosa.* The bilirubin and creatinine continued to rise over the subsequent week.

What is the patient's diagnosis on hospital day 10?

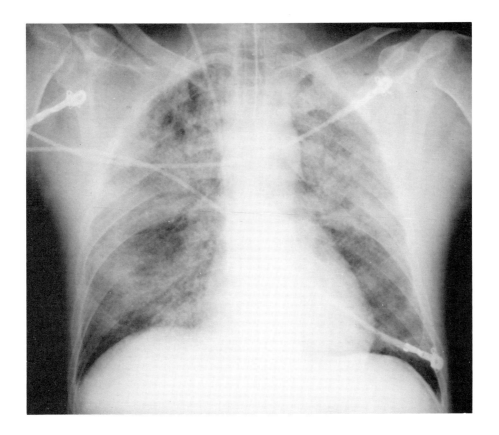

Diagnosis: Multiple organ failure syndrome (MOFS).

Discussion: MOFS is defined by both clinical and laboratory parameters. Clinically, an initiating event, either sepsis, trauma, hypotension, or persistent inflammation, results in sequential pulmonary, hepatic, and renal failure. The lungs fail first, causing profound hypoxic ventilatory failure (ARDS) that requires mechanical ventilation. After several days, initial stabilization is followed by the clinical picture of hypermetabolism with increased urine output, high cardiac index, low systemic vascular resistance, hyperglycemia, increased blood lactate levels, increased oxygen consumption, and urea nitrogen excretion exceeding 15 g/day.

Laboratory features of MOFS develop over the next 7 to 10 days; the bilirubin rises to levels > 3 mg/dl and renal failure follows (serum creatinine > 2 mg/dl). Gram-negative bacteremia with enteric organisms is common, as is the isolation of gram-negatives from tracheal aspirate. Inotropic agents and IV fluids to maintain an increased blood volume and cardiac preload are progressively required. Renal failure worsens and by 2 to 3 weeks a decision on dialysis needs to be made. Without dialysis, the patient usually dies 3 to 4 weeks following the initial insult. Renal failure can precede hepatic failure and, when this occurs, the etiology of the acute renal injury usually can be identified, with drugs or hypoperfusion being most frequent.

The onset of liver failure is the clinical marker of MOFS. Clinical settings commonly associated with MOFS include persistence of infection, tissue hypoperfusion, or inflammation (pancreatitis). The diagnosis of MOFS has major prognostic significance, as it is associated with a mortality risk of 40–60% in early MOFS and a risk approaching 100% in the latter stages. Late MOFS is characterized by deep coma, severe ARDS, autocannibalism, markedly increased BUN, creatinine > 2.5 mg/dl, bilirubin > 8 mg/dl, triglyceride > 250 mg/dl, and lactate > 3 mg/dl. Survivors of MOFS are markedly debilitated from prolonged hypermetabolism. Respiratory muscles, as well as total muscle groups, are affected and often necessitate prolonged ventilatory support until rehabilitation can be accomplished. A unique peripheral neuropathy of MOFS is characterized by both motor and sensory deficits; skeletal muscle denervation leads to severe muscle weakness and failure to wean from mechanical ventilation.

Effective therapy requires control of the source of injury, maintenance of oxygen transport to tissues, and metabolic support. The source of inflammation or infection needs to be removed early to prevent high mortality. Flow-dependent oxygen consumption needs to be assessed critically, as the usual clinical criteria of perfusion may have a decreased sensitivity in the settings of ARDS, sepsis, and pancreatitis. It is imperative to ensure adequate oxygen content and flow until excess lactate production has ceased.

Although patients with MOFS are malnourished, nutritional support does not alter the course of the disease. Nevertheless, a good nutritional program can limit loss of body mass and visceral malnutrition, both co-variables of mortality. General principles include: avoid excess total calories and glucose, titrate amino acids to achieve nitrogen equilibrium, and achieve normal hepatic protein synthesis. Using these principles over the past several years, there has been a reduction in the incidence and mortality of MOFS despite a lack of change in mortality of ARDS. The present patient, however, progressed and died within 23 days.

Clinical Pearls

1. The complex of injury, ARDS, and hypermetabolism followed by sequential liver and renal failure defines MOFS.

2. The initial injury in MOFS is usually sepsis, trauma, hypotension, or persistent inflammation.

3. Early recognition and control of the inciting cause, restoration and maintenance of oxygen transport, and metabolic support can reduce the mortality associated with MOFS. Persistence of the inciting source results in a high mortality.

REFERENCES
1. Hassett J, Cerra FB, Siegel JH, et al: Multiple systems organ failure: Mechanisms and therapy. Surg Annu 14:25–72, 1982.
2. Cerra FB: Hypometabolism, organ failure and metabolic support. Surgery 191:1–14, 1987.
3. Cerra FB, Siegel JH, Border JR, et al: Hepatic failure of sepsis: Cellular resubstrate. Surgery 86:409–422, 1979.

PATIENT 18

A 61-year-old man with COPD, hypercapnic respiratory failure, fever, pleurisy, and hemoptysis

A 61-year-old man with COPD and hypercapnic respiratory failure was transferred to the ICU from an outlying hospital for failure to wean from mechanical ventilation. His illness began with a URI and acute bronchitis that progressed to respiratory failure. He initially received therapy with IV aminophylline, an inhaled beta-agonist, a cephalosporin, and IV Solu-Medrol (30 mg q6h) that was rapidly tapered to 30 mg of prednisone daily. A tracheotomy was done and sufficient improvement occurred by the 23rd hospital day to allow weaning. He subsequently developed fever, pleuritic chest pain, worsening oxygenation, and brown, tenacious airway secretions intermixed with blood that prompted transfer after 26 days.

Physical Examination: Temperature 103°; pulse 120; respirations 32. Chest: bilateral rhonchi, rales on right. Cardiac: neck veins distended at 45°, increased P2. Extremities: 2+ edema. Neurologic: alert, no focal findings.

Laboratory Findings: Hct 50%, WBC 24,500/μl with 90% PMNs, 4% eosinophils. ABG (FiO$_2$ 0.55 on mechanical ventilation): pH 7.37, PCO$_2$ 43 mm Hg, PO$_2$ 65 mm Hg. Chest radiograph (below): diffuse alveolar infiltrates on the right, multiple cavitary lesions on the left. Sputum Gram stain: many PMNs, gram-positive diplococci and gram-negative coccobacilli. Bronchoscopy provided a presumptive diagnosis.

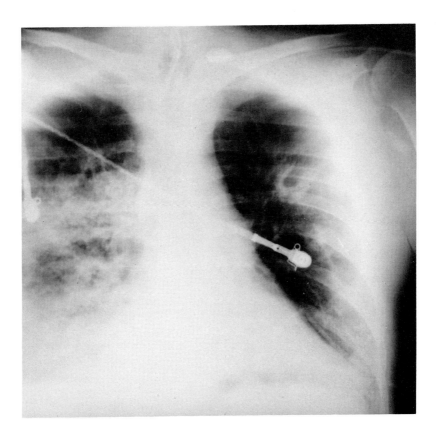

Diagnosis: Invasive aspergillosis. BAL fluid stain showed septate hyphae, and the culture demonstrated *Aspergillus fumigatus.*

Discussion: Most cases of invasive aspergillosis occur in severely immunocompromised patients, especially those with acute leukemia who have prolonged neutropenia from chemotherapy. Patients with solid tumors, lymphoma, and renal transplantation are affected less often. Other risk factors include corticosteroids, cytotoxic agents, and broad-spectrum antibiotics. Although invasive pulmonary aspergillosis has been reported in presumably immunocompetent hosts, most patients have subtle immunologic defects, neutrophil dysfunction, overwhelming inocula of aspergillus spores, interstitial lung disease, or alcoholism.

Chronic necrotizing aspergillosis is an alternate form of invasive aspergillus disease in which a nidus of infection progresses over weeks to months to a cavitary infiltrate involving a lobe or entire lung. Patients typically have underlying pulmonary disorders, such as COPD, sarcoidosis, or rheumatologic diseases, and have been receiving long-term low-dose corticosteroid therapy.

Corticosteroids are promoters of invasive aspergillus disease. In experimental animals, corticosteroids and antibiotics facilitate the growth of aspergillus in lung tissue. Corticosteroid-treated animals that inhale aspergillus spores develop hyphae in bronchial secretions and lung tissue quickly in association with an absent macrophage response, which may be responsible for the natural resistance to aspergillus infection.

Invasive aspergillosis should be considered in any patient with risk factors who develops fever, pleuritic chest pain, and cough with or without hemoptysis. Initially, the chest radiograph may be normal, but eventually it will show either multiple nodules with a predilection to cavitation, pleural-based infiltrates, or diffuse consolidation. Pleural effusions are uncommon.

A KOH stain of expectorated sputum that is positive for hyphal elements should suggest the diagnosis in the appropriate clinical setting. The finding of aspergillus in the sputum should not be dismissed simply as saprophytic colonization; multiple isolations should increase suspicion. A definitive diagnosis usually can be made by open lung biopsy, but even this procedure can give false-negative results. Bronchoscopy with BAL or bronchial washings with a plethora of hyphae that culture aspergillus establishes a presumptive diagnosis in the patient with risk factors for invasive disease; transbronchial lung biopsy may show tissue invasion with aspergillus but the false-negative rate can be high. Precipitating antibodies to aspergillus are found in only a few patients with rapidly invasive disease and become positive only late in the illness. Diagnostic utility is further limited by the delay in receiving results.

Amphotericin B is the drug of choice; total dose should be 2 to 2.5 g. Miconazole and ketoconazole do not appear to be effective nor is the combination of amphotericin B plus 5-fluorocytosine or rifampin better than amphotericin alone.

The present patient with underlying COPD developed rapidly invasive aspergillosis from corticosteroid therapy and broad-spectrum antibiotics. The disease simulated bacterial pneumonia, requiring bronchoscopy to confirm the diagnosis. The patient died from complications of tissue hypoxia after 7 days of amphotericin therapy.

Clinical Pearls

1. Rapidly progressive invasive aspergillosis can occur in patients receiving low-dose corticosteroid therapy with no other major risk factor.

2. Finding aspergillus in the sputum should raise the index of suspicion for invasive disease in any patient with a known risk factor(s).

3. The demonstration of tissue invasion with aspergillus establishes the diagnosis definitively; however, presence of aspergillus in BAL or bronchial washings in a patient with fever, pleuritic chest pain, and hemoptysis with pleural-based pulmonary infiltrates is justification for beginning amphotericin B therapy.

REFERENCES

1. Palmer LB, Schiff MJ: Rapidly progressive pneumonia in a patient with chronic obstructive pulmonary disease. Chest 1:179–180, 1989.
2. Karam GH, Griffin FM Jr: Invasive pulmonary aspergillosis in non-immunocompromised, non-neutropenic hosts. Rev Infect Dis 8:357–363, 1986.
3. Lake KB, Browne PM, Vandyke JJ, et al: Fatal disseminated aspergillosis in an asthmatic patient treated with corticosteroids. Chest 83:138–139, 1983.

PATIENT 19

A 70-year-old man with new onset of wheezing

A 70-year-old man was admitted to the hospital with a 2-day history of progressive dyspnea, fever, cough, and wheezing. He was a nonsmoker and did not have a history of asthma.

Physical Examination: Temperature 101°; pulse 120; respirations 32; blood pressure 130/85. Skin: no lesions. ENT: normal. Chest: diffuse wheezes and rhonchi. Cardiac: neck veins flat at 45°, heart sounds normal without gallops or murmurs. Extremities: no clubbing.

Laboratory Findings: Hct 44%, WBC 12,100/μl with 76% PMNs, 15% lymphocytes, 3% eosinophils. ABG (room air): pH 7.37, PCO_2 45 mm Hg, PO_2 59 mm Hg. Chest radiograph: normal.

Hospital Course: The patient was treated with IV aminophylline, inhaled beta-agonists, and IV corticosteroids but developed progressive hypoxia and hypercapnia, requiring intubation and mechanical ventilation. A bronchoscopy performed on the fourth hospital day showed marked erythema of the trachea and large bronchi with multiple mucosal ulcerations and a thick exudate partially obstructing both mainstem bronchi. Bronchial biopsy is shown below.

What is the most likely cause of the patient's new onset of wheezing and respiratory failure? What therapy should be recommended?

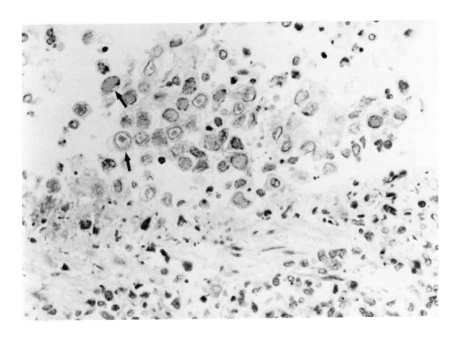

Diagnosis and Treatment: Herpetic tracheobronchitis. The patient should be treated with intravenous acyclovir.

Discussion: Herpetic tracheobronchitis has been documented in both immunocompromised (malignancy, organ transplants, and burns) and immunocompetent individuals. Normal hosts who develop herpetic tracheobronchitis typically are elderly individuals without herpes labialis or mucocutaneous lesions, suggesting that the pathogenesis of the illness is not extension of the virus from the upper to lower respiratory tract. Some patients with herpetic tracheobronchitis require ventilatory support, as the severe bronchospasm and airway obstruction leads to both hypoxic and hypercapnic respiratory failure. However, endotracheal intubation per se does not appear to be a predisposing factor for the development of herpes simplex virus infection. When the virus attacks the tracheobronchial mucosa, it results in necrotization, ulceration, and production of a fibrinopurulent exudate that at times causes partial obstruction of mainstem and lobar bronchi.

The indicated diagnostic procedure is bronchoscopy, which allows visualization of the characteristic lesions that involve primarily the trachea and mainstem and lobar bronchi. Endobronchial mucosal biopsy and cytology of bronchial washings typically show acute inflammation with intranuclear inclusions, as was demonstrated in the present patient (see figure, arrows). Culture of bronchial secretions documenting herpes simplex type I virus usually is positive in 2 to 5 days. Serology is only helpful in supporting the diagnosis retrospectively.

An elderly patient with new onset wheezing and a "normal" chest radiograph who is not responsive to standard bronchodilator therapy and corticosteroids should undergo fiberoptic bronchoscopy not only to exclude a tracheal carcinoma, laryngeal lesion, or a foreign body, but also to search for herpetic tracheobronchitis. On occasion, the patient with underlying asthma or COPD and an acute pulmonary embolism may present with wheezing and a normal chest radiograph. Patients with interstitial lung disease, especially sarcoidosis, congestive heart failure, gastric aspiration, Wegener's granulomatosis, and Churg-Strauss vasculitis may present with wheezing that is not classic asthma; the chest radiograph usually shows abnormalities in these conditions but may be unremarkable in Wegener's granulomatosis and Churg-Strauss disease. Patients with sarcoidosis, gastric aspiration, and Wegener's have characteristic airway findings at bronchoscopy.

Early detection of herpes simplex virus tracheobronchitis appears critical, so that acyclovir, a potent viral inhibitor specific for herpes simplex virus, can be given during the time of peak viral replication, which tends to coincide with symptomatic clinical illness. Repeat bronchoscopy as early as 3 weeks following diagnosis and institution of therapy usually shows complete epithelial regeneration with normal-appearing airways.

The patient received 10 days of IV acyclovir with improvement in airway obstruction. Mechanical ventilation was discontinued after 8 days.

Clinical Pearls

1. Herpetic tracheobronchitis should be considered in the differential diagnosis when an elderly patient presents with new onset wheezing unresponsive to conventional therapy.

2. At bronchoscopy, erythema, ulceration, and fibrinopurulent exudates in the trachea and large airways are typically seen. Bronchial biopsy and cytology of bronchial washings may show herpetic-type intranuclear inclusions. Bronchial secretions are culture-positive for herpes simplex virus type I.

3. Intravenous acyclovir for 7 to 10 days initiated at onset of symptomatic clinical illness usually is effective therapy.

REFERENCES
1. Sherry MK, Klainer AS, Wolff M, et al: Herpetic tracheobronchitis. Ann Intern Med 109:229–233, 1988.
2. Tuxen DV, Cade JF, McDonald MR, et al: Herpes simplex virus from the lower respiratory tract in adult respiratory distress syndrome. Am Rev Respir Dis 126:416–419, 1982.
3. Jordan SW, McLaren LC, Crosby JH: Herpetic tracheobronchitis: Cytologic and virologic detection. Arch Intern Med 135:784–788, 1975.

PATIENT 20

A 55-year-old man with epigastric pain, nausea, vomiting, and subsequent respiratory failure

A 55-year-old man with a history of alcohol abuse was admitted with a 2-day history of nausea, vomiting, and epigastric pain radiating to the chest. He denied hematemesis, melena, or diarrhea.

Physical Examination: Temperature 100.6°; pulse 120; respirations 28; blood pressure 110/65. Chest: basilar rales. Cardiac: regular tachycardia without gallops or murmurs. Abdomen: moderate abdominal distention, tenderness over the upper abdomen with muscle spasm, absent bowel sounds.

Laboratory Findings: Hct 50%, WBC 18,000/μl with 87% PMNs; glucose 185 mg/dl, Ca^{2+} 8.1 mg/dl, SGOT 220 IU/L (NL < 27), amylase 410 IU/L (NL < 115). ECG: ST and T wave abnormalities. Chest radiograph: small right pleural effusion and basilar atelectasis. Plain film of abdomen: minimal dilation of the small bowel without free air. Abdominal ultrasonography: normal biliary tree; cystic structure around the pancreas. ABG (room air): pH 7.49, PCO_2 32 mm Hg, PO_2 72 mm Hg.

Hospital Course: The patient was treated with IV fluids, analgesia, and nasogastric suction. Twenty-four hours later, he complained of dyspnea. Chest examination showed increased dullness to percussion at the right base and increased basilar rales. Repeat chest radiograph (below) showed bilateral alveolar infiltrates and a larger right pleural effusion. ABG (6 L O_2/min): pH 7.51, PCO_2 27 mm Hg, PO_2 55 mm Hg. Right thoracentesis: protein 4.2 g/dl, LDH 420 IU/L, WBC 8500/μl with 75% PMNs, glucose 70 mg/dl, pH 7.31, amylase 1800 IU/L.

What is the primary diagnosis and what complications have occurred?

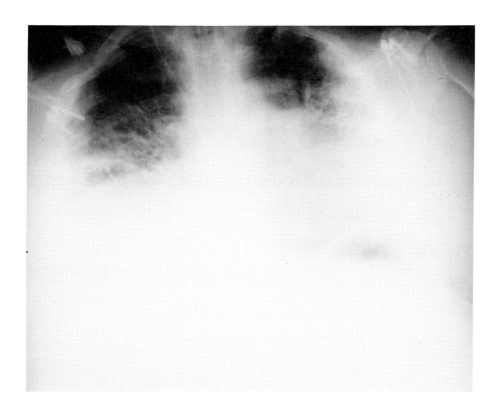

Diagnosis: Necrotizing pancreatitis with pseudocyst, pancreaticopleural fistula to the right pleural space with pleural effusion, and the adult respiratory distress syndrome.

Discussion: The diagnosis of acute pancreatitis should be considered when a patient presents with unremitting abdominal pain, nausea, vomiting, and an abnormal abdominal examination. The diagnosis is supported by an elevated serum amylase and/or lipase. The differential diagnosis includes ruptured viscus, acute cholecystitis, mesenteric vascular obstruction, diabetic ketoacidosis, acute intestinal obstruction, aortic dissection, and pneumonia. Several of these diagnoses can be excluded by a plain film of the abdomen, ultrasonography, chest radiograph, and routine blood chemistries.

The spectrum of pancreatic inflammation ranges from mild edematous pancreatitis to severe, necrotizing pancreatitis that is associated with local and systemic complications. Local complications include phlegmon, pseudocyst, abscess, and ascites. Systemic complications most prominently involve the lungs, cardiovascular system (hypotension), and GI tract (hemorrhage). Additional complications include metabolic derangements (hypocalcemia, hypertriglyceridemia) and hematologic abnormalities (DIC).

Pulmonary complications increase mortality and include atelectasis, pleural effusion, mediastinal abscess, pneumonia, and ARDS. Clinically occult, mild hypoxemia is common during the first 2 or 3 days of acute pancreatitis. Hypoxemia bears no relationship to patient age, serum amylase level, hypocalcemia, or the volume of intravenous fluids received. Patients with mild pancreatitis may manifest severe hypoxemia. Changes in oxyhemoglobin affinity during acute pancreatitis may further increase the physiologic consequences of hypoxemia and respiratory failure. While most patients' pulmonary dysfunction improves as their pancreatitis resolves, major progressive pulmonary disease develops in up to one-third of individuals; high initial serum amylase levels, early hypocalcemia, advanced age, and early fluid sequestration in large volumes appear to be risk factors for progressive pulmonary involvement.

Treatment of pancreatitis-induced ARDS is supportive with emphasis on limiting the persistent inflammatory response and the use of PEEP to reduce the risk of oxygen toxicity. Corticosteroids are not beneficial in treating these patients. Peritoneal lavage during the first few days of pancreatitis may be effective early treatment in patients with pulmonary complications.

Ten to fifteen percent of patients with acute pancreatitis develop pleural effusions. The effusions are generally small and left-sided and have a higher amylase concentration than in serum due to the clearance of amylase from the bloodstream by the kidney. Larger effusions result when a fistula develops between a pseudocyst and the mediastinum or either pleural space; these effusions may contain high concentrations of amylase, sometimes > 100,000 IU/L. Large pleural effusions interfere with ventilation and gas exchange and further aggravate respiratory failure.

The present patient was treated with mechanical ventilation and chest tube drainage of the pancreatico-pleural effusion; ARDS and the pleural effusion resolved over two weeks.

Clinical Pearls

1. Pulmonary complications of acute pancreatitis include atelectasis, pleural effusion, mediastinal abscess, pneumonia, and ARDS.

2. Pulmonary complications tend to occur more commonly in older patients and those with initially high serum amylase levels, early hypocalcemia, and early fluid sequestration.

3. Respiratory management of patients with pancreatitis-induced ARDS is similar to ARDS from other etiologies. Corticosteroids are of no benefit. Removal of intraperitoneal exudate by lavage may be an effective adjunct in the management of those with pulmonary complications.

REFERENCES
1. Hayes MF Jr, Rosenbaum RW, Zibelman M, et al: Adult respiratory syndrome in association with acute pancreatitis. Am J Surg 127:314–319, 1974.
2. Ranson JHC, Spencer FC: The role of peritoneal lavage in severe acute pancreatitis. Ann Surg 187:565–575, 1978.
3. Lee BC, Malik AB, Barie PS, et al: Effect of acute pancreatitis on pulmonary transvascular fluid and protein exchange. Am Rev Respir Dis 123:618–621, 1981.

PATIENT 21

A 23-year-old man with massive hemoptysis

A 23-year-old man with remote IV drug abuse came to the emergency room after expectorating a "basin of blood." He had been in good health without previous respiratory complaints until 2 weeks prior when he developed cough, dyspnea, and fatigue. He was a cigarette smoker who used marijuana frequently.

Physical Examination: Temperature 99.4°; pulse 100; respirations 32; blood pressure 125/75. Skin: normal. ENT: no lesions. Chest: bilateral rales most prominent in the bases. Cardiac: tachycardia with normal heart sounds without murmurs or gallops. Extremities: no cyanosis, clubbing, or edema.

Laboratory Findings: Hct 28%; WBC 12,000/μl with 80% PMNs, 3% eosinophils, platelet count 653,000/μl; PT 12 seconds, PTT 25 seconds; creatinine 0.9 mg/dl; ABG (6 L/min O_2): pH 7.48, PCO_2 32 mm Hg, PO_2 60 mm Hg. Urinalysis: normal. Chest radiograph (below): bilateral alveolar infiltrates with a predominance in the bases.

Hospital Course: During the first several hours in the ICU he had 300 ml of hemoptysis. He subsequently stabilized and the next day a diagnostic procedure was performed.

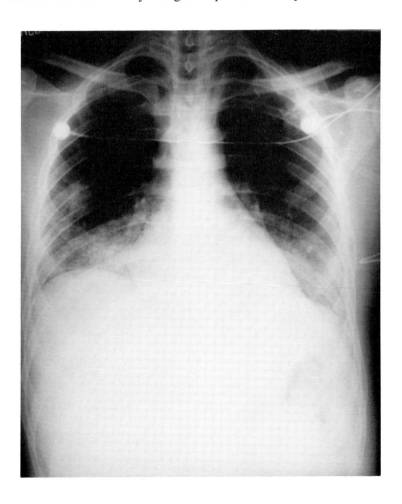

Diagnosis: Goodpasture's syndrome. Fiberoptic bronchoscopy (FOB) showed diffuse airway hemorrhage; BAL revealed hemosiderin-laden macrophages; and transbronchial lung biopsy demonstrated hemorrhage and linear deposition of IgG along the alveolar-capillary basement membrane.

Discussion: Patients with massive hemoptysis (100 to several hundred ml of blood/24 hours) require immediate evaluation and treatment. The most common causes of massive hemoptysis due to a focal lesion are tuberculosis, bronchiectasis, necrotizing pneumonia, lung abscess, aspergilloma, and lung cancer. Etiologies associated with diffuse alveolar hemorrhage include Goodpasture's syndrome, connective tissue disease (SLE), systemic vasculitides, and rapidly progressive glomerulonephritis. History and physical examination may suggest an etiology but are rarely definitive. Routine diagnostic studies should include CBC, coagulation profile, chest radiograph, sputum examination and ABGs. The chest radiograph may suggest the bleeding site and etiology; however, the radiographic lesion may be chronic and unrelated to the acute event. Bilateral alveolar infiltrates are typical of diffuse alveolar hemorrhage but can be seen with a focal lesion and aspiration of blood. A normal chest radiograph implies bleeding from the upper airway, large airways, or a radiographically occult pulmonary parenchymal focus. Sputum examination may reveal purulence, a predominant organism, a positive AFB smear, or malignant cells.

Bronchoscopy is the most useful procedure in defining bleeding sites and whether they are focal or diffuse; it should be performed as early in the patient's course as possible. FOB via the nasal route allows examination of the nasopharynx and larynx, in addition to the tracheobronchial tree. However, FOB may be inadequate for suctioning blood from the airways to allow a systematic examination. Rigid bronchoscopy provides better removal of endobronchial blood and together with FOB is often effective in identifying the site of hemorrhage.

Patients with massive hemoptysis should be managed emergently, because they have a high mortality when appropriate treatment is not given. A mortality rate of 75% has been reported in patients managed with medical therapy alone when hemoptysis totals 600 ml within 16 hours. Death from massive hemoptysis is rarely the result of exsanguination but is due to asphyxiation if blood occludes the major airways. Therefore, maintenance of airway patency is the first and most essential therapeutic maneuver. If the bleeding is focal and the site is known, the patient should be positioned with the bleeding lung dependent; if the site is unknown or the bleeding diffuse, the patient should be placed in the Trendelenburg position. An endotracheal tube and suction equipment should be available at the bedside. Airway protection can be afforded by insertion of a double-lumen endotracheal tube or placement of an endotracheal tube with bronchoscopic guidance into the nonbleeding mainstem bronchus. Previous pulmonary function tests and ABGs are invaluable in the decision concerning surgery.

Emergent resection is associated with a high mortality and should be avoided, if possible, if endobronchial tamponade or bronchial artery embolization can be instituted rapidly to temporarily control the bleeding while surgery is considered. In the non-operable patient with localized disease, endobronchial control measures followed by bronchial artery embolization controls hemorrhage in most patients; however, the recurrence rate approaches 20%. Other temporizing measures that have been reported to be successful include pulmonary artery occlusion with a Swan-Ganz catheter, IV vasopressin, iced saline lavage, and laser photocoagulation.

Goodpasture's is a disease of young, adult males who most commonly present with diffuse alveolar hemorrhage and glomerulonephritis; however, patients may present with alveolar hemorrhage up to 1 year before the onset of renal manifestations. Hemoptysis may be massive or absent despite severe diffuse alveolar hemorrhage. The chest radiograph typically shows bilateral symmetric alveolar infiltrates radiating from the hilum with a tendency to affect the middle and lower lung zones. Greater than 90% of patients with Goodpasture's have increased anti-GBM antibody in serum. In patients with diffuse alveolar hemorrhage, normal urinalysis, and normal serum creatinine, Goodpasture's can be diagnosed by lung biopsy that shows alveolar hemorrhage without necrosis, linear deposition of IgG along the alveolar or glomerular basement membrane, and elevated circulating anti-GBM antibody.

The patient was treated with corticosteroids, cyclosphosphamide, and plasmapheresis with resolution of the alveolar hemorrhage over 2 weeks.

Clinical Pearls

1. Massive hemoptysis from localized disease should be treated by surgery, if possible, because it is a lethal condition if medical therapy alone is used.

2. Patients with massive hemoptysis from a localized source should undergo endobronchial balloon tamponade or bronchial artery embolization until surgery can be accomplished, because the major cause of death is asphyxiation from blood occluding the major airways.

3. Patients with massive hemoptysis from diffuse alveolar hemorrhage require rapid diagnosis so that specific medical therapy can be instituted.

REFERENCES

1. Albelda SM, Gefter WB, Epstein DM, et al: Diffuse pulmonary hemorrhage: A review and classification. Radiology 154:289–297, 1985.
2. Conlan AA, Hurwitz SS, Krige L, et al: Massive hemoptysis: A review of 123 cases. J Thorac Cardiovasc Surg 85:120–124, 1983.
3. Teague CA, Doak PP, Simpson IJ, et al: Goodpasture's syndrome: An analysis of 29 cases. Kidney Int 13:492–504, 1978.

PATIENT 22

A 57-year-old man with failure to wean from mechanical ventilation because of persistent hypoxemia

A 57-year-old man with chronic bronchitis was in his usual state of health until he developed bilateral pneumonia and hypoxic respiratory failure. He was treated with antibiotics and mechanical ventilation requiring high FiO_2. He responded clinically with defervescence, normalization of WBC, and improvement in chest radiograph. However, he could not be weaned from mechanical ventilation because of persistent hypoxemia. He was transferred to our medical center 15 days after initial hospitalization. Admission complaints were substernal chest pain and cough.

Physical Examination: Temperature 98.5°; pulse 100; respirations 32 (on ventilator). Chest: bilateral crackles. Cardiac: normal. Neurologic: alert, no focal findings.

Laboratory Findings: Hct 35%; WBC 9600/μl with 72% PMNs, 0% bands, 20% lymphocytes, 4% eosinophils. Chest radiograph (below): bilateral alveolar-interstitial infiltrates. ABG (FiO_2 0.70, PEEP 8 cm H_2O): pH 7.47, PCO_2 32 mm Hg, PO_2 58 mm Hg.

What is the most likely cause for the persistent hypoxic respiratory failure?

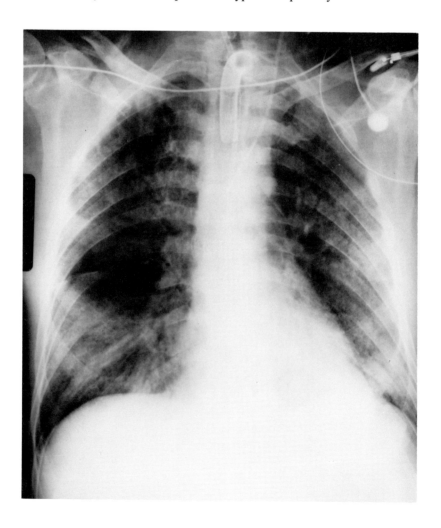

Diagnosis: Pulmonary oxygen toxicity.

Discussion: A review of the patient's records from the outlying hospital confirmed that he had been receiving inspired fractions of oxygen > 50% for 15 days. One hundred percent oxygen probably can be given safely to patients for up to 12 hours without clinical pulmonary damage; by 24 hours of 100% oxygen breathing, lung damage is almost assured. An FiO_2 of ≤ 0.50 can be continued for days or weeks without clinical toxicity. With concentrations of $O_2 > 50\%$, the time course of development of oxygen toxicity is unclear, but clinical toxicity can be anticipated within days of initiation of therapy and is related to the FiO_2 and duration of therapy.

Oxygen toxicity can be avoided by providing the lowest concentration of O_2 that will prevent tissue hypoxia. A clinical assessment of adequate tissue oxygenation can be performed at the bedside by monitoring mentation, urine output, blood pressure, and arterial pH; mixed venous oxygen tension also can be used when a Swan-Ganz catheter is in place, although values may be misleading in sepsis. In ARDS, when a high FiO_2 is required, the use of PEEP may allow a reduction in the FiO_2 below the critical toxic level by increasing FRC and decreasing the shunt fraction. Thus, one of the major impacts of PEEP in ARDS is the prevention of oxygen toxicity by allowing a reduction in FiO_2.

The diagnosis of oxygen toxicity is made clinically. Presently, there are no diagnostic tests that are useful. Oxygen toxicity develops insidiously after a variable latent period, depending upon individual susceptibility, duration and dose, changes in metabolic rate (oxygen tolerance decreases with fever and hyperthyrodism), and interaction with drugs and toxins (bleomycin, nitrofurantoin, adriamycin, and paraquat). Oxygen toxicity should be suspected in the proper clinical setting when the patient reports substernal chest pain associated with a nonproductive cough. Patients with oxygen toxicity show a deterioration in lung function characterized by progressive decrement in vital capacity, diffusing capacity, and lung compliance along with a widening of the alveolar-arterial oxygen tension gradient. However, the critically ill patient who is receiving a high concentration of oxygen usually has severe underlying pulmonary disease that is difficult to differentiate from oxygen toxicity.

Pulmonary oxygen toxicity occurs when toxic oxygen radicals, generated at an increased rate because of hyperoxia, overwhelm the antioxidant defense system. Damage to the alveolar-capillary membranes by oxygen radicals leads to increased capillary permeability with interstitial and alveolar edema and hemorrhage. Hyaline membranes are a prominent feature of this exudative stage. If hyperoxia continues, PMNs migrate into the interstitium and inflammation ensues. If the patient is removed from the high oxygen environment soon enough, healing results, leaving a variable degree of fibrosis.

Prevention is the key to management of pulmonary oxygen toxicity as no specific therapy is available. If the lowest concentration of oxygen is used to maintain adequate tissue oxygenation, then the syndrome probably will not develop. If oxygen toxicity occurs, the FiO_2 needs to be reduced to the lowest level that will prevent tissue hypoxia; this may require maintaining PaO_2 in the high 40s while monitoring indices of tissue oxygenation. The use of oxygen radical scavengers is currently not available.

The present patient died of complications of a massive myocardial infarction. Pathology of the lungs was compatible with oxygen toxicity without other lung disease.

Clinical Pearls

1. Pulmonary oxygen toxicity will develop in most patients who receive 100% oxygen for more than 24 hours but is unlikely to develop in those receiving $\leq$ 50% oxygen for weeks. Those receiving oxygen concentrations between 50 and 100% are at high risk for developing pulmonary toxicity after several days.

2. Patients with ARDS are at increased risk for developing pulmonary oxygen toxicity as they require a high FiO_2. PEEP should be used early to allow a reduction in the FiO_2 to $\leq$ 0.50; adequate tissue oxygenation should be monitored by clinical bedside observations.

3. Substernal chest pain and cough are the earliest symptoms of clinical pulmonary oxygen toxicity.

REFERENCES

1. Nash G, Blennerhassett JB, Pontoppidan H: Pulmonary lesions associated with oxygen therapy and artificial ventilation. N Engl J Med 276:368–374, 1967.
2. Davis WB, Rennard SE, Bitterman PB, et al: Pulmonary oxygen toxicity: Early reversible changes in human alveolar structures induced by hyperoxia. N Engl J Med 309:878–883, 1983.
3. Fisher AB: Pulmonary oxygen toxicity. In Fishman AP (ed): Pulmonary Diseases and Disorders, 2nd ed. New York, McGraw-Hill, 1988, pp 2332–2338.

CHAPTER 2

Cardiology

Blase A. Carabello, M.D.
Bruce W. Usher, M.D.
Nelson S. Gwinn, M.D.

PATIENT 1

A 55-year-old man with tachycardia and hypotension

A 55-year-old man was 2 days status post coronary artery bypass surgery; saphenous vein bypass grafts were placed to the left anterior descending artery, marginal of the circumflex coronary and distal right coronary artery. Before surgery the patient had suffered an anterior myocardial infarction and had moderate left ventricular dysfunction with an ejection fraction of 35%. He was observed in the CCU and noted to be having increasing ectopic beats followed by the paroxysmal development of a sustained tachycardia.

Physical Examination: Pulse 140 and regular; blood pressure 80/50. Neck: Cannon A waves in jugular venous pulses. Cardiac: S_1 variable in intensity.

Laboratory Findings: Na+ 137 mEq/L, CL⁻ 102 mEq/L, HCO₃⁻ 24 mEq/L, K+ 4.7 mEq/L; BUN 17 mg/dl. ECG: wide complex tachycardia. An intracardiac ECG was obtained via a previously placed pacing electrode (below).

What arrhythmia was occurring?

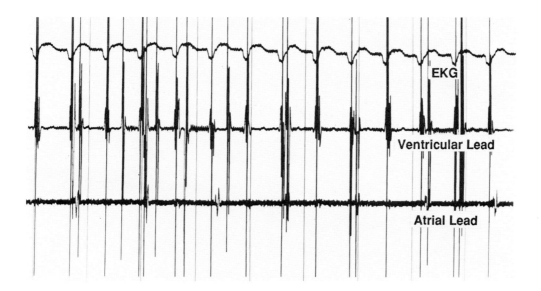

Diagnosis: Ventricular tachycardia.

Discussion: Making the distinction between supraventricular tachycardia and ventricular tachycardia is unimportant if the patient is severely hemodynamically compromised. In such cases immediate countershock is required. However, when the patient with a paroxysmal tachyarrhythmia is relatively stable, there is time to establish the specific diagnosis of the arrhythmia, which in turn influences management.

Narrow QRS complex tachycardias are easily identified as supraventricular. However, wide QRS-complex tachycardias are more difficult to diagnose and the distinction between ventricular tachycardia and supraventricular tachycardia with aberrancy may be difficult to make. The hallmark of ventricular tachycardia is atrioventricular dissociation; the impulse arises from the ventricle without relationship to the atria unless retrograde atrial conduction occurs. Physical examination for signs of atrioventricular dissociation may be as helpful as the electrocardiogram in establishing the diagnosis. The intensity of the first heart sound is dependent on the position of the mitral and tricuspid valves prior to ventricular systole. In ventricular tachycardia, atrial systole occurs at varying intervals with respect to ventricular systole. If atrial systole occurs just before ventricular systole, the mitral and tricuspid valves will be wide open and ventricular contraction will cause a loud first heart sound. If atrial systole occurs earlier, the atrioventricular valve leaflets will have had time to drift closed and ventricular systole will cause a soft first heart sound. Thus, variability in the intensity of the first heart sound is an important clue to the presence of ventricular tachycardia. Another sign of atrioventricular dissociation develops if right atrial contraction occurs while the tricuspid valve is closed during ventricular systole. In this situation a large A wave (Cannon A wave) will be seen in the jugular venous pulse.

Electrocardiographic distinctions between wide complex supraventricular versus ventricular tachycardia include: (1) the consistent presence of P waves prior to the QRS-complex in supraventricular tachycardia; (2) the resemblance of the tachycardia to previously documented premature atrial versus premature ventricular contractions; and (3) if the widened QRS-complex has a right bundle branch pattern, it is more likely to be supraventricular than ventricular tachycardia.

If the patient's condition is relatively stable but physical examination and the electrocardiogram have not yielded the diagnosis, an intra-atrial or intra-esophageal electrocardiogram will be diagnostic. If the patient already has external pacing leads such as are usually present following cardiac surgery, or if the patient has a central venous catheter in place, either can be used to record an intracardiac electrogram. If a central venous catheter is present, an electrode wire can be placed through the catheter to record the electrogram or the catheter itself can be converted to conductor by injecting it with 1 to 2 ml of sodium chloride or sodium bicarbonate. The electrocardiographic chest lead is then attached to a needle placed in the venous catheter or to the electrode wire to record the intraatrial electrogram.

The present patient was treated with intravenous lidocaine with resolution of his ventricular tachycardia and premature ventricular contractions.

Clinical Pearls

1. The distinction between supraventricular and ventricular wide complex tachycardia is irrelevant if the patient is severely compromised. Immediate countershock must be performed.

2. When the patient's condition permits it, careful physical examination may reveal the diagnosis by demonstrating classic signs of atrioventricular dissociation.

3. A central venous catheter, pacing electrode, or intraesophageal electrode can be used to make a definitive diagnosis.

REFERENCES

1. Gulamhusein S, Yee R, Ko PT, et al: Electrocardiographic criteria for differentiating aberrancy and ventricular extrasystole in chronic atrial fibrillation: Validation by intracardiac recordings. J Electrocardiol 18:41–50, 1985.
2. Dongas J, Lehmann MH, Mahmud R, et al: Value of preexisting bundle branch block in the electrocardiographic differentiation of supraventricular from ventricular origin of wide QRS tachycardia. Am J Cardiol 55:717–721, 1985.
3. Miles WM, Prystowsky EN, Heger JJ, et al: Evaluation of the patient with wide QRS tachycardia. Med Clin North Am 68:1015–1038, 1984.

PATIENT 2

A 46-year-old woman with coronary artery disease receiving quinidine found unresponsive

A 46-year-old woman with coronary artery disease was admitted to the hospital because of the new onset of angina at rest. Her medications at the time of admission included propranolol 40 mg q.i.d., and sublingual nitroglycerin. These medications were continued in the hospital, and diltiazem 60 mg t.i.d. was added to the regimen. Although her angina was controlled with these medications, she was noted to have several episodes of coupled and tripled premature ventricular contractions. She was begun on quinidine sulfate 300 mg q.i.d.

Physical Examination: Vital signs: normal. Neck: normal jugular venous pulsations. Chest: clear. Cardiac: occasional ectopic beats.

Laboratory Findings: CBC: normal. K^+ 4.7 mEq/L; quinidine level 2.6 μg/ml. Chest radiograph normal.

Hospital Course: On the third hospital day her QT-interval was noted to be 0.54 seconds. She was subsequently found to be unresponsive and hypotensive. Her ECG monitor printed the ECG shown below. Administration of DC countershock restored normal sinus rhythm.

Diagnose the arrhythmia.

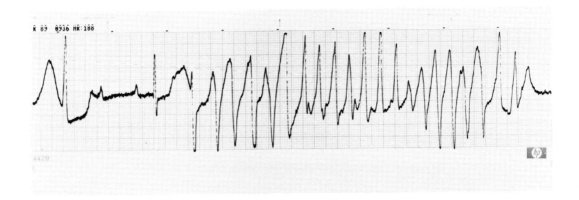

Diagnosis: Torsade de pointes.

Discussion: This variant of ventricular tachycardia literally means "revolution around a point." The axis and magnitude of the QRS-complex oscillate over time, going first positive, then negative, then positive again, and so on. Its electrophysiologic mechanism is uncertain. Torsade de pointes occurs in conjunction with a prolonged QT-interval that was present prior to the onset of the tachycardia. Exact definition of what constitutes a prolongation of the QT-interval is unclear because the QT-interval varies with heart rate. In general, a QT-interval of longer than 0.44 seconds is considered prolonged. The extent of QT-prolongation required to cause torsade de pointes is also uncertain, although QT-intervals ≥ 0.60 seconds are particularly dangerous. Prolongation of the QT-interval is frequently induced by class IA or class III antiarrhythmic drugs, including quinidine, procainamide, disopyramide, and amiodarone.

Other causes of prolonged QT-interval include congenital prolongation of the QT-interval, hypokalemia, hypocalcemia, hypomagnesemia, use of tricyclic antidepressants, or extended use of liquid protein diets. Episodes of torsade de pointes may be self-terminating or may be sustained and can degenerate into ventricular fibrillation. Although the initial episode can frequently be terminated by countershock, the tachycardia is likely to recur unless successful definitive therapy is employed.

Therapy depends on whether the QT-interval prolongation is congenital or acquired. Torsade de pointes in conjunction with congenital QT-prolongation often occurs secondary to increased sympathetic activity such as might develop with exercise or emotional upset. Beta-adrenergic blockade is frequently successful in controlling an arrhythmia due to congenital QT-prolongation. In acquired QT-prolongation the rhythm is often triggered by bradycardia or an electrocardiographic pause. Therapy includes discontinuing the offending agent responsible for the QT-interval prolongation, correcting electrolyte abnormalities and increasing the heart rate with atrial pacing or isoproterenol infusion. Intravenous infusion of 1 to 2 gm of magnesium sulfate may also successfully prevent recurrence of the arrhythmia.

The present patient recovered after DC countershock. With discontinuation of quinidine, she had no recurrence of the arrhythmia.

Clinical Pearls

1. Torsades de pointes is a serious side effect of agents that prolong the QT-interval. As such, it may limit the overall efficacy of these agents.

2. No numerical prolongation of the QT-interval is specific for torsade de pointes, but a QT-interval > 0.60 seconds is especially dangerous.

3. Therapy for torsade de pointes differs from that for usual ventricular tachycardia. For torsade de pointes associated with congenital QT-prolongation, beta-blockade is the therapy of choice. For acquired prolonged QT-interval torsade de pointes, removal of the offending agent and acceleration of the sinus rate or magnesium infusion are the mainstays of therapy.

REFERENCES

1. Kay GN, Plumb VJ, Arciniegas JG, et al: Torsade de pointes: The long-short initiating sequence and other clinical features. Observations in 32 patients. J Am Coll Cardiol 2:806–817, 1983.
2. Bhandari AK, Scheinman M: The long QT syndrome. Mod Concepts Cardiovasc Dis 54:45–50, 1985.
3. Tzivoni D, Keren A, Cohen AM, et al: Magnesium therapy for torsade de pointes. Am J Cardiol 53:528–530, 1984.

PATIENT 3

A 30-year-old man on renal dialysis with a history of congestive heart failure

A 30-year-old man had been on dialysis 6 months for chronic renal failure resulting from uncontrolled severe hypertension and nephrosclerosis. He had previously been treated for congestive heart failure thought to be secondary to hypertensive heart disease combined with volume overload from renal failure. In the week before admission, he had noted occasional inspiratory chest pain; 24 hours before admission he had progressively worsening dyspnea on exertion, culminating in dyspnea at rest. At admission, he denied chest pain but did complain of orthopnea.

Physical Examination: Temperature 36.5°; pulse 110; respirations 28; blood pressure 90/70 during expiration and 86/66 during inspiration. Neck veins: distended; estimated CVP 18 cm H_2O. Cardiac: point of maximal impulse not palpable; S_1 and S_2 normal; no rubs, gallops, or murmurs.

Laboratory Findings: Hct 25%, WBC 8,900/μl, normal differential; K+ 5.5 mEq/L, Na+ 135 mEq/L, Cl− 107 mEq/L; HCO_3^- 18 mEq/L; BUN 110 mg/dl, creatinine 8.9 mg/dl. Chest radiograph: enlarged cardiac silhouette with CT ratio of 0.6; pulmonary vascular redistribution. ECG: low voltage in limb leads with electrical alternans. Echocardiogram is displayed below. Swan-Ganz catheterization: RAP 20 mm Hg, PCWP 20 mm Hg, cardiac output 2.8 L/min.

What is your diagnosis?

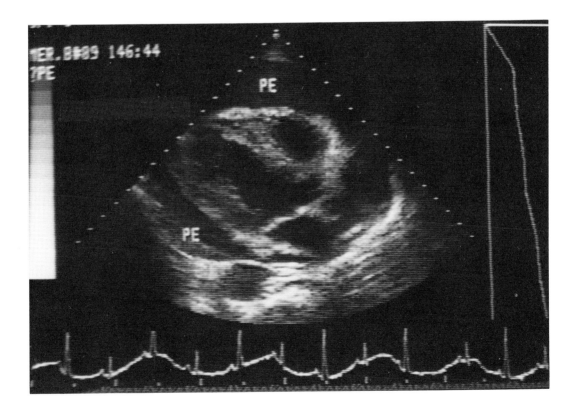

Diagnosis: Pericardial tamponade.

Discussion: While tamponade can occur in any condition that produces a pericardial effusion, it is the rapidity with which the effusion develops that determines whether or not ventricular filling is compromised. In myxedema, for example, the effusion develops slowly and a large effusion may exist without tamponade. Conversely, in cardiac trauma the rapid leakage of blood into the pericardial space can produce cardiac tamponade after accumulation of only 50 to 100 ml of blood.

Pericardial tamponade classically presents with signs of reduced systemic cardiac output, muffled heart tones, pulsus paradoxus, jugular venous distention, and a narrowed pulse pressure. However, in an individual patient, any of these signs may be absent. Although pulsus paradoxus is the most reliable sign of pericardial tamponade, it may also be present in obstructive airway disease, in constrictive pericarditis, and in hypovolemic shock. Although the exact pathophysiology of pulsus paradoxus is uncertain, it is believed to occur secondary to differential filling of the two ventricles during inspiration. Inspiration enhances filling of the right ventricle, causing a shift of the intraventricular septum toward the left ventricle; increased right ventricular filling also produces increased occupancy of the pericardial space by the right ventricle. Both limit left ventricular filling and left ventricular stroke volume, thereby reducing systemic cardiac output and blood pressure during inspiration. Increased lung capacity with decreased venous return to the left ventricle during inspiration, together with an increase in left ventricular transmural pressure (afterload) due to negative inspiratory thoracic pressure, may further reduce inspiratory systemic cardiac output.

Pulsus paradoxus was absent in the present patient. Pulsus paradoxus will be absent when differential filling of the two ventricles during respiration fails to occur. Absence of differential filling occurs when an antecedent atrial septal defect or ventricular septal defect produces equal filling of both ventricles. Pulsus paradoxus may also be absent when severe left ventricular failure is present coincidentally with tamponade. With left ventricular failure, the enlarged left ventricle together with its high diastolic filling pressure resists the inspiratory effects of increased right ventricular filling.

Jugular venous distention is another sign usually seen in pericardial tamponade. Jugular venous distention is usually present secondary to the increase in intrapericardial pressure reflected upon all chambers of the heart, including the right atrium. However, jugular venous distention may be absent if the patient is volume-depleted at the time tamponade occurs.

The diagnosis of pericardial tamponade should be suspected by the clinical presentation together with an echocardiogram that demonstrates pericardial effusion. The echocardiographic signs of right atrial and/or right ventricular collapse serve to heighten suspicion that tamponade is present. Right heart catheterization, which demonstrates equalization of the filling pressures in all chambers, helps to confirm the diagnosis. However, diagnosis of pericardial tamponade is only certain when relief of the tamponade produces an increase in cardiac output. Although tamponade always constitutes a medical emergency, some cases are less acute than others. If time permits, hemodynamic monitoring of filling pressures and cardiac output can be measured before and after pericardiocentesis to confirm the diagnosis.

The only effective therapy for pericardial tamponade is drainage of the pericardial sac either by needle pericardiocentesis or surgical pericardiotomy. Medical therapy such as volume expansion or the use of pressor agents may help to stabilize the patient while preparing for mechanical relief of the tamponade, but these therapies are unsatisfactory for long-term management and are no substitute for pericardial drainage.

The present patient was diagnosed as having pericardial tamponade related to uremic pericarditis. He underwent pericardiocentesis with relief of symptoms.

Clinical Pearls

1. The most reliable sign of pericardial tamponade is pulsus paradoxus; this sign may be absent, however, in the presence of an atrial septal defect, a ventricular septal defect, or if left ventricular failure is present.

2. Jugular venous distention is usually present with pericardial tamponade. However, this sign may also be absent if the patient is volume-depleted at the time tamponade develops.

3. The only absolute proof of the presence of tamponade is improvement in hemodynamics following removal of the pericardial fluid.

4. There is no effective medical therapy for pericardial tamponade. Drainage is the only definitive treatment.

REFERENCES

1. McGregor M: Current concepts: Pulsus paradoxus. N Engl J Med 301:480–482, 1979.
2. Reddy PS, Curtiss EI, O'Toole JD, et al: Cardiac tamponade: Hemodynamic observations in man. Circulation 58:265–272, 1978.
3. Shabetai R, Fowler NO, Guntheroth WG: The hemodynamics of cardiac tamponade and constrictive pericarditis. Am J Cardiol 26:480–489, 1970.

PATIENT 4

A 45-year-old woman with migraine headaches and nocturnal chest pain

A 45-year-old woman with a 3-year history of migraine headaches developed early morning chest pain during the previous 3 weeks that caused her to awaken from sleep. The pain lasted 10 to 15 minutes and frequently radiated to the left arm. In the emergency room, the patient was without chest pain and her ECG was within normal limits. She was admitted to the CCU for observation. On the following evening she again noted chest pain.

Physical Examination (during the painful episode): Temperature 36.8°; pulse 80; respirations 22; blood pressure 160/90. The patient was in distress with chest pain. Cardiac: S_4 present; no murmurs or rubs.

Laboratory Findings: CBC, electrolytes, BUN, and creatinine: normal. Serial ECGs (limb leads): shown below.

What is the etiology of the patient's chest pain?

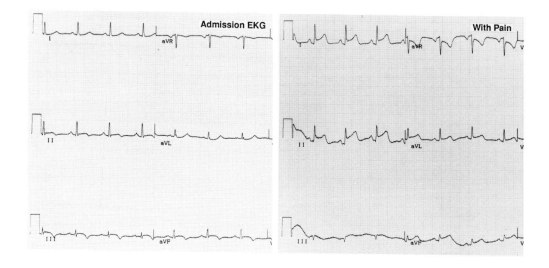

Diagnosis: Variant (Prinzmetal's) angina.

Discussion: Angina develops when myocardial oxygen demand exceeds supply, thereby causing myocardial ischemia. Classic angina occurs when exertion increases myocardial oxygen demands beyond the oxygen supply that can be delivered by diseased coronary arteries. Conversely, variant angina typically occurs at rest and results from a reduction in myocardial oxygen supply with little increase in demand. This reduction in supply is due to coronary vasospasm, which may occur in relatively "normal" coronary arteries or in conjunction with severe atherosclerotic coronary disease. The spasm results in temporary total occlusion of the affected coronary, producing transmural ischemia.

The resultant transmural ischemia is reflected in the ECG as ST segment elevation (the hallmark of variant angina) instead of ST segment depression seen in typical angina. Thus during the attack of angina, the ECG is consistent with an acute transmural myocardial infarction, but spontaneous release of the spasm results in coronary reperfusion and normalization of the ECG before significant myocardial damage occurs.

Variant angina is distinguished from other causes of ST segment elevation (left ventricular aneurysm, pericarditis, and normal variants) by its transient nature and the usual presence of "reciprocal" ST segment depression in opposing ECG leads. The diagnosis of variant angina is most easily made by recording an ECG during the patient's episode of chest pain. While classic angina may occur without ECG changes, variant angina is by definition associated with ST segment elevation during the episode.

Occasionally patients with variant angina will have rest pain associated with both ST segment elevations as well as ST segment depression. Electrocardiographic Q waves may develop during angina and disappear when the pain is relieved. Episodes of variant angina may also be associated with malignant ventricular arrhythmias, including sustained ventricular tachycardia. Antiarrhythmic drugs are usually unsuccessful in treating these arrhythmias. The key to arrhythmia therapy in this disease is relief of the spasm and ischemia with reperfusion of the affected area of the myocardium.

If there has been no chance to observe the patient and to obtain an ECG during an episode of angina, provocation of an attack by infusion of intravenous ergonovine can be performed. This is done with great caution, usually in the catheterization laboratory. Small doses of ergonovine (50 μg) are infused while monitoring for changes in the ECG together with angiographic examination of the coronary arteries for spasm. If spasm is precipitated, it is reversed by sublingual, intravenous, or intracoronary infusion of nitroglycerin.

The cause of spasm in variant angina is unknown. In some cases, variant angina is part of a diffuse, vasospastic process that may be associated with migraine headaches and Raynaud's phenomenon. Supersensitivity of the vascular smooth muscle to circulating humoral agents or secretion of some as yet unidentified vasoconstrictor substance are postulated mechanisms for the vasospasm.

Acute episodes of variant angina are usually treated successfully with sublingual administration of nitroglycerin. While long-acting nitrates may also provide prophylaxis against repeated episodes, calcium channel blockers are considered the long-term therapy of choice. All currently available calcium blockers—nifedipine, verapamil, and diltiazem—have been shown to be effective in the treatment of variant angina. Revascularization as a therapy for variant angina is considered only if severe obstructive coronary disease underlies the vascular spasm. In general, surgery or percutaneous transluminal angioplasty has the same indications and limitations for variant angina associated with underlying obstructive coronary disease as for chronic stable angina.

The present patient was placed on therapy with diltiazem, and no future episodes of angina occurred during 3 months of follow-up.

Clinical Pearls

1. Transient ST segment elevation during the attack of pain establishes the diagnosis of variant angina.

2. Arrhythmias occurring during vasospastic angina are usually refractory to antiarrhythmic agents but respond to relief of the vasospasm.

3. Variant angina may be part of a generalized vasospastic tendency associated with migraine headaches or Raynaud's phenomenon.

REFERENCES

1. Oliva PB, Potts DE, Pluss RG: Coronary arterial spasm in Prinzmetal angina: Documentation by coronary arteriography. N Engl J Med 288:745–751, 1973.
2. Waters DD, Szlachcic J, Theroux P, et al: Ergonovine testing to detect spontaneous remissions of variant angina during long-term treatment with calcium antagonist drugs. Am J Cardiol 47:179–184, 1981.
3. Prida XE, Gelman JS, Feldman RL, et al: Comparison of diltiazem and nifedipine alone and in combination in patients with coronary artery spasm. J Am Coll Cardiol 9:412–419, 1987.
4. Corcos T, David PR, Bourassa MG, et al: Percutaneous transluminal coronary angioplasty for the treatment of variant angina. J Am Coll Cardiol 5:1046–1054, 1985.

PATIENT 5

A 76-year-old man presenting with congestive heart failure and shock

A 76-year-old man was in his usual state of health until 48 hours before admission when he noted increasing dyspnea, orthopnea, and paroxysmal nocturnal dyspnea. He became lightheaded with minimal exertion. Two years earlier he had suffered an episode of syncope after climbing two flights of stairs. During the ensuing 2 years he noted gradually progressive limitation of exercise tolerance due to dyspnea. He denied a history of angina pectoris.

Physical Examination: Temperature 36.7°; pulse 100; respirations 28; blood pressure 70/50. Carotid pulses: normal upstroke but diminished in volume. Chest: bibasilar rales. Cardiac: forceful left ventricular precordial impulse; I/VI systolic ejection murmur that radiated weakly to the carotids; single S_2; S_3 gallop over the cardiac apex.

Laboratory Findings: CBC: normal; Na+ 141 mEq/L; Cl⁻ 102 mEq/L, HCO_3^- 18 mEq/L, K+ 4.2 mEq/L; BUN 35 mg/dl, creatinine 2.5 mg/dl. Chest radiograph: mild cardiomegaly and interstitial edema. ECG: normal sinus rhythm with left ventricular hypertrophy. Echocardiogram: severe restriction of aortic valve motion; concentric left ventricular hypertrophy with reduced ejection performance; estimated ejection fraction 35%. Doppler interrogation of aortic valve (below): transvalvular gradient 137 mm Hg.

What is the cause of this patient's shock?

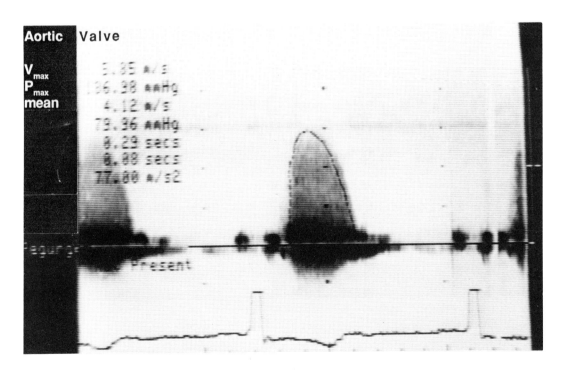

Diagnosis: Shock secondary to aortic stenosis.

Discussion: The most common cause of adult aortic stenosis is senile calcification of the aortic valve. Calcification may occur on a tricuspid aortic valve where is presents as aortic stenosis in the seventh through ninth decades of life, or on a previously bicuspid aortic valve where it typically presents in the fifth or sixth decades. Pressure-overload imposed on the left ventricle by aortic stenosis is compensated for by concentric left ventricular hypertrophy.

Typically the adult patient with aortic stenosis enjoys a long latent period during which there are no symptoms associated with this compensatory hypertrophy. During this asymptomatic phase, life span is nearly normal and there is little risk of sudden death. However, once angina develops, 50% of such patients will be dead within 5 years; once syncope develops, 50% will be dead in 2 to 3 years; and once symptoms of congestive heart failure develop, 50% will be dead within 1 to 2 years. Thus the development of symptoms requires immediate mechanical correction of the stenotic valve.

The diagnosis of aortic stenosis is usually apparent at the bedside in the classic case. The presence of delayed carotid upstrokes, a systolic ejection murmur of moderate intensity that radiates to the carotid arteries, and a single second heart sound (only the P2 component) usually leads to the diagnosis. Once pump failure ensues, however, the intensity of the murmur decreases as less flow crosses the aortic valve. Further, as the carotid arteries lose their elastic recoil with age, the delayed quality of the aortic pulse may become pseudonormalized. Thus, the classic findings on physical examination may be absent in some patients with advanced disease. In such patients, ECG evidence of left ventricular hypertrophy together with a chest radiograph that shows a relatively small heart despite the present of congestive heart failure helps to raise suspicion that aortic stenosis is present. A cardiac echo Doppler study will demonstrate that the aortic valve fails to open normally and that a pressure gradient exists across its orifice.

The diagnosis of aortic stenosis is usually confirmed at cardiac catheterization; however, the elderly patient described above may not tolerate this procedure. A combination of the clinical picture together with dense calcification of an aortic valve that moves poorly on echocardiogram and a significant transvalvular gradient may be enough to proceed with therapy.

The only effective therapy for aortic stenosis is mechanical relief of the obstruction accomplished by replacing the aortic valve. Because elderly patients with poor left ventricular function are at increased risk during aortic valve replacement, some investigators have advocated balloon aortic valvuloplasty as a temporizing measure. This procedure allows for partial correction of the obstruction and stabilization of the hemodynamics. While cases of reversal of cardiogenic shock from aortic stenosis have been reported following balloon valvuloplasty, the role of valvuloplasty versus surgery for this situation is still unclear.

The present patient underwent cardiac surgery with replacement of a stenotic aortic valve.

Clinical Pearls

1. In advanced aortic stenosis in the elderly, the classic murmur may be of reduced intensity, and the delay of the carotid upstrokes may be absent.

2. An echo Doppler study will usually help to confirm the diagnosis once the question has been raised.

3. Mechanical intervention to relieve the obstruction is the only successful therapy for this disease. Aortic valve replacement may be beneficial even in moribund patients.

REFERENCES

1. Lombard JT, Selzer A: Valvular aortic stenosis. A clinical and hemodynamic profile of patients. Ann Intern Med 106:292–298, 1987.
2. Carabello BA, Green LH, Grossman W, et al: Hemodynamic determinants of prognosis of aortic valve replacement in critical aortic stenosis and advanced congestive heart failure. Circulation 62:42–48, 1980.
3. Schwarz F, Baumann P, Manthey J, et al: The effect of aortic valve replacement on survival. Circulation 66:1105–1110, 1982.
4. McKay RG, Safian RD, Lock JE, et al: Assessment of left ventricular and aortic valve function after aortic balloon valvuloplasty in adult patients with critical aortic stenosis. Circulation 75:192–203, 1987.

PATIENT 6

A 50-year-old woman with massive hemoptysis following placement of a Swan-Ganz catheter

A 50-year-old woman with a history of idiopathic hypertrophic subaortic stenosis (IHSS) and mitral regurgitation developed progressive dyspnea on exertion, orthopnea, and paroxysmal nocturnal dyspnea in the 48 hours before admission. Because maneuvers that made the IHSS better made the mitral regurgitation worse and vice versa, she was admitted to the CCU for placement of a Swan-Ganz catheter to guide therapy.

Physical Examination: Pulse 110; respirations 28; blood pressure 100/74. Chest: bibasilar rales. Cardiac: systolic murmur.

Laboratory Findings: Hct 35%. ECG: left ventricular hypertrophy and sinus rhythm.

Hospital Course: The Swan-Ganz catheter was placed and initial hemodynamic findings were: PAP 50/30 mm Hg, PCWP 25 mm Hg, and cardiac output 3.0 L/min. Twenty-four hours later, the patient developed massive hemoptysis of approximately 1 liter of blood. A chest radiograph demonstrated the Swan-Ganz catheter in the right lower lobe with the balloon inflated.

What is the cause of the patient's hemoptysis?

Diagnosis: Swan-Ganz catheter–induced pulmonary artery rupture.

Discussion: Pulmonary artery catheterization, which has become commonplace in modern intensive care, can yield invaluable information about left and right ventricular filling pressures and cardiac output and is thus an aid in managing fluids and in gauging the effect of cardiovascular drugs. Although this procedure has been reported to cause several different types of complications, most are rare and avoidable by scrupulous attention to safe catheter manipulation. Complications of Swan-Ganz catheterization fall into two categories: those produced while gaining venous access for catheter insertion, and those due to the presence of the catheter itself.

The Swan-Ganz catheter may be inserted from the subclavian, internal jugular, brachial, and femoral approaches. Complications of insertion primarily occur during insertion into the subclavian and internal jugular veins. These complications include pneumothorax, inadvertent puncture of the subclavian artery producing hemothorax, and inadvertent puncture of the carotid artery producing cerebrovascular compromise.

Complications from the catheter itself include: (1) ventricular arrhythmias during catheter manipulation, (2) knotting of catheter, (3) right bundle branch block (this will result in complete heart block if antecedent left bundle branch block also happened to be present), (4) pulmonary infarction, (5) infection and endocarditis, (6) disruption of the tricuspid valve with tricuspid insufficiency, and (7) rupture of the pulmonary artery.

Pulmonary artery rupture occurs when the catheter has been left constantly in the wedge position (either with the balloon inflated or deflated) or when the balloon is inflated while the catheter is positioned in a small distal pulmonary artery. This latter complication can be avoided by ensuring that it takes exactly 1.5 ml of air to inflate the balloon to the point at which it enters the wedge position. If wedging occurs prior to full balloon inflation, it indicates that the catheter tip has migrated distally. In this situation the catheter should be withdrawn until the balloon accepts 1.5 ml of air coincident with wedging. Persistent wedging of the catheter is recognized by the characteristic wave form seen in the wedged position. These characteristics include: (1) a bifid wave form displaying A and V waves, (2) the mean pulmonary wedge pressure is less than the mean pulmonary artery pressure, and (3) the V wave in the wedge pressure tracing occurs after the T wave of the electrocardiogram. If it is suspected that the catheter is wedged, it should be withdrawn slightly. A change in wave form or a rise in the mean pressure indicates that the catheter was wedged and has now been withdrawn to the pulmonary artery position. Fluoroscopy is useful in confirming the position of the distal tip of the catheter.

The present patient became hypotensive and required transfusion. Hemoptysis ceased spontaneously but recurred 1 week later, necessitating a right lower lobectomy.

Clinical Pearls

1. Pulmonary artery rupture occurs from persistent or improper wedging of a Swan-Ganz catheter. Wedging of a pulmonary artery catheter should always require the full 1.5 cc of air.

2. The wedge pressure tracing, especially one with a high V wave, can be confused with a pulmonary artery pressure. However, mean pulmonary pressure will be greater than the mean wedge pressure and the V wave in the wedged tracing will always follow the T wave of the electrocardiogram; conversely, the peak of the pulmonary artery tracing will occur before or coincident with the T wave of the electrocardiogram.

3. If Swan-Ganz catheterization is performed in a patient with left bundle branch block, all equipment needed to perform temporary pacing should be readily available in case complete heart block occurs.

4. Because ventricular tachycardia and ventricular fibrillation are complications of Swan-Ganz catheterization, the procedure must always be performed in the presence of a cardiac defibrillator.

REFERENCES
1. Carabello BA, Grossman W: Bedside hemodynamic monitoring, cardiac catheterization, and pulmonary angiography. In Cohn PF, Wynne J (eds): Diagnostic Methods in Clinical Cardiology. Boston, Little, Brown & Co., 1982, pp 235–269.
2. Boyd KD, Thomas SJ, Gold J, et al: A prospective study of complications of pulmonary artery catheterizations in 500 consecutive patients. Chest 84:245–249, 1983.
3. Kelly TF Jr., Morris GC Jr, Crawford ES, et al: Perforation of the pulmonary artery with Swan-Ganz catheters: Diagnosis and surgical management. Ann Surg 193:686–692, 1981.

PATIENT 7

A 52-year-old man with inferior myocardial infarction, a new holosystolic murmur, and congestive heart failure

A 52-year-old man was in his usual state of health until he developed substernal chest pain associated with nausea and diaphoresis. In the emergency room his blood pressure was 110/70, his pulse 60 and regular, and there were no signs of congestive heart failure. His ECG demonstrated an acute inferior myocardial infarction. The patient was admitted to the CCU. The first 2 days in the hospital were uneventful. On the third hospital day he noted lethargy, dyspnea, and orthopnea.

Physical Examination: Pulse 100; respirations 27; blood pressure 95/70. Cardiac: III/VI holosystolic murmur heard best at left lower sternal border with radiation toward sternum.

Laboratory Findings: Hct 43%, WBC 12,000/μl, normal differential. Serum electrolytes and BUN: normal. Chest radiograph: borderline cardiomegaly and pulmonary vascular redistribution. ECG: ST segment elevation and Q waves in leads II, III, and AVF consistent with acute inferior myocardial infarction. Swan-Ganz catheterization data are shown below.

Hemodynamic measurement	Pressure (mm Hg)	Oxygen saturation (%)
Right atrium	9	62
Right ventricle	40/10	84
Pulmonary artery	40/20	85
Pulmonary capillary wedge	21	95
Radial artery	95/70	95

Estimated shunt ratio 3.3:1

What complication of myocardial infarction has developed?

Diagnosis: Myocardial infarction (MI) complicated by ventricular septal defect (VSD).

Discussion: Rupture of the interventricular septum occurs in approximately 4% of all MIs. Because the left anterior descending artery gives off a large number of septal perforating arteries, VSD might be anticipated to occur primarily in anterior infarction. However, the posterior descending artery from the right coronary also gives off septal perforators and thus one third of VSDs occur following inferior MI. Following MI, necrosis and liquefaction of the infarcted tissue begin rapidly. Liquefaction peaks between the second and fifth days following the infarct, and it is during this time when ventricular septal rupture usually occurs.

In acute ventricular septal rupture, the left ventricle, already compromised by MI, now "wastes" a significant portion of its cardiac output through intracardiac shunting. Congestive heart failure and circulatory shock develop as a result. While the left ventricle is the primary chamber affected, coexistent right ventricular dysfunction, if present, further compromises cardiac output. Indeed, right ventricular function may be as important a determinant of outcome as left ventricular function.

Ventricular septal defect is suspected when a new holosystolic murmur develops following MI. Echocardiography may demonstrate the actual defect, and color-flow Doppler studies have a high sensitivity in detecting the left to right shunt.

The magnitude of the shunt and the resultant hemodynamic compromise are quantified during right heart cardiac catheterization. A step-up in oxygen saturation at the level of the right ventricle confirms the presence of the VSD. The typical Swan-Ganz catheter has a proximal port located in the right atrium (above the VSD) and a distal port in the pulmonary artery (distal to the VSD) from which blood for oxygen saturation determination can be obtained. Saturations from these two positions together with an arterial saturation can be used to instantaneously calculate the shunt ratio using the following formula:

$$Qp/Qs = \frac{ART\ sat - RA\ sat}{ART\ sat - PA\ sat}$$

where Qp/Qs = the shunt ratio, RA sat = oxygen saturation in the right atrium, PA sat = the oxygen saturation in the pulmonary artery, and ART sat = the oxygen saturation in the systemic artery. This formula can be used to evaluate the change in the shunt ratio produced by therapeutic interventions.

Pulmonary capillary wedge (P_{CW}) pressure is almost always elevated in the acute VSD. Large V waves may be present in the P_{CW} tracing because increased venous return to the left atrium produced by the shunt increases left atrial filling. Thus, although large P_{CW} V waves are usually associated with mitral regurgitation, they may also be seen in acute VSD.

The ultimate therapy for VSD is surgical correction. However, systemic afterload reduction is useful in stabilizing the patient until surgery can be performed. Pharmacologically, this is best achieved with infusion of nitroprusside, but many patients are already in shock following the development of a VSD and will not tolerate vasodilator therapy. Intraaortic balloon pumping is the temporizing therapy of choice when shock complicates VSD. Aortic balloon pumping augments systemic pressure by counterpulsation and also increases forward cardiac output by reducing left ventricular afterload, which in turn reduces the magnitude of the shunt.

The present patient stabilized with intra-aortic balloon therapy for 4 days but eventually cardiac output deteriorated and he died before surgery.

Clinical Pearls

1. Ventricular septal defect complicates inferior as well as anterior infarctions.

2. A Swan-Ganz catheter may be used to obtain blood oxygen saturations, enabling calculation of the shunt ratio.

3. Giant V waves, thought to be a sign of acute mitral regurgitation, may also occur in acute VSD.

4. Intraaortic balloon pumping is the temporizing therapy of choice until surgery can be performed.

REFERENCES

1. Radford MJ, Johnson RA, Daggett WM, et al: Ventricular septal rupture: A review of clinical and physiologic features and an analysis of survival. Circulation 64:545–553, 1981.
2. Matsui K, Kay JH, Mendez M, Zubiate P, et al: Ventricular septal rupture secondary to myocardial infarction. Clinical approach and surgical results. JAMA 245:1537–1539, 1981.
3. Edwards BS, Edwards WD, Edwards JE: Ventricular septal rupture complicating acute myocardial infarction: Identification of simple and complex types in 53 autopsied hearts. Am J Cardiol 54:1201–1205, 1984.

PATIENT 8

A 40-year-old woman with malaise, weight loss, and sudden claudication of the right hand

A 40-year-old woman was in her usual state of health until 6 weeks before admission when she noted the gradual onset of malaise, anorexia, and a 5-pound weight loss. On the morning of admission, she noticed her right hand becoming first cold and then painful. She had no history of antecedent heart disease.

Physical Examination: Temperature 37.2°; pulse 90; respirations 20; blood pressure 100/70. Thin woman with pain in her right hand. Cardiac: right ventricular sternal tap; P_2 component of S_2 increased; I/VI diastolic rumble at the apex. Extremities: absent right brachial, radial, and ulnar pulses.

Laboratory Findings: Hct 30.2%, WBC 10,200/μl, differential normal, ESR 57 mm hr. Chest radiograph: straightening of left heart border. ECG: normal sinus rhythm with left atrial abnormality. Echocardiogram: shown below.

What diagnosis underlies the patient's constitutional and peripheral vascular symptoms?

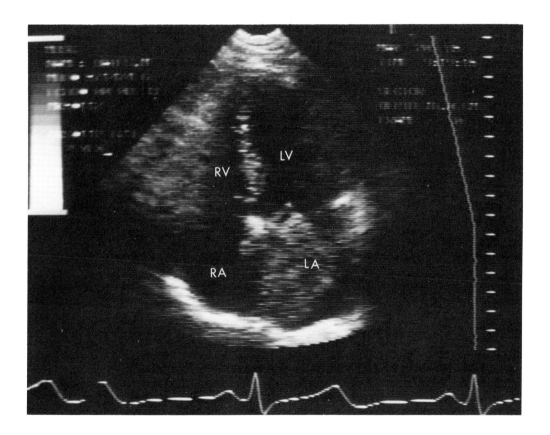

Diagnosis: Left atrial myxoma.

Discussion: Of the primary tumors of the heart, myxoma is the most common, constituting approximately 50% of all primary cardiac tumors. Of myxomas, 90% arise in the left atrium. The manifestations of left atrial myxoma fall into three categories: systemic, embolic, and hemodynamic.

Left atrial myxoma may present as a systemic illness. Patients may report malaise, weight loss, fever, and arthralgias. Laboratory examination may demonstrate anemia, leukocytosis, and an elevated erythrocyte sedimentation rate. Because the tumors are friable, they may frequently be the source of systemic emboli. As such, the disease masquerades as subacute bacterial endocarditis.

If the tumor obstructs left ventricular inflow, it may simulate mitral stenosis. A loud first heart sound, a diastolic rumble, signs of pulmonary hypertension, and an early diastolic sound (tumor plop), which may mimic an opening snap, can fool the best diagnostician. Occasionally, limitations of mitral valve inflow by the tumor may vary with the patient's position. In such cases, patients may note worsening symptoms when they sit upright.

The most sensitive technique for the detection of left atrial myxoma is echocardiography. Provided the patient has an adequate sonographic window, echocardiography can demonstrate almost all left atrial myxomas. Because of the potential for embolization, all left atrial myxomas should be removed surgically. Thus, the amount of hemodynamic derangement caused by the tumor is less important than it is in mitral stenosis in deciding upon therapy. Although cardiac catheterization may yield important data about the presence of other valvular lesions or of incidental coronary disease, catheterization is generally not necessary before surgical removal of the left atrial myxoma. On the other hand, if an adequate echocardiogram cannot be performed, cardiac catheterization may be useful in establishing the diagnosis. In such cases a pulmonary arteriogram with followthrough of contrast into the left atrium usually demonstrates the mass. Because the tumor may damage the mitral valve, rendering it incompetent, left ventriculography should usually be performed to evaluate the amount of mitral regurgitation present.

Surgical removal of myxoma is generally curative. Recurrence, however, is a problem in about 5% of cases and occurs most commonly in familial myxoma. In this condition, a second primary (as opposed to recurrence of the original tumor) may result in a tumor being discovered at late follow-up.

The present patient was diagnosed as having an atrial myxoma on the basis of her typical clinical presentation and echocardiographic findings. She underwent surgical resection of the tumor with complete resolution of symptoms.

Clinical Pearls

1. Left atrial myxoma may masquerade as subacute bacterial endocarditis, presenting with fever, malaise, heart murmur, and evidence of systemic emboli.

2. Echocardiography is the diagnostic modality of choice; cardiac catheterization is usually unnecessary in the diagnostic workup of such patients.

3. Sudden changes in cardiovascular status associated with changes in position should raise the suspicion of left atrial myxoma.

REFERENCES
1. MacGregor GA, Cullen RA: The syndrome of fever, anaemia and high sedimentation rate with an atrial myxoma. Br Med J 2:991–993, 1959.
2. Charuzi Y, Bolger A, Beeder C, Lew AS: A new echocardiographic classification of left atrial myxoma. Am J Cardiol 55:614–615, 1985.
3. Smith C: Tumors of the heart. Arch Pathol Lab Med 110:371–374, 1986.

PATIENT 9

A 62-year-old man with hypotension following an acute inferior myocardial infarction

A 62-year-old man was well until 2 days prior to admission when he developed anterior chest pain with radiation to the left arm. He was seen in the emergency room where an ECG revealed an acute inferior myocardial infarction. He was admitted to the CCU. Over the next 24 hours the patient's blood pressure gradually decreased to 80/50 and urinary output decreased to less than 20 ml/hr.

Physical Examination: Temperature 37°; pulse 68; respirations 22; blood pressure 80/50. Neck: estimated CVP 15 cm H_2O; neck vein distention increased during inspiration. Cardiac: PMI difficult to palpate, normal S_1 and S_2, no murmurs, gallops or rubs.

Laboratory Findings: Chest radiograph: normal. ECG: ST segment elevations in leads II, III and AVF with T waves in the same leads consistent with acute inferior myocardial infarction. Echocardiogram: akinesis of left ventricular inferior wall, and hypokinesis of right ventricle. Swan-Ganz catheter: data shown below.

Hemodynamic measurement	Pressure (mm Hg)	Oxygen saturation (%)
Right atrium	11	58
Right ventricle	30/11	59
Pulmonary artery	30/18/24	59
Pulmonary capillary wedge	19	95

What is the patient's cardiac diagnosis?

Diagnosis: Inferior myocardial infarction with concomitant right ventricular infarction.

Discussion: Occlusion of a dominant right coronary artery may result in infarction of the left ventricular inferior wall. In approximately 40% of inferior myocardial infarctions, some degree of right ventricular infarction also occurs. However, right ventricular infarction is manifested clinically only in approximately one quarter of all right ventricular infarctions. Thus, inferior left ventricular myocardial infarction can be expected to be complicated by clinically important right ventricular infarction in approximately 10% of all cases of inferior myocardial infarction.

The right ventricle's main function is to fill the left ventricle. In inferior myocardial infarction, left ventricular function is impaired. Compensation for this dysfunction is derived by increased filling of the left ventricle to maximize use of the Frank-Starling mechanism. However, when the right ventricle is also infarcted, its ability to fill the left ventricle becomes impaired and Frank-Starling compensation does not occur, resulting in reduced systemic cardiac output and shock. The inability of the right ventricle to fill the left ventricle in right ventricular infarction is further compounded as the right ventricle becomes distended secondary to right ventricular failure. Distention of the right ventricle takes up room inside the pericardial sac and also displaces the interventricular septum into the left ventricle. Both of these effects decrease left ventricular compliance and make it more difficult for the right ventricle to fill the left ventricle, further reducing left ventricular output.

Dominant right ventricular infarction presents with signs of reduced systemic output (reduced urinary output and/or shock) together with signs of isolated right ventricular failure. Jugular venous distention may be present with little evidence of left-sided congestion; thus pulmonary rales or a left ventricular S_3 is typically absent.

The diagnosis should be suspected in any inferior myocardial infarction complicated by shock and right ventricular failure. The diagnosis is confirmed by echocardiography, which shows a poorly contractile right ventricle, and right heart catheterization, which demonstrates increased right atrial pressure, a steep right atrial y descent, narrowed pulmonary artery pulse pressure without pulmonary hypertension, and only modest elevation of left ventricular filling pressure. Right and left atrial pressure may even be identical, and the condition may mimic pericardial tamponade. The distinction between dominant right ventricular infarction and tamponade can be made echocardiographically on the basis of the presence or absence of pericardial effusion. Occasionally, equalization of right and left atrial filling pressure in conjunction with a previously patent foramen ovale may cause a right-to-left shunt with subsequent cyanosis.

Standard therapy for right ventricular infarction includes volume expansion to increase right ventricular filling pressure and right ventricular cardiac output. While this is usually successful, it may also have the effect of further distending the right ventricle, causing it to take up additional space inside the pericardium further compromising left ventricular filling. In such cases, the addition of a pressor agent, such as dobutamine, is successful in restoring forward output.

The present patient responded to volume expansion with improvement in hemodynamic parameters.

Clinical Pearls

1. Right ventricular infarction is a frequent and, most importantly, a reversible cause of shock following inferior myocardial infarction. Recognition of right-sided failure (neck vein distention) out of proportion to left-sided failure is a key to the diagnosis.

2. The occasional coexistence of a patent foramen ovale with right ventricular infarction may result in severe right-to-left shunting and cyanosis.

3. Although volume expansion is the treatment of choice, this is frequently counterproductive, as it further limits left ventricular filling. In such instances, pressor agents such as dobutamine are indicated.

REFERENCES
1. Lorell B, Leinbach RC, Pohost GM, et al: Right ventricular infarction. Clinical diagnosis and differentiation from cardiac tamponade and pericardial constriction. Am J Cardiol 43:465–471, 1979.
2. Dell'Italia LJ, Starling MR, Crawford MH, et al: Right ventricular infarction: Identification by hemodynamic measurements before and after volume loading and correlation with noninvasive techniques. J Am Coll Cardiol 4:931–939, 1984.
3. Dell'Italia LJ, Starling MR, Blumhardt R, et al: Comparative effects of volume loading, dobutamine, and nitroprusside in patients with predominant right ventricular infarction. Circulation 1327–1335, 1985.

PATIENT 10

A 57-year-old man with longstanding hypertension presenting with severe chest pain

A 57-year-old man with long-term, poorly controlled hypertension developed severe precordial chest pain radiating to the back while doing garden work. There was no previous history of chest pain, dyspnea, or orthopnea.

Physical Examination: Temperature 37.4°; pulse 110; respirations 20; blood pressure 200/100. The patient was in severe distress with chest pain. Eyes: normal. Pharynx: normal palate. Neck: carotid upstrokes normal; left brachial and radial pulses decreased. Cardiac: forceful PMI in fifth interspace 2 cm to the left of midclavicular line; II/VI diastolic blowing murmur along left sternal border. Extremities: no arachnodactyly.

Laboratory Findings: Hct 43%, WBC 13,300/μl, differential normal. Chest radiograph: borderline cardiomegaly with a widened mediastinum. ECG: normal sinus rhythm and left ventricular hypertrophy. Echocardiogram: shown below. Doppler interrogation of the aorta: mild to moderate aortic insufficiency.

Consider the patient's diagnosis and therapy.

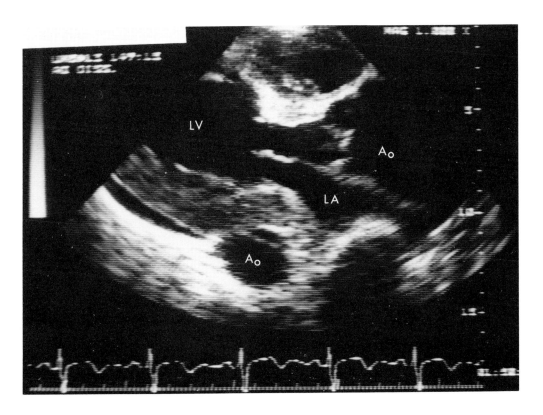

Diagnosis: Aortic dissection.

Discussion: Aortic dissection occurs when a sudden tear in the aortic intima allows blood, under the force of systemic pressure, to be driven between the intima and media, disrupting the integrity of the aorta. The intimal tear usually occurs in the presence of cystic medial necrosis. While cystic medial necrosis is part of the normal aging process, it appears as an accelerated and severe form in patients with Marfan's syndrome and those with long-term, poorly controlled systemic hypertension. Other conditions that predispose to an increased risk of aortic dissection include Ehlers-Danlos syndrome, Turner's syndrome, coarctation of the aorta, and pregnancy.

Many classification schemes for aortic dissection have been proposed. Practically, classification of aortic dissection as either proximal (arising in the ascending aorta near the aortic valve) or distal (arising in the descending aorta distal to the left subclavian artery) is most useful because this simple division also relates to prognosis and therapy.

Typically, aortic dissection presents as severe chest pain that is often described as tearing or stabbing in nature. The pain may radiate to the back, particularly in distal dissections. Occasionally, dissections are painless and are discovered fortuitously by chest radiography or at the time of cardiac catheterization. Other presentations for acute aortic dissection stem from vascular compromise to various parts of the body as the dissection proceeds to include arteries branching from the aorta. Thus, myocardial infarction or cerebrovascular accident may occur. Aortic dissection may render the aortic valve incompetent, producing aortic insufficiency, which may be severe. Rupture of the dissection into the pericardial space produces pericardial tamponade and shock.

The hallmarks of aortic dissection on physical examination include aortic insufficiency, neurologic disorders, and pulse deficits. The latter may wax and wane as the dissection progresses. Horner's syndrome, pulsation of one of the sternoclavicular joints, evidence of pleural effusion, and pericardial tamponade occur less frequently.

As in the case of meningitis, once the suspicion of an aortic dissection is raised, the diagnosis must be thoroughly evaluated and definitively established or excluded. The diagnosis is frequently considered in the patient presenting with severe chest pain who only has minor nonspecific changes on ECG. A chest radiograph is abnormal in approximately 90% of cases of aortic dissection. It usually reveals widening of the aortic contour and may demonstrate separation of existent calcium in the aortic knob from the other soft tissues of the aorta (calcium sign). Echocardiography of the proximal aorta may detect a false channel in proximal dissections. CT scan with contrast and MRI usually reveal the dissection and have supplanted aortography in some institutions. However, contrast aortography is still considered the gold standard for establishing the definitive diagnosis.

Initial management of aortic dissection involves supportive care for congestive heart failure and hypotension if these complications are present. However, most patients with aortic dissection are hypertensive, and reduction of arterial pressure is the cornerstone of medical therapy. A combination of beta-blockade and nitroprusside, combined alpha- and beta-blockade with labetalol, or use of a ganglionic blocker such as trimethaphan are all effective. An important caveat is that nitroprusside alone may actually worsen the dissection by increasing aortic outflow velocity. Addition of beta-blockade prevents this unwanted hemodynamic effect.

The prognosis of proximal dissection treated medically is poor; thus proximal dissection is considered an indication for surgery in most centers. Conversely, surgery has not improved the expected 80% survivorship of distal dissections where medical therapy is generally the treatment of choice. Distal dissection should be treated surgically, however, if the dissection shows evidence of progression to involve new vital organs or develops a saccular aneurysm, which may in turn rupture.

The present patient was considered on the basis of physical findings and echocardiographic results to have an ascending aortic dissection with resultant aortic valvular insufficiency. He received intravenous nitroprusside and beta-blockade with control of his hypertension. An aortic valve replacement was required in addition to surgical repair of the dissection.

Clinical Pearls

1. The diagnosis of aortic dissection is facilitated if the examiner recognizes that longstanding hypertension or Marfan's syndrome is present.

2. The chest radiograph shows some abnormality in almost every patient with aortic dissection.

3. Nitroprusside as initial therapy for aortic dissection should be used in conjunction with beta-blockade because nitroprusside alone may increase aortic outflow velocity and worsen the dissection.

4. Because of the consequences of aortic dissection, aortic dissection must be established or excluded definitively once the diagnosis is considered.

REFERENCES

1. Slater EE, DeSanctis RW: The clinical recognition of dissecting aortic aneurysm. Am J Med 60:625–633, 1976.
2. Wheat MW Jr. Acute dissecting aneurysms of the aorta: Diagnosis and treatment–1979. Am Heart J 99:373–387, 1980.
3. Granato JE, Dee P, Gibson RS: Utility of two-dimensional echocardiography in suspected ascending aortic dissection. Am J Cardiol 56:123–129, 1985.
4. Doroghazi RM, Slater EE, DeSanctis RW, et al: Long-term survival of patients with treated aortic dissection. J Am Coll Cardiol 3:1026–1034, 1984.

PATIENT 11

A 52-year-old woman with congestive heart failure developing anorexia, nausea, and palpitations

A 52-year-old woman noted increasing anorexia and nausea with sensations of a rapid heart beat over the previous 1 week. Vomiting in the preceding 24 hours prompted emergency room evaluation. She had a history of orthopnea and dyspnea on exertion that was diagnosed 1 year earlier as idiopathic cardiomyopathy. A gated nuclear cardiac scan at that time demonstrated an ejection fraction of 24%; hepatic and renal function had remained normal. She was treated with digoxin 0.25 mg q.d. plus furosemide 40 mg p.o. q.d. Recently, quinidine sulfate 300 mg q.i.d. had been added to her regimen to treat ventricular ectopy.

Physical Examination: Temperature 36.7°; pulse 110; respirations 20; blood pressure 110/70. Neck veins: prominent pulsations; estimated CVP 8 cm H_2O. Chest: bibasilar rales. Cardiac: PMI enlarged in the sixth interspace 2 cm left of the midclavicular line; S_4 present; no S_3; II/VI holosystolic apical murmur.

Laboratory Findings: CBC normal; K+ 3.6; digoxin level 5.2 ng/ml. Chest radiograph: cardiomegaly and mild vascular redistribution. ECG: shown below.

What is the diagnosis?

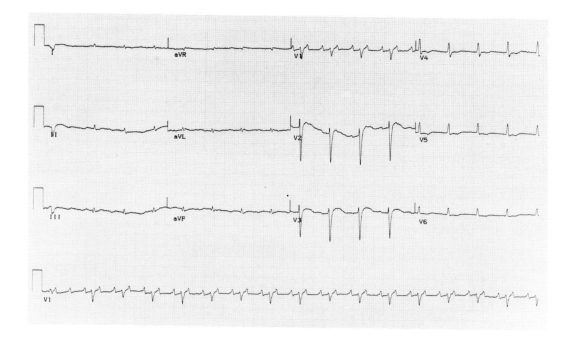

Diagnosis: Digitalis intoxication.

Discussion: It is estimated that digitalis intoxication occurs in 10 to 20% of hospitalized patients receiving the drug. Frequently, intoxication occurs when a nontoxic drug-dosing schedule becomes toxic secondary to a change in the patient's condition that decreases digitalis excretion. Approximately two-thirds of digoxin (by far the most widely prescribed preparation) is excreted by the kidney, whereas one-third is excreted by the liver. Thus, a reduction in renal or hepatic function will have the net effect of increasing digitalis concentration and predisposing the patient to digitalis intoxication. Another cause of digitalis intoxication is the coincident use of other cardiac drugs that affect digitalis excretion. The most prominent among these are quinidine, amiodarone, and verapamil, whose addition to a patient's drug regimen may increase digoxin concentrations by as much as 100%.

The basic mechanisms of digitalis intoxication revolve around the drug's direct effects on cardiac muscle together with its action on the central nervous system. Digitalis reduces myocardial conduction and increases refractory period in the AV node. The drug increases excitability and automaticity in the Purkinje's fibers. Thus, in high concentrations, digitalis may be responsible for heart block and ventricular tachyarrhythmias. Digitalis increases cardiac sympathetic nerve activity, augmenting its arrhythmogenic potential. Concordantly, it has been shown that digitalis preparations that do not cross the blood–brain barrier have substantially less arrhythmogenic potential than those that do.

Clinically, the major effects of digitalis intoxication are on cardiac rhythm, the gastrointestinal tract, and the central nervous system. While digitalis intoxication can produce almost any cardiac arrhythmia, common arrhythmias include increased ventricular ectopy, paroxysmal atrial tachycardia with block, and nonparoxysmal junctional tachycardia. The gastrointestinal effects of digitalis intoxication include anorexia, nausea, and vomiting. Neurologic symptoms include disorientation, confusion, delirium, seizures, and visual disturbances. The visual disturbances include scotomas, halos, and changes in color perception.

Blood digoxin levels provide a rough guide to help confirm the diagnosis. However, it must be emphasized that some patients can be digitalis intoxicated even though blood levels are within the "normal" range, whereas other patients are not intoxicated even though the blood level is increased above this range.

Therapy for most cases of digitalis intoxication is simply to withhold the drug until excretion renders the patient no longer toxic. Since myocardial digitalis concentrations decrease as serum potassium increases, hypokalemia, if present, should be aggressively treated. If life-threatening arrhythmias complicate digitalis intoxication, phenytoin sodium or lidocaine are the drugs of choice for treatment. Propranolol may also be of use in treating digitalis intoxication if the situation is not complicated by bradyarrhythmia. Conversely, bretylium, which after infusion increases norepinephrine levels, may transiently worsen digitalis-induced arrhythmia, and this drug should be avoided. In the case of massive digitalis intoxication, such as might occur with a suicide attempt, infusion of digitalis-specific antibodies is the treatment of choice.

The present patient's digoxin level was in the toxic range. The drug was withheld and she spontaneously converted to normal sinus rhythm soon after initial evaluation. The addition of therapy with quinidine was considered the cause of digitalis toxicity.

Clinical Pearls

1. Addition of quinidine, verapamil, or amiodarone to a patient's therapeutic regimen may increase digitalis concentration by 100% if the digitalis dose is not decreased.

2. Bretylium should be avoided in the treatment of digitalis-induced ventricular arrhythmias.

3. The effects of digitalis on the central nervous system augment its intoxication potential.

4. Administration of digitalis specific antibody is the treatment of choice in life-threatening digitalis intoxication.

5. Digitalis intoxication is defined by a clinical syndrome, not by the blood level of the drug.

REFERENCES

1. Antman EM, Smith TW: Drug interactions with digitalis glycosides. In Smith TW (ed): Digitalis Glycosides. Orlando, Grune and Stratton, 1985, pp 65–81.
2. Blatt CM, March JD, Smith TW: The role of neural factors in digitalis intoxication. In Smith TW (ed): Digitalis Glycosides. Orlando, Grune and Stratton, 1985, pp 227–293.
3. Friedman PL, Antman EM: Electrocardiographic manifestations of digitalis toxicity. In Smith TW (ed): Digitalis Glycosides. Orlando, Grune and Stratton, 1985, pp 241–275.

PATIENT 12

A 40-year-old woman with a history of mitral valve prolapse presents with acute dyspnea

A 40-year-old woman had carried the diagnosis of mitral valve prolapse for 8 years. She was asymptomatic until the evening of admission when she developed severe dyspnea and orthopnea, causing her to come to the emergency room. She had no previous history of congestive heart failure or chest pain.

Physical Examination: Temperature 37°; pulse 110; respirations 32; blood pressure 140/90. The patient is in acute distress with dyspnea. Chest: bibasilar rales. Cardiac: PMI normal location; thrill palpated in apical area, S_3 gallop; IV/VI holosystolic murmur radiating to the axilla. Extremities: no edema.

Laboratory Findings: CBC and electrolytes normal. Chest radiograph: pulmonary edema without cardiomegaly. ECG: nonspecific ST and T wave abnormalities. Echocardiogram: hyperkinetic left ventricle, mildly enlarged left atrium. LV and Pcw pressure tracings: shown below.

What is the cause of the patient's pulmonary edema?

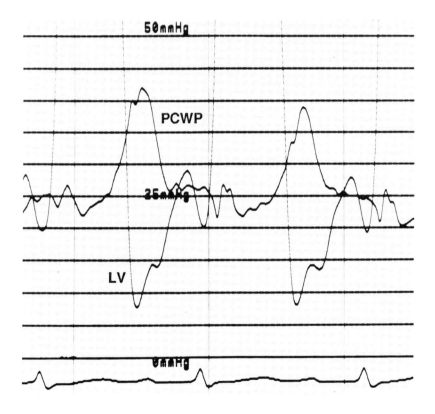

Diagnosis: Acute pulmonary edema secondary to mitral chordal rupture.

Discussion: Chordal rupture is an important cause of acute mitral regurgitation. In general the posterior leaflet is involved more frequently than the anterior leaflet. The amount of mitral regurgitation produced is related to the number and size of the chordae that have ruptured. In the present patient, the degree of mitral regurgitation was severe, producing acute pulmonary edema.

In severe acute mitral regurgitation, the relatively noncompliant left atrium is presented with an extreme volume overload, producing consequent elevation in left atrial pressure. This increased atrial pressure is transmitted to the pulmonary vessels where it produces pulmonary edema. Acute mitral regurgitation causes important alterations in left ventricular mechanics. The volume overload increases left ventricular sarcomere stretch (increased preload). The new pathway for ejection into the left atrium reduces overall left ventricular afterload, thereby reducing end-systolic volume. The resultant increased preload and decreased afterload increase ejection fraction and *total* stroke volume. However, in severe mitral regurgitation more than half of the stroke volume is ineffective (ejected backward into the left atrium), and thus *forward* stroke volume is severely reduced, effectively decreasing cardiac output.

In acute severe mitral regurgitation, the patient typically complains of acute shortness of breath and orthopnea. In 5% of instances of chordal rupture, the patient may note chest pain. On physical examination, the hallmark of mitral regurgitation, a holosystolic murmur, will be found in virtually every patient. The murmur is usually loudest at the apex and often radiates toward the axilla. A third heart sound is also usually present. The ECG often remains normal or may show nonspecific ST and T wave abnormalities. The chest radiograph shows pulmonary congestion but the heart is not greatly enlarged because compensatory eccentric hypertrophy has not yet had time to develop.

An echo/Doppler study is the procedure of choice to confirm the diagnosis. The echocardiogram may demonstrate the ruptured chorda itself. The Doppler portion of the examination demonstrates the regurgitant jet and may be useful in helping to approximate the amount of mitral regurgitation present. Because such patients are usually severely ill with both congestive heart failure and an element of circulatory shock, insertion of a Swan-Ganz catheter is usually helpful in patient management. During placement of the catheter, oxygen saturations are determined in the right atrium and pulmonary artery to rule out an acute ventricular septal rupture as the cause of the new holosystolic murmur. Classically, in acute mitral regurgitation a large V wave is demonstrated in the pulmonary capillary wedge pressure tracing.

Therapy for severe acute mitral regurgitation usually requires mitral valve repair or replacement. Medical therapy prior to surgery is aimed at reducing left ventricular afterload, thereby preferentially increasing forward output while decreasing the amount of mitral regurgitation. Afterload reduction may be effected by the use of a potent vasodilator such as nitroprusside. If the patient is in shock and will not tolerate a vasodilator, insertion of an intraaortic balloon pump will help to both reduce left ventricular afterload and increase systemic blood pressure. Diuretics are an important adjunct to therapy to help lower left ventricular filling pressure.

In less severe cases of acute mitral regurgitation, medical therapy with diuretics and vasodilators may result in greatly reducing the patient's symptoms. The eventual development of eccentric cardiac hypertrophy of the left ventricle increases forward stroke volume toward normal. Left atrial enlargement allows the volume overload to be present at reduced filling pressure, lessening symptoms of pulmonary congestion. These changes allow for the development of chronic compensated mitral regurgitation, which may be tolerated for several years before the onset of left ventricular dysfunction necessitates mitral valve repair or replacement.

Recently, surgical mitral valve repair has gained wider recognition in the United States as an alternative to mitral valve replacement. Because this technique avoids leaving the patient with the potential risks of a prosthesis, it may be advisable to proceed with repair in significant but less severe amounts of mitral regurgitation.

Clinical Pearls

1. Afterload reduction therapy with vasodilators or intraaortic balloon pumping is the initial therapy of choice for acute nonischemic mitral regurgitation.

2. If patients can tolerate the acute phase of the disease with the help of medical management, they may enter a chronic compensated phase that may be tolerated for years without the need for valve replacement.

3. Mitral valve repair, because of its reduced morbidity, may become the therapy of choice for significant mitral regurgitation.

REFERENCES

1. Carabello BA, Grossman W: Effects of acute and chronic mitral regurgitation on left ventricular mechanics and contractile muscle function. In Recent Progress in Mitral Valve Disease. London, Butterworth Publishing, pp 181–192, 1984.
2. Hickey AJ, Wilcken DE, Wright JS, et al: Primary (spontaneous) chordal rupture: Relation to myxomatous valve disease and mitral valve prolapse. J Am Coll Cardiol 5:1341–1346, 1985.
3. Yoran C, Yellin EL, Becker RM, et al: Mechanism of reduction of mitral regurgitation with vasodilator therapy. Am J Cardiol 43:773–777, 1979.

PATIENT 13

A 25-year-old man with dyspnea and a heart murmur of varying intensity

A 25-year-old previously healthy man noticed progressive dyspnea on exertion during jogging. Because of this symptom, he reduced his jogging from several miles to one mile a day. He denied orthopnea, paroxysmal nocturnal dyspnea, chest pain, or edema. His brother was known to have congestive heart failure and a heart murmur.

Physical Examination: Vital signs: normal. Cardiac: forceful PMI located in fifth interspace in midclavicular line; S_1 normal; S_2 physiologically split; II/VI systolic ejection murmur along left sternal border—murmur decreases when patient lies down but increases to grade III with Valsalva maneuver. Extremities: normal.

Laboratory Findings: CBC: normal. Chest radiograph: normal. ECG: probable left ventricular hypertrophy and strain. Echocardiogram: asymmetric septal hypertrophy, systolic anterior motion of mitral valve during Valsalva maneuver.

What cardiac abnormality explains the patient's clinical presentation?

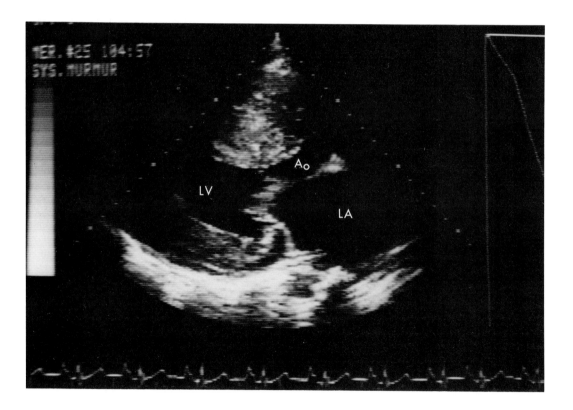

Diagnosis: Idiopathic hypertrophic subaortic stenosis (IHSS).

Discussion: IHSS is a disease in which asymmetric hypertrophy of the interventricular septum leads to left ventricular outflow obstruction. The disorder is usually inherited in an autosomal dominant pattern but may also occur sporadically.

In the normal heart, the interventricular septum lies in close proximity to the anterior leaflet of the mitral valve. In IHSS, the septum becomes thickened, thereby decreasing the narrow separation from the anterior leaflet. During left systole the anterior leaflet moves even closer to the septum, obstructing the left ventricular outflow tract. However, the septum in IHSS is abnormal (catenoid shape) and does not shorten or thicken normally during systole. Thus it is the anterior leaflet of the mitral valve which plays the active role in causing obstruction.

The left ventricular outflow gradient and degree of obstruction in IHSS are labile. Circumstances that diminish the size of the left ventricle bring the anterior leaflet of the mitral valve and the septum in closer contact, worsening the obstruction. Conditions that enlarge the left ventricle, such as assuming the recumbent position, reduce the obstruction. Additionally, maneuvers that increase myocardial contractility, thereby accelerating blood-flow through the outflow tract, augment obstruction by sucking the anterior leaflet against the septum by the Bernoulli principle.

The classic symptoms of IHSS are angina, syncope, and CHF. Angina probably occurs because limited coronary blood flow reserve present in hypertrophied states is insufficient to maintain myocardial oxygen demands. Syncope usually occurs after exercise. Decreased venous return to the heart, increased contractile function from increased circulating catecholamines, and reduced afterload due to vasodilatation all contribute after exercise to reduced left ventricular size. Reduced left ventricular size in turn increases obstruction with a resultant decrease in left ventricular outflow, leading to syncope. CHF results from the reduced compliance (diastolic dysfunction) of the hypertrophied left ventricle.

The classic physical findings in IHSS are a carotid upstroke with a spike and dome pattern and a systolic ejection murmur. Maneuvers that reduce cardiac size, such as the Valsalva maneuver, increase the intensity of the murmur and accentuate the spike and dome pattern of the carotid pulse. Maneuvers that increase cardiac size, such as squatting, have the opposite effect.

The ECG in IHSS usually demonstrates left ventricular hypertrophy and is seldom normal. Provided the patient has an adequate sonographic window, echocardiography is usually diagnostic, showing the increased septal thickness. If obstruction is present, systolic anterior motion of the mitral valve will also be seen. If not present at rest, maneuvers that decrease heart size or increase contractility may cause systolic anterior motion to develop.

Therapy for IHSS differs greatly from that for fixed aortic stenosis. In contrast to aortic stenosis, the mortality in IHSS does not correlate well with the measured pressure gradient. Thus, myomectomy for high-grade obstruction in IHSS does not clearly reduce mortality.

Usual therapies for CHF such as digitalis and diuretics may cause dramatic deterioration in the patient with IHSS, since both maneuvers increase outflow obstruction. Treatment with beta-blockers, which decrease cardiac contractility and also increase cardiac size, decrease the gradient and reduce symptoms. Calcium blockers may also be effective by the same mechanism. Additionally, calcium blockers may enhance diastolic relaxation and assist reduction of left ventricular filling pressures. However, verapamil may cause intractable pulmonary edema when given to patients with IHSS if filling pressures are elevated or if overt CHF is present. Surgery in IHSS is performed only when medical therapy fails to relieve symptoms. Myomectomy to reduce septal thickness or mitral valve replacement (to remove the anterior leaflet of the mitral valve) both will diminish left ventricular outflow obstruction and improve symptoms.

The present patient received therapy with verapamil with improvement of symptoms.

Clinical Pearls

1. Mortality in IHSS, unlike in fixed aortic stenosis, is related to the muscle disease and not the outlfow gradient.

2. Therapeutic modalities that reduce left ventricular size (such as diuretics) or that increase myocardial contractility (such as digitalis) should generally be avoided in IHSS.

3. Verapamil may be effective in reducing symptoms but may also precipitate congestive heart failure in patients with known elevation in left ventricular filling pressure.

REFERENCES

1. Epstein SE, Henry WL, Clark CE, et al: Asymmetric septal hypertrophy. Ann Intern Med 81:650–680, 1974.
2. Gardin JM, Dabestani A, Glasgow GA, et al: Echocardiographic and Doppler flow observations in obstructed and nonobstructed hypertrophic cardiomyopathy. Am J Cardiol 56:614–621, 1985.
3. Epstein SE, Rosing DR: Verapamil: Its potential for causing serious complications in patients with hypertrophic cardiomyopathy. Circulation 64:437–441, 1981.

PATIENT 14

A 36-year-old man with hypercholesterolemia and acute chest pain

A 36-year-old man was awakened from sleep with substernal, nonradiating chest pain that improved slightly when he sat up in bed. The patient noted diaphoresis but denied nausea or vomiting. The patient's two older brothers had myocardial infarctions early in their fifth decades. The patient denied hypertension, but had a recent blood cholesterol level of 312 mg/dl.

Physical Examination: Temperature 37.5°; pulse 70; respirations 18; blood pressure 160/90. Neck: normal arterial and venous pulsations. Cardiac: normal PMI; no murmurs, gallops or rubs.

Laboratory Findings: Hct 36%, WBC 12,200/μl, 53% PMNs, 44% lymphocytes (atypical lymphocytes noted), 3% monocytes. CPK, SGOT, and LDH: normal. ECG: shown below.

What is your initial diagnostic impression?

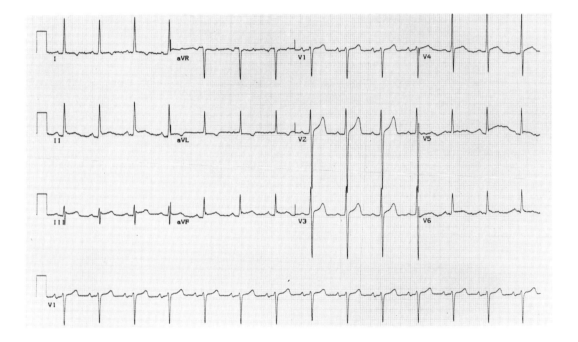

Diagnosis: Acute pericarditis.

Discussion: Acute pericarditis may commonly mimic myocardial infarction. In the current era of thrombolytic therapy for acute coronary occlusion, the distinction between these two disorders is crucial. If pericarditis is misdiagnosed as myocardial infarction, thrombolytic agents may cause pericardial hemorrhage and cardiac tamponade.

The patient's presentation can often assist in the diagnosis of acute pericarditis. Although the chest pain may be similar to that of myocardial infarction, there is usually a pleuritic component in pericarditis and the pain is often relieved when the patient sits up and leans forward. The clinician may or may not detect a pericardial friction rib; this physical finding is evanescent and may not exist during the brief period of cardiac examination. The presence of a rub facilitates the diagnosis.

The ECG in pericarditis may demonstrate diffuse ST segment elevation, which at first glance may suggest an acute myocardial infarction. Unlike acute myocardial infarction, however, pericarditis does not produce reciprocal ST segment depression. If the distinction between acute myocardial infarction and acute pericarditis remains uncertain and thrombolytic therapy is still contemplated, an urgent echocardiogram should be performed. If cardiac wall motion is completely normal, the diagnosis of acute myocardial infarction is excluded. The echocardiogram may demonstrate a small pericardial effusion, thereby leading to the diagnosis of pericarditis.

Specific etiologies of pericarditis include: (1) idiopathic (often suspected but rarely proven to be viral), (2) post myocardial infarction (early and late), (3) infectious (most commonly tuberculosis), (4) neoplastic, (5) uremic, (6) pericarditis associated with collagen vascular disease, (7) post irradiation, and (8) drug-induced.

Therapy includes general measures that combat the inflammation and specific measures directed at the underlying etiology of pericarditis. Nonsteroidal anti-inflammatory agents such as aspirin or indomethacin are usually effective in relieving the inflammation and pain of pericarditis. If the pericarditis is due to early inflammation following acute myocardial infarction, anti-inflammatory drugs such as indomethacin must be given with caution because these agents have produced impaired scar formation following experimental myocardial infarction in animals. If the nonsteroidal agents are ineffective in relieving the pain, prednisone may be employed. In such instances, however, discontinuing steroids may result in recrudescence of the disease.

The present patient was considered to have pericarditis on the basis of his typical ECG with diffuse ST segment elevation and the description of the pain. He was treated with indomethacin with gradual resolution of symptoms. Medical evaluation determined that his pericarditis was idiopathic in etiology.

Clinical Pearls

1. It is imperative that thrombolytic therapy not be administered for pericarditis masquerading as a myocardial infarction.

2. Reciprocal ST segment depression is absent in acute pericarditis.

3. An urgent echocardiogram may help to make the distinction between acute myocardial infarction and pericarditis.

4. Nonsteroidal anti-inflammatory drugs are the treatment of choice. However, these should be given with caution during acute myocardial infarction because they may reduce scar formation.

REFERENCES
1. Lorell BH, Braunwald E: Pericardial disease. In Braunwald E (ed): Heart Disease, 3rd ed. Philadelphia, W.B. Saunders Co., 1988, pp 1484–1534.
2. Spodick DH: Pericardial rub: Prospective, multiple observer investigation of pericardial friction in 100 patients. Am J Cardiol 35:357–362, 1975.
3. Spodick DH: Diagnostic electrocardiographic sequences in acute pericarditis. Significance of PR segment and PR vector changes. Circulation 48:575–580, 1973.

PATIENT 15

A 45-year-old man with headache and flank pain

A 45-year-old man with a 10-year history of hypertension presented with severe flank pain radiating to the left groin and gross hematuria developing over the previous 4 hours. He also noted a headache.

Physical Examination: Temperature 36.8°; pulse 68; respirations 20; blood pressure 240/140. Patient was in distress with flank pain. Fundi: arteriolar narrowing without papilledema. Cardiac: forceful PMI in the normal position; S_1 normal; increased intensity of A2; loud S_4; no murmurs.

Laboratory Findings: Hct 42%, electrolytes normal; BUN 37 mg/dl, creatinine 2.0 mg/dl. Urinalysis: 1+ proteinuria with gross hematuria. Chest: borderline cardiomegaly; normal lung fields. ECG: sinus rhythm; left ventricular hypertrophy with strain. Abdominal radiograph: radiopaque calculus in left ureter.

What would you do about this patient's blood pressure?

Diagnosis: Pseudohypertensive crisis.

Discussion: Hypertensive crisis with sustained diastolic blood pressures above 140 mm Hg is a major cause of organ vascular damage, which most commonly develops in the brain and kidney. Manifestations of injury to the brain include headache, confusion, somnolence, delirium, and focal neurologic deficits. Renal vascular damage results in hematuria, proteinuria, and a rise in serum creatinine and BUN. The acute increase in left ventricular afterload may also result in acute congestive heart failure.

True hypertensive crises are associated with marked, sustained increases in blood pressure that require urgent therapy to prevent end-organ injury. As such, they must be distinguished from a pseudohypertensive crisis that occurs in patients experiencing extremely painful conditions. These patients develop profound degrees of hypertension as a physiologic response to pain. Therapy in pseudohypertensive crisis is directed primarily at pain relief and correction of the underlying condition rather than at modalities to directly treat the hypertension itself.

Therapy for true hypertensive crisis requires immediate but controlled lowering of the blood pressure. This goal is most easily accomplished by infusion of sodium nitroprusside, beginning at low doses. The dose is then gradually increased until the blood pressure is controlled. Many patients with hypertension may have significant atherosclerotic arterial occlusion; excessive reduction of blood pressure into normal range may result in reduced organ perfusion. In general, a target diastolic pressure of 90 to 100 mm Hg is desirable for the initial treatment of hypertensive crisis. Trimethaphan or labetalol are suitable alternatives to nitroprusside. Because labetalol is a beta-blocker, it must be used with caution in heart failure and avoided if there is a history of bronchospasm.

The present patient suffered from a renal calculus. He received morphine sulfate intravenously, which decreased his pain. The blood pressure decreased to 170/90 and required no additional therapy.

Clinical Pearls

1. Hypertensive crisis must be distinguished from pseudohypertensive crisis caused by severe pain.

2. Therapy for a hypertensive crisis should not reduce diastolic pressure to the normal range but should target a diastolic pressure of 90 to 100 mm Hg.

REFERENCES
1. Ferguson RK, Vlasses PH: Hypertensive emergencies and urgencies. JAMA 255:1607–1613, 1986.
2. Anderson RJ, Reed WG: Current concepts in treatment of hypertensive urgencies. Am Heart J 111:211–219, 1986.

PATIENT 16

A 61-year-old woman with chest pain and hypotension three days after a laparotomy

A 61-year-old woman developed abdominal pain and distention followed by nausea and vomiting 24 hours before admission. She was admitted with a small bowel obstruction and underwent a laparotomy when nasogastric suction failed to eliminate her symptoms. The patient had a history of an acute inferior myocardial infarction 3 months earlier and had occasional episodes of exertional angina subsequently. Her medications included propranolol 40 mg q.i.d. and sublingual nitroglycerin. She had stopped all medications with the recent onset of nausea and vomiting. On the third postoperative day, the patient developed severe precordial chest pressure and diaphoresis.

Physical Examination: Temperature of 37°; pulse 90; respirations 24; blood pressure 80/50. The patient was in distress from chest pain and appeared pale and clammy. Neck: jugular venous distention; estimated CVP 9 cm H_2O. Cardiac: S_4 present. Abdomen: hypoactive bowel sounds: normally healing incision.

Laboratory Findings: Hct 36%, WBC 12,300/μl, normal differential. Electrolytes and BUN normal. ECG: acute anterior myocardial infarction.

What factors contributed to this patient's postoperative complication? What preventive measures could have been employed?

Diagnosis: Myocardial infarction following noncardiac surgery.

Discussion: Serious cardiovascular complications occur in approximately 5% of all patients undergoing noncardiac surgery. The risk of cardiac complications, however, varies widely in individual patients, from low frequencies in the young previously healthy patient without cardiovascular disease to markedly increased risk in the elderly patient with coronary disease. The two major challenges confronting the physician managing patients undergoing surgery are preoperative recognition of the high-risk patient and avoidance of complications intra- and postoperatively.

The history of angina or even of remote myocardial infarction does not necessarily increase the risk of surgery. Goldman and colleagues and others have helped to elucidate some of the risk factors that indicate the potential for postoperative cardiac complications: (1) myocardial infarction during the 6 months before surgery; (2) congestive heart failure present immediately prior to surgery; (3) significant ventricular ectopy recorded in the 24 hours preceding surgery; (4) cardiac rhythm other than sinus; (5) age greater than 70; (6) an emergency operation; (7) poor overall condition indicated by abnormalities in renal function, pulmonary function and/or hepatic function; and (8) operations involving the thorax, abdomen, or aorta. Although these factors are useful in helping to evaluate the operative candidate, they are generally specific but not sensitive.

Other patients at particularly high risk are those with unstable angina and those with peripheral vascular disease and a positive preoperative thallium scintillation scan who undergo vascular surgery.

If the patient is at high risk but still requires noncardiac surgery, what can be done to reduce the incidence of cardiovascular complications? Recognition of the time periods when patients are at highest risk is useful to increase vigilance in avoiding complications. The patient is at particularly high risk for a complication during tracheal intubation immediately before surgery; the peak incidence of postoperative complications is on the third day after surgery.

Recognition of antecedent cardiac dysfunction also helps to forewarn the physician of potential complications. In patients whose history and physical examination suggest the presence of left ventricular dysfunction, confirmation may be obtained by echocardiography. If cardiac dysfunction exists, preoperative insertion of a Swan-Ganz catheter is useful in managing the patient's fluid status. If the patient has been on beta-blockers prior to surgery, the drugs should be continued up until the time of surgery to prevent beta-blockade withdrawal syndrome. Postoperatively, beta-blockers should be continued. If the patient is unable to take medication orally, the constant infusion of esmolol can provide beta-blockade until oral medications are resumed. Careful attention to postoperative volume status and the control of pain are also important adjuncts in reducing cardiovascular complications.

The present patient was diagnosed as having acute myocardial ischemia probably secondary to the stress of surgery and the effects of beta-blockade withdrawal.

Clinical Pearls

1. Patients with a recent myocardial infarction, congestive heart failure, or peripheral vascular disease are particularly high risk for noncardiac surgery.

2. The peak incidence of cardiac complications following noncardiac surgery is on the third postoperative day.

3. Patients receiving beta-blockers should be maintained on these agents preoperatively and postoperatively. Intravenous infusion of esmolol is useful in patients who cannot receive oral postoperative beta-blocker medication.

REFERENCES
1. Goldman L, Caldera DL, Nussbaum SR, et al: Multifactorial index of cardiac risk in noncardiac surgical procedures. N Engl J Med 297:845–850, 1977.
2. Boucher CA, Brewster DC, Darling RC, et al: Determination of cardiac risk by dipyridamole-thallium imaging before peripheral vascular surgery. N Engl J Med 312:389–394, 1985.
3. Foster ED, Davis KB, Carpenter JA, et al: Risk of noncardiac operation in patients with defined coronary disease: The Coronary Artery Surgery Study (CASS) registry experience. Ann Thorac Surg 41:42–50, 1986.

PATIENT 17

A 25-year-old woman with palpitations, lightheadedness, and electrocardiographic abnormalities

A 25-year-old woman presented with a history of transient palpitations. She denied loss of consciousness but noted lethargy and a feeling of lightheadedness. She had two previous episodes of palpitations, both resolving spontaneously. The current episode persisted for 1 hour, causing her to seek medical attention. She was taking no medications. There was no history of congestive heart failure, congenital heart disease, or chest pain.

Physical Examination: Temperature 36.8°; pulse 105 and regular; respirations 18; blood pressure 100/60. Cardiac: tachycardia, otherwise normal.

Laboratory Findings: CBC and electrolytes normal. Chest radiograph: normal. ECG: shown below.

What is the etiology of the patient's arrhythmias?

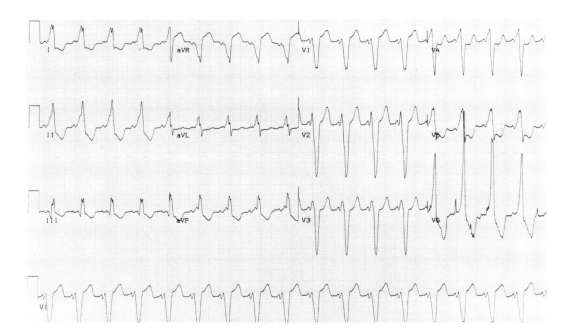

Diagnosis: Wolff-Parkinson-White syndrome (WPW).

Discussion: In WPW, a bundle of cardiac muscle (sometimes called the bundle of Kent) connects with the atria and ventricles. This tract bypasses the normal conduction delay provided by the AV node and also produces an abnormality in the sequence of depolarization of the interventricular septum. Electrocardiographically, this anatomic situation results in a shortened PR interval and a slur in the upstroke of the QRS (delta wave). These ECG manifestations are demonstrated only when the impulse is conducted antegrade through the bypass tract.

Alternatively, the impulse may be conducted normally through the AV node while the bypass tract allows for a reentrant pathway that helps to promote the occurrence of supraventricular tachyarrhythmias. In fact, conduction in WPW usually occurs over the normal pathway because although conduction velocity is faster in the accessory pathway, the refractory period of this pathway is longer, blocking accessory pathway antegrade conduction. Frequently a premature atrial contraction produces a pause that allows the accessory pathway to become responsive, leading to a reciprocating tachycardia with conduction antegrade down the normal pathway and completion of the circuit back to the atria through the accessory pathway. When patients with an accessory tract conduct antegrade through the accessory tract during the tachycardia, the widened QRS from the abnormal septal depolarization may mimic ventricular tachycardia. In sinus rhythm, the abnormal septal depolarization may cause the ECG to resemble the patterns seen in either inferior or anterior myocardial infarction.

Medical therapy for WPW is aimed at increasing the refractory period of the AV node, increasing the refractory period of the accessory pathway or slowing conduction in the accessory pathway. Verapamil and propranolol both increase the refractory period of the AV node and are useful in the treatment of tachyarrhythmias when antegrade conduction is down the normal pathway. Class IA drugs such as quinidine or procainamide, and Class IC drugs such as flecainide or encainide increase the refractory period of the accessory pathway and are also effective. Amiodarone is also effective in the therapy of the syndrome but is usually reserved until failure of the other drugs has been demonstrated, because of its high toxicity.

Although digitalis increases the refractory period of the AV node and may help to control arrhythmias through this mechanism, the drug also increases conduction through the accessory pathway. Should the patient develop atrial fibrillation in the course of his arrhythmias, the presence of digitalis could accelerate the heart rate and lead to hypotension and ventricular fibrillation. For this reason, digitalis is generally avoided in all patients with WPW. Likewise, verapamil may also increase the rate in atrial fibrillation in WPW, and caution should be used when this drug is given intravenously.

If medical therapy is ineffective in controlling the arrhythmias, electrical ablation using a transvenously placed catheter or surgery to sever the bundle are effective alternatives.

The present patient was treated with various antiarrhythmic drugs during the subsequent 6 months. Quinidine proved to be the most effective agent in preventing recurrence of tachycardias.

Clinical Pearls

1. Wolff-Parkinson-White syndrome may cause misinterpretation of the electrocardiogram as showing the presence of myocardial infarction or ventricular tachycardia.

2. The presence of very rapid atrial arrhythmias should suggest the presence of an accessory pathway.

3. Digitalis should be avoided in all patients with Wolff-Parkinson-White syndrome. Intravenous verapamil should be given with caution.

REFERENCES
1. Wolff L, Parkinson J, White PD: Bundle branch block with short P-R interval in healthy young people prone to paroxysmal tachycardia. Am Heart J 5:685–704, 1930.
2. Bardy GH, Packer DL, German LD, et al: Pre-excited reciprocating tachycardia in patients with Wolff-Parkinson-White syndrome: Incidence and mechanisms. Circulation 70:377–391, 1984.
3. Gulamhusein S, Ko P, Carruthers SG, et al: Acceleration of the ventricular response during atrial fibrillation in the Wolff-Parkinson-White syndrome after verapamil. Circulation 65:348–354, 1982.

PATIENT 18

A 65-year-old man with unstable angina referred for cardiac catheterization

A 65-year-old man with a history of chronic stable angina experienced an increased frequency of chest pain to one to two episodes each day during the 2 weeks before admission. The angina, characterized as a substernal pressure with radiation to the left arm, was precipitated by exercise until the day before admission when an episode occurred during rest. There was no history of congestive heart failure.

Physical Examination: Normal.

Laboratory Findings: Normal.

Hospital Course: The patient was begun on diltiazem and intravenous nitroglycerin for unstable angina, but chest pain recurred on the evening of admission. An ECG taken during the episode revealed ST segment depression in leads V1, V2, and V3, which resolved following the attack. The patient was referred for cardiac catheterization on the following day. Catheterization demonstrated a normal left ventriculogram. There was an 80% narrowing of the left main coronary artery with a 90% proximal stenosis of the left anterior descending artery. The catheterization was uneventful and the patient was returned to the CCU. Four hours later he again developed chest pain. The patient became progressively hypotensive and an intraaortic balloon pump was inserted, stabilizing the patient's condition. A repeat ECG showed diffuse ST-T wave abnormalities.

What aspects of this patient's cardiac disease predisposed him to this complication?

Diagnosis: Myocardial infarction following cardiac catheterization in a patient with a left main coronary artery disease.

Discussion: Cardiac catheterization has evolved into a highly accurate and relatively safe procedure with a risk of death of approximately 0.1%. However, patients who subsequently are discovered to have significant disease in the left main coronary artery compose a group in which a disproportionate number of serious complications occur. While disease of the left main coronary artery is present in only 7% of patients undergoing cardiac catheterization, it accounts for approximately 90% of all serious complications. Thus, the incidence of death or life-threatening complications following catheterization in which left main coronary artery disease is subsequently discovered is approximately 1%.

The importance of the left main coronary artery is obvious: approximately 85% of all left ventricular coronary blood flow must pass through this vessel. However, the mechanism by which catheterization of patients with disease in this artery leads to a 10-fold increase in complications is currently unknown. The complication frequently does not occur in the catheterization laboratory itself but may occur in the 6 hours following the procedure.

Risk factors for the development of a life-threatening complication following catheterization in which significant left main coronary disease is demonstrated include angina in the 24 hours prior to the procedure and positioning the catheter in close proximity (6 mm or less) to the lesion during the procedure. While this last factor might appear to be avoidable by careful catheter positioning, unfortunately the catheterizing physician usually is unaware that the lesion is present. Further, the catheter must often be positioned close to the lesion in order to get adequate opacification of the vessels to produce an accurate study.

Noninvasive studies prior to catheterization, including a markedly positive exercise test or an echocardiogram, that suggest the presence of left main disease may be useful in warning of the presence of left main disease. However, these tests are not sensitive or specific enough for the accurate precatheterization detection of left main coronary disease.

Currently, the best way of avoiding complications of cardiac catheterization in patients with left main coronary artery disease is unknown. Admission to the CCU for close observation following catheterization, limitation of the number of injections performed, and avoidance of a left ventriculogram (if one has not already been performed) all seem prudent but are without known benefit. If hypotension or severe angina occurs during the procedure, urgent surgery is probably indicated. Insertion of an intraaortic balloon pump may help to temporize and stabilize the patient's condition until surgery can be performed.

The present patient stabilized with placement of the intraaortic balloon pump and underwent urgent coronary artery bypass surgery. He had sustained a massive myocardial infarction, however, and did not survive the postoperative period.

Clinical Pearls

1. When cardiac catheterization demonstrates ≥ 50% narrowing of the left main coronary artery, close supervision of the patient following the procedure is indicated.

2. Angina in the 24 hours before the catheterization and close proximity of the catheter to the lesion during the procedure are associated with increased risk.

3. Complications, when they occur, frequently occur 1 to 6 hours *after* termination of the cardiac catheterization.

REFERENCES
1. Davis K, Kennedy JW, Kemp HG Jr, et al: Complications of coronary arteriography from the Collaborative Study of Coronary Artery Surgery (CASS). Circulation 59:1105–1112, 1979.
2. Cabin HS, Roberts WC: Fatal cardiac arrest during cardiac catheterization for angina pectoris: Analysis of 10 necropsy patients. Am J Cardiol 48:1–8, 1981.
3. Gordon PR, Abrams C, Gash AK, et al: Pericatheterization risk factors in left main coronary artery stenosis. Am J Cardiol 59:1080–1083, 1987.

PATIENT 19

A 31-year-old drug addict with fever and shortness of breath

A 31-year-old abuser of intravenous drugs was in his usual state of health until 1 week before admission. The patient, who habitually injected drugs with dirty needles, began to notice chills, fever, anorexia, and weight loss. On the day before admission, he noted mild dyspnea on exertion and that evening developed two-pillow orthopnea.

Physical Examination: Temperature 38.2°; pulse 120; respirations 24; blood pressure 100/60. Skin: occasional petechiae. Cardiac: normal heart size; S_1 diminished in intensity; II/VI long diastolic blowing murmur along left sternal border. Extremities: splinter hemorrhages under nail bed of third finger on left hand.

Laboratory Findings: Hct 34%, WBC 14,200/μl, normal differential; electrolytes normal. Urinalysis: microscopic hematuria. ECG: normal. M-mode echocardiogram (below): preclosure of the mitral valve. Doppler interrogation of aortic valve: severe aortic insufficiency.

What is the patient's diagnosis and what is the optimal therapy?

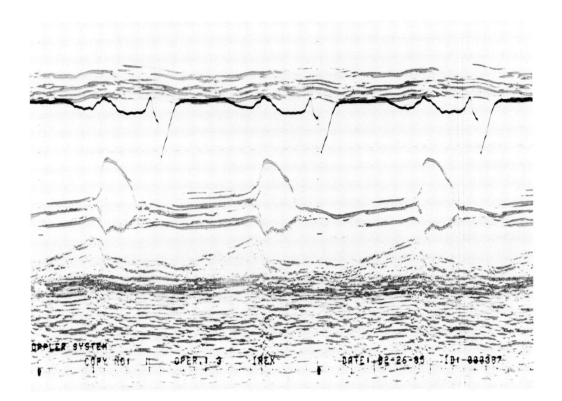

Diagnosis: Acute aortic insufficiency due to bacterial endocarditis.

Discussion: Acute aortic insufficiency constitutes a medical emergency once even mild signs or symptoms of congestive heart failure appear. The most common cause of acute aortic regurgitation is infective endocarditis. The mortality of acute aortic regurgitation in which congestive heart failure has developed is as high as 75% when treated medically but mortality is reduced to 25% with surgical therapy. The cause of this high mortality is uncertain but is probably due to the severe hemodynamic disruption caused by acute aortic insufficiency.

In acute aortic regurgitation, blood is driven back into the left ventricle from the aorta in diastole under relatively high pressure, resulting in a severe fall in forward cardiac output and very high left ventricular filling pressures. Coronary blood flow occurs primarily in diastole. The reduction in driving pressure in aortic insufficiency (aortic diastolic pressure) and the increase in myocardial compressive forces produced by the increased filling pressure may severely limit coronary blood flow. Reduction in coronary blood flow may produce severe subendocardial ischemia and cause further ventricular compromise. It is possibly this chain of events which produces the downward spiral of worsening left ventricular function and eventual cardiovascular collapse.

The consequences of severe aortic insufficiency may be remarkably hard to detect on physical examination. With the exception of the diastolic murmur, most of the signs thought to be typical of aortic insufficiency are absent when the condition is acute. Most of the signs of chronic aortic insufficiency revolve around the large stroke volume and widened pulse pressure that develop as eccentric cardiac hypertrophy and left ventricular dilatation occur. However, these processes are not present acutely but take time to develop. Thus the widened pulse pressure and the signs that follow it (e.g., Corrigan's pulse, de Rossier's sign, de Musset's sign) will be absent. A sign that may be present in acute aortic insufficiency is reduction in intensity of S_1. A soft S_1 occurs as the high diastolic left ventricular pressure closes the mitral valve early in diastole, reducing the intensity of the first heart sound.

When acute aortic insufficiency with heart failure is suspected, an urgent echo/Doppler study is indicated. This study may demonstrate the vegetations on the aortic valve consistent with endocarditis. The most important finding, however, is preclosure of the mitral valve (shown on preceding page). While mitral valve preclosure helps to protect the pulmonary vasculature from the high left ventricular filling pressures, this finding indicates that left ventricular diastolic pressures are extremely high and that the aortic insufficiency is severe. Most cases in which this sign is present will eventually decompensate and require surgery. Insertion of a Swan-Ganz catheter helps to confirm the severity of the hemodynamic abnormalities present and may be useful in guiding early medical therapy of the disease. In the young patient in whom the physical examination and echo/Doppler findings are consistent with isolated severe aortic insufficiency, left-sided cardiac catheterization, although safe to perform, is usually unnecessary prior to aortic valve replacement.

Therapy with vasodilators such as nitroprusside are useful in temporarily decreasing left ventricular filling pressure and increasing forward cardiac output. However, it must be emphasized that once even mild signs of symptoms of congestive heart failure develop in the patient with acute aortic insufficiency, aortic valve replacement is urgent. Frequently, delay in surgery with the hope of improving the patient's condition with medical therapy only results in further deterioration and increases the urgency and risk of valve replacement.

The present patient underwent urgent aortic valve replacement the evening of hospital admission. He subsequently completed an 8-week course of intravenous antibiotics.

Clinical Pearls

1. Acute aortic insufficiency complicated by even mild heart failure mandates urgent aortic valve replacement.

2. Most signs of chronic aortic insufficiency are absent in the acute condition.

3. Mitral valve preclosure serves to protect the lungs from the high left ventricular filling pressure present in acute aortic insufficiency. This sign in turn indicates that severe hemodynamic abnormalities are present.

REFERENCES

1. Mann T, McLaurin L, Grossman W, et al: Assessing the hemodynamic severity of acute aortic regurgitation due to infective endocarditis. N Engl J Med 293:108–113, 1975.
2. Meyer T, Sareli P, Pocock WA, et al: Echocardiographic and hemodynamic correlates of diastolic closure of mitral valve and diastolic opening of aortic valve in severe aortic regurgitation. Am J Cardiol 59:1144–1148, 1987.
3. Sareli P, Klein HO, Schamroth CL, et al: Contribution of echocardiography and immediate surgery to the management of severe aortic regurgitation from active infective endocarditis. Am J Cardiol 57:413–418, 1985.

PATIENT 20

A 72-year-old woman with syncope

A 72-year-old woman was admitted because of syncope. She had been previously well but suddenly lost consciousness during two separate episodes in the preceding 24 hours. One episode occurred during rest, the other while doing housework. There was no previous history of syncope, chest pain, or congestive heart failure. An ECG performed 5 years earlier showed left bundle branch block.

Physical Examination: Temperature 36.3°; pulse 36; respirations 24; blood pressure 120/40. Head: contusion over right eye. Neck: Cannon A waves in jugular venous pulse. Cardiac: variability in intensity of S_1; no gallops or murmurs. Neurologic: somnolent, no focal signs.

Laboratory Findings: CBC, electrolytes, BUN, and creatinine normal. Chest radiograph: normal. ECG: shown below.

Hospital Course: Intravenous atropine failed to increase the patient's heart rate. Transcutaneous pacing successfully restored a normal heart rate and the patient became more alert. A transvenous temporary ventricular pacemaker was inserted.

What therapeutic options would you consider in this patient?

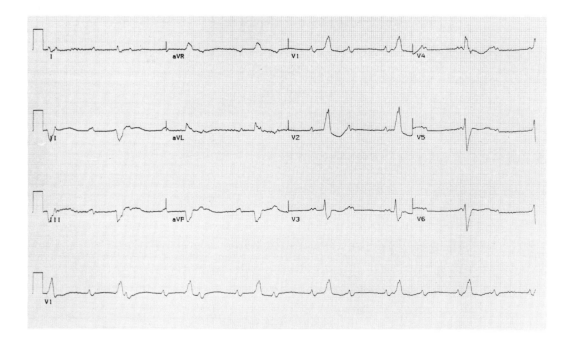

Diagnosis: Complete heart block (CHB).

Discussion: CHB has three major etiologies: (1) isolated disease of the conducting system, (2) infiltrative or degenerative myocardial diseases that affect the conducting system, and (3) acute myocardial infarction. Since CHB diminishes both determinants of cardiac output (heart rate and stroke volume), syncope occurs because of the hypotension that follows the sudden fall in cardiac output. Heart rate is decreased in CHB because the escape rate of the ventricles is substantially slower than the intrinsic rate of the sinus node. Stroke volume is reduced because atrioventricular dissociation produced by CHB desynchronizes atrial contraction from ventricular contraction, leading to the loss of that part of the stroke volume contributed by atrial systole.

Besides bradycardia and hypotension, salient features on physical examination are those of atrioventricular dissociation. A variation in intensity of the first heart sound and Cannon A waves may lead to the diagnosis even before the ECG is taken.

Therapy is aimed at restoration of effective heart rate and stroke volume. The site of CHB may be either at or below the AV node in the bundle of His or the ventricular bundle branches. It is usually impossible, however, to localize the block from the scalar ECG. Because the AV node has significant parasympathetic input, atropine may restore conduction in AV nodal block. Because small doses of atropine may produce paradoxic bradycardia due to direct (nonautonomic) effects, at least 0.5 mg should be given intravenously, followed by a second dose if unsuccessful. If atropine fails to increase the heart rate, infusion of isoproterenol may increase the automaticity of the ventricular escape site and increase the heart rate. Infusion of isoproterenol may produce serious ventricular ectopy, however, and the drug must be administered with caution.

A third temporizing measure is transcutaneous pacing, wherein cutaneous electrodes placed over the heart apply a synchronized discharge, thereby increasing heart rate. Transcutaneous pacing is usually effective in restoring rate but may be painful and poorly tolerated. Heart rate is usually more easily controlled by a temporary transvenous pacemaker, which is considered the best short-term therapy for CHB. Ventricular pacing usually restores adequate cardiac output; however, in patients with antecedent severe myocardial disease, atrioventricular pacing may be necessary.

The need for a permanent pacemaker is determined by the etiology of the CHB. Heart block occurring during an acute inferior myocardial infarction is almost always transient and does not require a permanent pacemaker. Chronic conducting system disease that has progressed to CHB or acute anterior myocardial infarction associated with CHB, however, usually requires implantation of a permanent pacemaker. In acute anterior myocardial infarction, even a short episode of second or third degree heart block is treated with permanent pacing because of a higher incidence of late sudden death in untreated patients.

Progression of conducting system disease in the absence of acute myocardial infarction is slow and unpredictable. The incidence of progression of CHB even in the face of antecedent bifascicular block is less than 1% per year. In such cases the risks of pacemaker implantation outweigh any gain from prophylactic pacing and a permanent pacemaker should not be placed.

In acute anterior myocardial infarction, the new appearance of right bundle branch block with either left anterior hemiblock or left posterior hemiblock is associated with a high incidence of progression (40 to 50%) to CHB. These conditions, therefore, are indications for prophylactic placement of a temporary pacemaker. The new appearance of isolated left bundle branch block or isolated right bundle branch block during acute anterior myocardial infarction has an incidence of progression to CHB of approximately 15 to 20%. In this instance more controversy surrounds the placement of a temporary transvenous pacemaker.

Clinical Pearls

1. Temporary transvenous pacemaking is the definitive short-term therapy of choice for CHB. Infusion of atropine or isoproterenol, or the use of transcutaneous pacemaking may be adequate temporizing measures. Small doses of atropine (< 0.5 mg) may produce paradoxical bradycardia.

2. Prophylactic pacemaker insertion is not indicated for asymptomatic chronic conducting system disease that has not progressed to CHB.

3. Even if the AV conduction disturbance is transient in acute anterior myocardial infarction, implantation of a permanent pacemaker is indicated because of the high incidence of recurrence of CHB and sudden death in untreated patients.

REFERENCES

1. Frye RL, Collins JJ, DeSanctis RW, et al: Guidelines for permanent cardiac pacemaker implantation, May 1984. A report of the Joint American College of Cardiology/American Heart Association Task Force on Assessment of Cardiovascular Procedures (Subcommittee on Pacemaker Implantation). J Am Coll Cardiol 4:434–442, 1984.
2. Hindman MC, Wagner GS, JaRo M, et al: The clinical significance of bundle branch block complicating acute myocardial infarction. II. Indications for temporary and permanent pacemaker insertion. Circulation 58:689–699, 1978.
3. Zoll PM, Zoll RH, Falk RH, et al: External noninvasive temporary cardiac pacing: Clinical trials. Circulation 71:937–944, 1985.
4. Atkins JM, Leshin SJ, Blomqvist G, et al: Ventricular conduction blocks and sudden death in acute myocardial infarction. N Engl J Med 288:281–284, 1973.

CHAPTER 3

Renal and Electrolytes

Robert J. Anderson, M.D.
Randy L. Howard, M.D.

PATIENT 1

A 72-year-old woman with azotemia after sustaining a hip fracture

A 72-year-old woman was found by a neighbor lying on the floor of her apartment. She had fallen 2 days previously and had been unable to move because of severe hip pain. Her medical history was unremarkable except for hypertension managed with hydrochlorothiazide.

Physical Examination: Temperature 99°; pulse 124; respirations 24; blood pressure 110/60 (85/50 sitting). Thin, elderly woman with dry mucous membranes and pain in the right hip, which had limited range of motion.

Laboratory Findings: Hct 52%; albumin 4.5 gm/dl; BUN 90 mg/dl, creatinine 2.6 mg/dl. UA: normal; spot urinary Na+: 5 mEq/L. Renal ultrasound: normal-sized kidneys without evidence of obstructive uropathy. Hip radiograph: intertrochanteric fracture.

What is the likely cause of the increased BUN and creatinine?

Diagnosis: Prenal azotemia from intravascular volume depletion after an intertrochanteric fracture.

Discussion: The evaluation of a patient with azotemia is assisted by an understanding of the pathophysiology of raised BUN and creatinine. Blood urea nitrogen is formed from protein delivered to the liver and is then excreted by the kidneys. An elevated BUN can occur as a result of a high protein load delivered to the liver, as is seen with high dietary protein intake, gastrointestinal bleeding, and a catabolic state (sepsis, corticosteroid therapy, and necrotic tissue). An elevated BUN can also occur by diminished renal excretion, as occurs with either a decreased glomerular filtration rate (GFR) or increased tubular reabsorption of nitrogen. Such increased tubular reabsorption develops in low urinary flow states, as in dehydration or obstructive uropathy.

Serum creatinine is formed by the nonenzymatic hydrolysis of creatine released from muscle and is eliminated from the blood by glomerular filtration. High serum creatinine can thus be due to muscle crush injury or impaired renal function. In some assays, ketones and medications, such as cefoxitin, trimethoprim, and cimetidine, falsely elevate serum creatinine. Elevation of both BUN and serum creatinine, however, usually indicates impaired GFR.

In patients with diminished GFR as demonstrated by increased BUN and serum creatinine, three major causes should be considered: prerenal azotemia (renal hypoperfusion), postrenal azotemia (obstruction of urine flow), and renal azotemia (renal parenchymal disorders and acute tubular necrosis). Prerenal azotemia is the most common cause of an abrupt decline in renal function, constituting 50 to 80% of all cases. Either extracellular fluid volume loss (such as diarrhea, burns, vomiting, GI hemorrhage, or diuretic therapy) or sequestration (such as pancreatitis, peritonitis, or muscle crush injury) leads to diminished renal perfusion and impaired glomerular filtration. Occasionally, prerenal azotemia is due to a marked impairment in cardiac output, as occurs with severe congestive cardiac failure. In patients with intravascular volume depletion, prompt fluid administration can reverse prerenal azotemia even when BUN and serum creatinine are markedly elevated, as in the present patient. Delays in therapy can lead to ischemic acute tubular necrosis, which carries a mortality of 25 to 75%.

Early recognition of prerenal azotemia is thus critical. Clues to this condition include: (1) a history compatible with extracellular fluid volume loss, fluid sequestration, or impaired cardiac output; (2) physical findings compatible with extracellular fluid deficits (such as orthostatic hypotension, tachycardia, dry mucous membranes, absence of moisture in the axillae, decreased skin turgor, and weight loss) or impaired cardiac output (such as an S_3 or elevated JVP); (3) normal urinalysis; and (4) low Na+ concentration on a spot urinalysis.

The low spot urinary Na+ in patients with prerenal azotemia indicates that the renal tubules are avidly reabsorbing Na+ in an attempt to improve renal perfusion. Thus, it is an indicator of intact tubular function and potentially reversible prerenal azotemia. By contrast, in acute tubular necrosis, impaired renal tubules no longer avidly reabsorb Na+, resulting in a spot Na+ concentration that usually exceeds 40 mEq/L. Recently, some investigators have proposed that either a renal failure index (spot urine Na+ divided by the spot urine to plasma creatinine ratio, i.e., $U_{Na}/[U_{Cr}/P_{Cr}]$) or a fractional excretion of Na+ ($[U_{Na}/P_{Na}]/[U_{Cr}/P_{Cr}] \times 100$) of less than 1 may provide a sensitive indicator of prerenal azotemia when the spot Na+ concentration is > 20 mEq/L.

In the present patient, chronic diuretic use plus immobilization with inability to maintain salt and water intake led to intravascular volume depletion and renal hypoperfusion. The normal urinalysis suggested no renal cause of azotemia and the normal renal ultrasound excluded obstructive uropathy. Cautious administration of 2 liters of normal saline restored her hemodynamic parameters and normalized the BUN and creatinine.

Clinical Pearls

1. Prerenal azotemia is the most common setting of acute renal failure and is usually responsive to therapy.
2. A normal urinalysis and a low (< 20 mEq/L) spot urinary Na+ are highly suggestive of prerenal azotemia.

REFERENCES

1. Badr K, Ichikawa I: Prenal failure: A deleterious shift from renal compensation to decompensation. N Engl J Med 319:623–629, 1988.
2. Shapiro JI, Anderson RJ: Sodium depletion states. In Brenner BM, Stein JH (eds): Contemp Issues Nephrol 16:245–276, 1987.

PATIENT 2

A 29-year-old man with depression developed altered mental status and metabolic acidosis

A 29-year-old man had been hospitalized on the psychiatry service with depression for 2 months. He left the hospital on a pass and upon returning complained of abdominal pain and vomiting. Over the next several hours he became more agitated and was then found unarousable with decerebrate posturing.

Physical Examination: Temperature 102°; pulse 120; respirations 35; blood pressure 160/100. No odors were noted on the breath. Fundi: normal. Neurologic: unresponsive to pain without focal findings.

Laboratory Findings: Serum Na+ 142 mEq/L, K+ 4.7 mEq/L, Cl⁻ 111 mEq/L, HCO_3^- 10 mEq/L, anion gap 21 mEq/L. Ca^{2+} 9.4 mg/dl, BUN 12 mg/dl, creatinine 1.3 mg/dl, glucose 100 mg/dl. ABG (room air): pH 7.20, PCO_2 13 mm Hg, PO_2 100 mm Hg. Measured plasma osmolality: 347 mOsm/kg H_2O. Serum salicylate, ethanol, and ketones: negative. UA: pH 5.0, specific gravity 1.010, 1+ protein, 3+ heme, 20 to 30 RBC/hpf, hyaline casts and crystals (shown below).

Your initial differential diagnosis should encourage urgent consideration of what disorder?

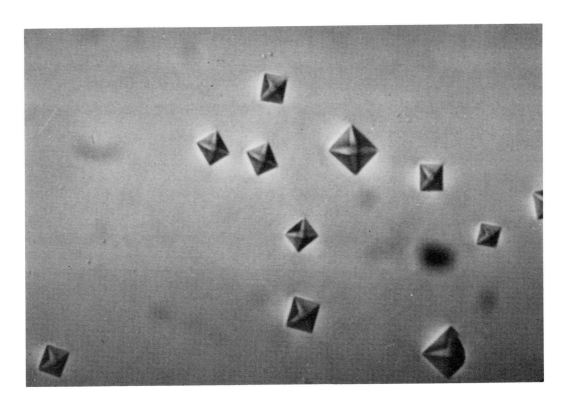

Diagnosis: Anion gap metabolic acidosis secondary to ethylene glycol ingestion.

Discussion: Reduced serum HCO_3^- occurs through either buffering of an organic acid (metabolic acidosis) or its loss via the gastrointestinal tract or kidneys. Bicarbonate loss from the gastrointestinal tract leads to metabolic acidosis, whereas loss from the kidney may be due to either renal tubular disease (renal tubular acidosis) or renal compensation for respiratory alkalosis. Thus a low serum HCO_3^- may be found both in metabolic acidosis and respiratory alkalosis. The present patient had a metabolic acidosis because depressed levels of HCO_3^- in respiratory alkalosis almost always exceed 15 to 16 mEq/L and are associated with an alkaline pH.

Causes of metabolic acidosis can be categorized as normal anion gap (hyperchloremic) or increased anion gap. The normal serum anion gap (calculated by subtracting serum Cl^- and HCO_3^- from $Na+$) ranges between 8 and 16 mEq/L. In general, the higher the anion gap, the more likely the diagnosis of organic acidosis.

Normal anion gap acidosis usually results from gastrointestinal (diarrhea and small bowel drainage or fistulae) or renal losses of HCO_3^-. The most common cause of renal HCO_3^- losses is proximal or distal renal tubular acidosis (RTA). Proximal RTA involves defective HCO_3^- reabsorption in the proximal tubule, and distal RTA results from defective H+ secretion by the distal tubule.

Increased anion gap acidosis results from three major processes: (1) decreased renal acid excretion during renal failure; (2) increased endogenous acid production; and (3) ingestion of toxic substances that are metabolized to organic acids. Increased endogenous acid production occurs most commonly in diabetic ketoacidosis (DKA), alcoholic ketoacidosis (AKA), and lactic acidosis.

Toxic substances that are metabolized to organic acids to form an anion gap acidosis include salicylate, methanol, and ethylene glycol. Salicylic acid and its acid intermediates result in the increased anion gap of salicylate poisoning. The major acids associated with methanol and ethylene glycol poisonings are formic acid and glycolic acid, respectively. In both of these toxic ingestions, lactic acidosis may also be present. Methanol is currently found as a de-icing agent in windshield fluid and ethylene glycol in antifreeze. Both agents cause mental status abnormalities after ingestion. A laboratory characteristic of methanol and ethylene glycol poisonings that aids diagnosis is the presence of an increase in the osmolal gap, which is the difference between measured and calculated serum osmolality. Osmolality can be calculated with the equation: 2[Na+] + [glucose]/18 + [BUN]/2.8 + [ethanol]/4.5. A normal osmolal gap is less than 15 mOsm/kg. In the present patient, calculated osmolality was 293 mOsm/kg H_2O. Another diagnostic clue to ethylene glycol intoxication is the presence of calcium oxalate crystals in the urine, as in the present patient.

Neither intact ethylene glycol nor methanol is intrinsically toxic; their metabolic products generate acids and cause the tissue damage. Treatment of both types of ingestion, therefore, involves ethanol infusions (serum ethanol of 100 to 200 mg/dl) to retard metabolism and production of toxic substances. Because the enzyme that metabolizes methanol and ethylene glycol (alcohol dehydrogenase) has a higher affinity for ethanol than for the toxins, maintenance of high blood ethanol prevents metabolism of ethylene glycol and methanol. Once an adequate ethanol level is achieved, hemodialysis can increase clearance of these substances.

In the present patient, an anion gap metabolic acidosis, a marked increase in osmolar gap, and urine calcium oxalate crystals strongly suggested the presence of ethylene glycol intoxication, which was confirmed by direct analysis. This patient was placed on an ethanol infusion and hemodialysis was initiated. He subsequently developed oliguric acute renal failure. After 10 days, urine output returned. Dialysis was discontinued 12 days after the ingestion, and the patient was left with chronic renal insufficiency (creatinine 5.0 mg/dl).

Clinical Pearls

1. The presence of both an elevated osmolal and anion gap should raise suspicion of methanol or ethylene glycol ingestion.

2. Diagnosis of methanol or ethylene glycol intoxication requires prompt initiation of ethanol infusion and hemodialysis.

REFERENCES

1. Kaehny WD, Gabow PA: Pathogenesis and management of metabolic acidosis and alkalosis. In Schrier RW (ed): Renal and Electrolyte Disorders. Boston, Little, Brown and Co., 1986, pp 141–186.
2. Gabow PA: Disorders associated with an altered anion gap. Kidney Int 27:472–483, 1985.

PATIENT 3

A 64-year-old man with congestive heart failure, bursitis, and oliguria

A 64-year-old man was being treated with digoxin and furosemide for an exacerbation of congestive heart failure due to coronary artery disease. Several days after the initiation of diuresis and weight loss, he had pain on movement of his right shoulder that improved with indomethacin.

Physical Examination: Pulse 90; respirations 24; blood pressure 100/60. Chest: bibasilar rales. Cardiac: elevated jugular venous pressure; S_3 gallop. Extremities: 2+ pedal edema; tenderness over the right shoulder bursa with limited range of motion.

Laboratory Findings: Serum Na+ 132 mEq/L, K+ 3.8 mEq/L; BUN 30 mg/dl, serum creatinine 1.9 mg/dl. UA: normal. Chest radiograph: cardiomegaly with vascular redistribution.

Hospital Course: The patient's cardiac condition continued to improve with therapy. Six days after admission, however, he became oliguric and diuretic-resistant in the absence of clinical signs of intravascular volume depletion.

What is your clinical suspicion regarding the patient's changed renal status?

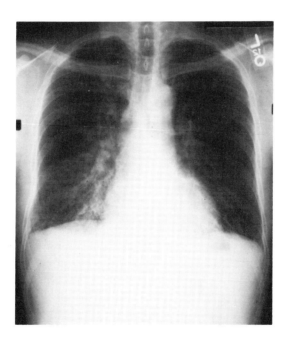

Diagnosis: Acute renal failure due to therapy with the nonsteroidal anti-inflammatory drug indomethacin.

Discussion: Nonsteroidal anti-inflammatory drugs (NSAIDs) are among the most commonly prescribed medications in the United States, and many of these agents are available without a prescription. They exert their anti-inflammatory and analgesic effects by inhibition of cyclo-oxygenase enzymes, thereby preventing the formation of inflammatory mediators, such as prostaglandins and prostacyclin. In the kidney, prostaglandins and prostacyclin are critical messengers in the maintenance of normal renal blood flow and tubular function. Removal of these renal products of cyclo-oxygenase can, under certain circumstances, have profound adverse influences on renal function and electrolyte balance.

Normally, renal blood flow is maintained by a balance between renal vasoconstrictor (angiotensin II, norepinephrine, and renal adrenergic tone) and vasodilator (prostaglandin E and prostacyclin) influences. In clinical settings associated with an increase in circulating angiotensin II and norepinephrine, administration of an NSAID can remove renal vasodilator influences and result in profound renal vasoconstriction and acute renal failure. Clinical settings associated with enhanced renal vasoconstrictors include intravascular volume depletion (such as with diuretic use, diarrhea, vomiting, and gastrointestinal bleeding) and disorders associated with a decreased effective circulating volume, and thus renal hypoperfusion (such as in cardiac failure, hypoalbuminemia, and hepatic cirrhosis). In these settings, NSAIDs often result in intense renal vasoconstriction with oliguria. Elderly patients and patients with underlying chronic renal failure may also be particularly predisposed to nonsteroidal-induced acute renal failure. If stopped quickly, the renal failure usually reverses. If the drug is continued, however, renal ischemia with acute tubular necrosis may develop. Rarely, NSAIDs can result in a hypersensitivity reaction with acute renal failure and heavy proteinuria due to interstitial nephritis.

In addition to occasionally inducing acute renal failure, NSAIDs exert several potential effects on electrolyte balance. These agents generally cause a modest amount of salt retention even in healthy individuals. This occasionally (5 to 10% of cases) leads to edema formation. In patients with advanced age, underlying renal failure, hypertension, or an underlying edematous disorder, salt retention can be more pronounced and have adverse clinical consequences. Several investigators have noted that NSAIDs significantly inhibit the diuretic effect of most commonly used diuretic agents. Finally, NSAIDs are capable of inhibiting renal renin secretion and aldosterone biosynthesis. Because the hormone aldosterone is important in regulating renal tubular secretion and thereby excretion of K+, NSAIDs can induce dangerous hyperkalemia. A hyperkalemic response to NSAIDs usually occurs in patients with underlying renal disease or in patients being concomitantly treated with a potassium-sparing diuretic (spironolactone, dyrenium, or amiloride).

In the present patient, underlying congestive heart failure had resulted in a mild form of prerenal azotemia. The administration of an NSAID caused a profound fall in renal function. Fortunately, cessation of the offending agent was accompanied by improvement in the oliguria within 24 hours. The patient was advised to avoid NSAIDs in the future unless absolutely necessary, at which time sulindac (Clinoril) would be recommended, because it is considered the least likely drug in this group to be nephrotoxic.

Clinical Pearls

1. Nonsteroidal anti-inflammatory drugs can cause acute renal failure in patients with advanced age, underlying intravascular volume depletion, or an edematous disorder.
2. Nonsteroidal anti-inflammatory agents can induce salt and water retention, diuretic resistance, and hyperkalemia.
3. Clinoril is the least likely in this class of drugs to be nephrotoxic.

REFERENCES
1. Blackshear JL, David M, Stillman T: Identification of risk for renal insufficiency from nonsteroidal anti-inflammatory drugs. Arch Intern Med 143:1130–1134, 1983.
2. Adam DN, Howie AJ, Micheal J, et al: Nonsteroidal anti-inflammatory drugs and renal failure. Lancet 1:57–60, 1986.

PATIENT 4

A 60-year-old man with cough, weight loss, confusion, and hyponatremia

A 60-year-old man with a long smoking history presented with a 20-pound weight loss. His chronic cough had recently increased in severity. Family members noted episodes of confusion during the several days before admission.

Physical Examination: Temperature 102.1°; pulse 80 without orthostatic changes; respirations 20; blood pressure 120/80. Skin: normal turgor. Mucous membranes: well hydrated. Cardiac: normal jugular venous pressure. Extremities: no edema. Neurologic: intermittent confusion without focal findings.

Laboratory Findings: CBC: normal. Serum Na+ 114 mEq/L, K+ 3.8 mEq/L, Cl⁻ 84 mEq/L, HCO_3^- 22 mEq/L; BUN 4 mg/dl; glucose 86 mg/dl. Serum Ca^{2+}, albumin, and liver function tests: normal. Spot urinary Na+: 69 mEq/L. Urinary osmolality: 340 mOsm/kg H_2O. Plasma osmolality: 240 mOsm/kg H_2O. Chest radiograph: left hilar mass. Head CT scan: unremarkable.

Based on the clinical presentation and laboratory studies, what is the cause of the patient's low serum Na+?

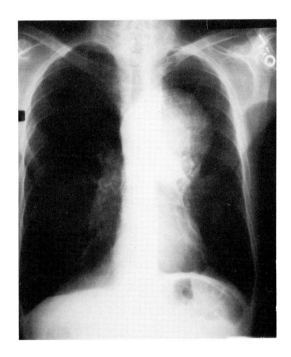

Diagnosis: Hyponatremia due to syndrome of inappropriate secretion of antidiuretic hormone (SIADH) resulting from small-cell lung cancer.

Discussion: When evaluating a low serum Na+ concentration, laboratory error and the effects of hyperglycemia are primary considerations. Hyperglycemia lowers the Na+ concentration by acting as an osmotic agent, drawing water into the extracellular space. Repeat serum Na+ in the present patient was 115 mEq/L, thereby excluding laboratory error, and hyperglycemia was not present.

It is important to recall that the serum Na+ concentration reflects the ratio of the relative amount of Na+ to water in the blood. Nearly all hyponatremia is due to a relative excess of water, thereby diluting the normal Na+ concentration. A relative excess of water occurs by continued water intake (thirst or intravenous administration) in the presence of compromised renal capacity for the excretion of water. Under normal circumstances, the kidneys are able to eliminate 20 liters of free water each day. Factors that limit renal water excretion are either severe renal failure (which is not present in this patient) or the action of the posterior pituitary hormone vasopressin (or antidiuretic hormone, sometimes abbreviated ADH) that causes the kidneys to avidly retain water.

Factors that result in persistent secretion of ADH include hypovolemia and disorders associated with a decreased effective circulating blood volume, such as heart failure, cirrhosis, and nephrosis. If such patients drink excess water or receive it intravenously, it will be retained, thereby lowering their serum Na+ concentration.

The present patient had no evidence to suggest the presence of either volume depletion or a decrease in effective circulating blood volume. He appeared clinically normovolemic, which was confirmed by the relatively high spot urinary Na+ concentration. These findings classify the patient as having normovolemic hyponatremia, a condition that most clinicians refer to as SIADH. The patient had impaired renal water excretion, as evidenced by a urinary osmolality higher than serum values. Such an inappropriately high urine osmolality occurs in all patients with true hyponatremia and is not diagnostic of any specific category of hyponatremia.

Several clinical conditions can cause SIADH, including medications (chlorpropamide, thiazide diuretics, tricyclics), intracranial pathology, the postoperative state, hormonal deficiency states (adrenal and thyroid insufficiency), decompensated psychosis, and all types of cancer.

A variety of pulmonary/intrathoracic processes are increasingly associated with SIADH. Such conditions include severe acute and chronic respiratory failure, mechanical ventilation, severe bronchospasm, and intrathoracic infectious and neoplastic disorders. The exact mechanism whereby these disorders induce SIADH remains unknown. However, small-cell lung cancer cells are known to synthesize ADH de novo. Although SIADH is a common complication of small-cell lung cancer, it is occasionally seen with other histologic types of bronchogenic carcinomas and rarely with pulmonary metastases.

In the present patient, neurologic symptoms due to hyponatremia were present but mild. He was treated with water restriction alone, which resulted in a slow increase in his serum Na+ concentration while a histologic diagnosis was made. Alternatively, either a small amount of hypertonic saline alone or the administration of furosemide (1 mg/kg body weight, which induces a diuresis approximately equivalent to one-half normal saline) with replacement of urinary electrolyte loss with 3% saline could have been used to raise his serum Na+ concentration to the 120 to 125 mEq/L range more rapidly. Chronic treatment modalities consist of water restriction, antitumor therapy, and rarely demeclocycline. Demeclocycline impairs the renal collecting tubular water permeability response to ADH by an unknown mechanism, thereby increasing renal water elimination and elevating the serum Na+ concentration.

Clinical Pearls

1. Hyponatremia associated with normovolemia as assessed by clinical criteria and confirmed by a spot urinary Na+ concentration > 40 mEq/L is due to SIADH.

2. Several intrathoracic/pulmonary processes, including respiratory failure, bronchospasm, mechanical ventilation, and intrathoracic infections and tumors, can cause SIADH.

3. Demeclocycline assists the management of SIADH by impeding the renal water permeability response to ADH of the collecting tubule, thereby increasing renal water elimination.

REFERENCES

1. Dreyfuss D, Leviel F, Paillard M, et al: Acute infectious pneumonia is accompanied by a latent vasopressin-dependent impairment of renal water excretion. Am Rev Respir Dis 138:583–589, 1988.
2. Dixon BS, Anderson RJ: Pneumonia and the syndrome of inappropriate antidiuretic hormone secretion: Don't pour water on fire. Am Rev Respir Dis 183:512–513, 1988.
3. Anderson RJ, Chung HM, Kluge R, et al: Hyponatremia: A prospective analysis of its epidemiology and the pathogenetic role of vasopressin. Ann Intern Med 102:164–168, 1985.

PATIENT 5

A 50-year-old woman with fever, rash, myalgia, and oliguria following a herpes labialis infection

A 50-year-old woman developed a herpetic lesion on her lower lip. After several days her lip became red, warm, and swollen, and her physician suspected secondary bacterial infection with cellulitis. She was placed on a regimen that included warm compresses, topical acyclovir, and antibiotic therapy (dicloxacillin). Five days later she noted a generalized maculopapular rash, diffuse arthralgias, low-grade fever, and bilateral flank pain.

Physical Examination: Temperature 100.1°; pulse 90. Skin: fine maculopapular rash on the back and chest; edematous and erythematous lower lip with a crusting lesion. Cardiac: no murmurs. Thorax: moderate bilateral costovertebral angle tenderness.

Laboratory Findings: Hct 35%; WBC 10,400/μl with 8% eosinophils. UA: 20 to 30 white cells per high powered field and white blood cell casts. Hansel's stain (below) of the urinary sediment: positive for eosinophils. Serum creatinine: 3.4 mg/dl. Electrolytes: normal.

What is the most likely diagnosis?

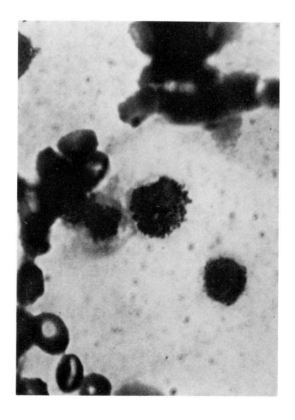

Diagnosis: Acute renal failure due to dicloxacillin-induced hypersensitivity nephritis.

Discussion: In recent years acute interstitial nephritis in the setting of drug hypersensitivity has been recognized as an important cause of reversible acute renal failure. Histologically, interstitial nephritis is characterized by interstitial edema and infiltration with mononuclear cells consisting of lymphocytes, monocytes, plasma cells, and eosinophils. The glomeruli and vessels are usually normal. This renal lesion has been reported to occur in idiosyncratic fashion with a wide variety of drugs that include penicillin, cephalosporins, sulfonamides, thiazide diuretics, furosemide, rifampin, vancomycin, minocycline, allopurinol, nonsteroidal anti-inflammatory agents, sulfinpyrazone, phenytoin, azathioprine, phenobarbital, carbamazepine, cimetidine, and captopril.

In the initial description of hypersensitivity nephritis, the diagnosis was suspected clinically because of the association between acute renal failure and evidence of a systemic allergic reaction, such as fever, skin rash, arthralgias, and peripheral eosinophilia. Subsequent reports, however, demonstrate that many or all of these clinical features may be absent. Indeed, the clinical presentation of hypersensitivity nephritis may be nonspecific with oliguric or nonoliguric renal failure, microhematuria, low-grade proteinuria, and pyuria. In recent series, hypersensitivity nephritis was identified by renal biopsy in 10 to 15% of patients with unexplained acute renal failure. Therefore, the diagnosis of drug-induced hypersensitivity nephritis should be considered in any instance of renal failure of uncertain etiology. Early diagnosis is important because discontinuation of the offending drug may be followed by rapid recovery of renal function. Furthermore, corticosteroid therapy may improve the outcome.

Because the majority of clinical and laboratory features in hypersensitivity nephritis are nonspecific, a simple screening test has been sought. Following the classic description of methicillin-induced hypersensitivity nephritis in which urinary eosinophils were found by Wright's stain, this technique came to be regarded as a sensitive and specific screening test for the diagnosis of drug-induced interstitial nephritis of any cause. However, it has recently been shown that the Wright's stain has technical difficulties that limit its sensitivity for detecting eosinophiluria. Hansel's stain has been shown to be a more sensitive technique. Unfortunately, eosinophiluria itself does not confirm the diagnosis of acute interstitial nephritis. Although eosinophiluria is absent in ischemic/nephrotoxin-induced acute tubular necrosis, it can occur with rapidly progressive glomerulonephritis, postinfectious glomerulonephritis, chronic interstitial nephritis, prostatitis, obstructive uropathy, acute transplant rejection, and other acute and chronic disorders of the genitourinary tract. Thus, the finding of eosinophiluria must be interpreted in light of the clinical situation. The absence of eosinophiluria by Hansel's stain in the setting of unexplained acute renal failure, however, provides strong evidence against the diagnosis of hypersensitivity nephritis.

[67]Gallium scintigraphy is also a sensitive screen for drug-induced interstitial nephritis. In this disorder, intense, diffuse, bilateral renal ^{67}Ga uptake is found. In contrast, there is no significant renal ^{67}Ga uptake in acute tubular necrosis. Unfortunately, ^{67}Ga uptake is also seen in other causes of acute renal failure such as glomerulonephritis. Thus, like the Hansel stain, ^{67}Ga scanning appears to differentiate hypersensitivity nephritis from acute tubular necrosis but does not exclude other causes of renal insufficiency. Renal biopsy remains the gold standard for the diagnosis of hypersensitivity nephritis.

In the present patient, cessation of dicloxacillin did not result in dramatic clinical improvement and the serum creatinine increased further to 5.2 mg/dl. At that point, prednisone (60 mg/day) was instituted, resulting in a rapid resolution of symptoms and a return of normal renal function.

Clinical Pearls

1. Many drugs can result in acute renal failure due to hypersensitivity interstitial nephritis, which may or may not be associated with systemic symptoms.

2. Hansel's stain of the urine for eosinophils is a sensitive test for hypersensitivity nephritis and, in the appropriate clinical setting, can be used to make a presumptive diagnosis; eosinophiluria does not occur in ischemic/nephrotoxin-induced acute tubular necrosis but may be present in other causes of renal insufficiency.

3. Corticosteroid therapy can hasten recovery from hypersensitivity interstitial nephritis.

REFERENCES

1. Nolan CR, Anger MS, Kelleher SP: Eosinophiluria: A new method of detection and definition of a clinical spectrum. N Engl J Med 315:1516–1519, 1986.
2. Galpin JE, Shinaberger JH, Stanley TM, et al: Acute interstitial nephritis due to methicillin. Am J Med 65:756–764, 1978.

PATIENT 6

A 54-year-old man with chronic pancreatitis, diabetes, abdominal pain, and severe vomiting

A 54-year-old man with a history of chronic pancreatitis and resultant diabetes mellitus presented with abdominal pain and severe vomiting of 1 week's duration. The patient had consumed up to one gallon of milk daily and sodium bicarbonate for the abdominal pain.

Physical Examination: Temperature 98.2°; pulse 100 (130 sitting); respirations 18; blood pressure 132/95 (100/65 sitting). Skin: decreased turgor. Mucous membranes: dry. Abdomen: epigastric tenderness; no stool occult blood.

Laboratory Findings: Na+ 140 mEq/L, K+ 3.4 mEq/L, Cl⁻ 69 mEq/L, HCO_3^- 40 mEq/L, creatinine 2.6 mg/dl, glucose 108 mg/dl. UA: normal. ABG (room air): pH 7.86; PCO_2 23 mm Hg, PO_2 81 mm Hg. Chest radiograph: normal.

Characterize the patient's acid-base disturbance and consider the pathogenesis.

Answer: Triple acid-base disturbance with metabolic alkalosis (secondary to vomiting and alkali ingestion), anion gap metabolic acidosis, and respiratory alkalosis.

Discussion: Metabolic alkalosis occurs when a primary increase in the serum HCO_3^- concentration causes a rise in blood pH. The causes of metabolic alkalosis are divided into three major categories: (1) sodium chloride-responsive alkalosis occurring in volume-contracted conditions (urinary $Cl^- < 10$ mEq/L); (2) sodium chloride-resistant alkalosis occurring in normal or volume expanded conditions (urinary $Cl^- > 20$ mEq/L); and (3) an unclassified category. By far, sodium chloride-responsive alkalosis with volume contraction is the most commonly encountered form.

In most instances, the development of metabolic alkalosis involves two stages. The first, or generation, stage can result from three processes: (1) net loss of H+ ion in extracellular fluid eliminated either through the gastrointestinal tract (vomiting) or kidneys (diuretics) with a concomitant rise in the serum HCO_3^- concentration; (2) net addition of HCO_3^- from either exogenous or endogenous substances that the liver converts to HCO_3^- (lactate, citrate, acetate); and (3) external loss of fluid containing high concentrations of Cl^- and low concentrations of HCO_3^-, as occurs with diuretics and certain gastrointestinal tract diseases, such as villous adenoma.

The second, or maintenance, stage of metabolic alkalosis develops when certain factors constrain the kidney's normal corrective role of excreting HCO_3^- in the face of rising blood pH. Extracellular volume depletion acts as one of the most important of these factors by stimulating increased Na+ reabsorption and HCO_3^- reclamation in the proximal tubule. Increased aldosterone, which occurs in volume depletion, stimulates exchange of Na+ for either H+ ion or K+ in the distal tubule—H+ exchange promotes HCO_3^- generation in the serum. Serum Cl^- concentration is another important factor in the maintenance of metabolic acidosis because it is the only anion other than HCO_3^- that can accompany Na+ tubular reabsorption. Since serum Cl^- concentration falls as the HCO_3^- concentration rises, less Cl^- is available in metabolic alkalosis to allow HCO_3^- excretion. Potassium depletion and hypercapnia, which develop in compensation for metabolic alkalosis, may also increase the renal HCO_3^- reabsorption threshold.

Sodium chloride-responsive metabolic alkalosis usually occurs in the setting of gastrointestinal disorders or diuretic therapy. Vomiting and gastric drainage generate metabolic alkalosis by eliminating H+ ions and maintain alkalosis through extracellular volume depletion, decreased Cl^- concentration, and hypokalemia, thereby preventing the kidney from dumping the excess HCO_3^-. In the conditions of chloride diarrhea and villous adenoma, Cl^- losses from the colon generate metabolic alkalosis while volume depletion and hypokalemia maintain the metabolic disturbance. Potent diuretics generate metabolic alkalosis through volume and K+ depletion in the setting of dietary Cl^- restriction. Continued diuretic-initiated delivery of Na+ to the distal tubule combine with these factors to increase H+ ion secretion, thus generating and maintaining the metabolic alkalosis.

Sodium chloride-resistant metabolic alkalosis usually develops with profound K+ depletion or excess mineralocorticoid activity, as occurs in primary hyperaldosteronism, Bartter's syndrome, and Cushing's syndrome. The ingestion of glycyrrhizic acid, which is present in English licorice and is structurally and functionally similar to aldosterone, can also induce metabolic alkalosis.

Although the clinical manifestations of metabolic alkalosis are nonspecific, severe alkalemia can cause serious cardiac arrhythmias and decrease the concentration of serum ionized Ca^{2+} by increasing binding of Ca^{2+} to albumin. The resultant hypocalcemia can provoke tetany, carpal-pedal spasm, and rarely seizures or laryngeal spasm.

The treatment of metabolic alkalosis in all cases involves correction of the underlying disorder that generated the metabolic disturbance. This condition, however, may have previously resolved and other factors may be maintaining the alkalosis. Therapy should then be directed at these aggravating disorders. In sodium chloride-responsive metabolic alkalosis, volume depletion and Cl^- losses are important factors that can be treated with saline solutions. Excess mineralocorticoid activity can be treated by volume expansion, which suppresses mineralocorticoid secretion, or rarely by blocking the renal effects of aldosterone with spironolactone. In some patients who are unable to tolerate volume administration, acetazolamide may be beneficial by increasing renal HCO_3^- excretion.

Patients with serious arrhythmias or neuromuscular complications of alkalemia may improve with a rebreathing mask, although they may rarely require intubation with mechanical hypoventilation to increase PCO_2. Also, intravenous infusion of 0.1 N hydrochloric acid can rapidly lower blood pH. Finally, in patients undergoing nasogastric suctioning, prophylactic administration of H_2 blockers can prevent loss of H+ ion and attenuate the development of metabolic alkalosis.

The present patient's alkalemic pH and elevated serum HCO_3^- confirmed the presence of alkalosis.

The decreased PCO_2 indicated a concurrent respiratory alkalosis, and the increased anion gap indicated the presence of metabolic acidosis. This constellation of metabolic disturbances represents the so-called triple acid-base disorder. The patient was treated with normal saline and potassium chloride replacement, and a contrast study subsequently revealed a peptic ulcer with gastric outlet obstruction.

Clinical Pearls

1. A "triple acid-base disturbance" is identified by the presence of a high serum HCO_3^-, a low PCO_2, and an abnormally large anion gap.

2. The ingestion of English licorice can induce metabolic alkalosis through the effects of glycyrrhizic acid, which is functionally similar to aldosterone.

3. The most common factor involved in the maintenance phase of metabolic alkalosis is extracellular volume depletion.

REFERENCES

1. Kaehny WD, Gabow PA: Pathogenesis and management of metabolic acidosis and alkalosis. In Schrier RW (ed): Renal and Electrolyte Disorders. Boston, Little, Brown and Co., 1986, pp 141–186.
2. Gabow PA: Metabolic alkalosis. In Fluid and Electrolytes: Clinical Problems and Their Solutions. Boston, Little, Brown and Co., 1983, pp 43–55.

PATIENT 7

A 64-year-old woman with renal insufficiency, hypotension, and an abnormal electrocardiogram

A 64-year-old woman with chronic renal insufficiency and congestive heart failure secondary to amyloidosis from longstanding rheumatoid arthritis presented to the emergency room feeling poorly. She noted a decreased urine output the day of admission. Medications included digoxin, salicylic acid, bumetanide, prazosin hydrochloride, and potassium supplements.

Physical Examination: Temperature 98.7°; pulse 72; respirations 16; blood pressure 94/48. Chronically ill-appearing woman. Chest: normal. Cardiac: grade II/VI holosystolic murmur at apex radiating to axillae. Abdomen: normal without hepatosplenomegaly or ascites. Extremities: severe deformities from rheumatoid arthritis; 2+ edema of both legs. Neurologic: normal motor strength.

Laboratory Findings: Electrocardiogram shown below.

What is your clinical impression based on the initial available data?

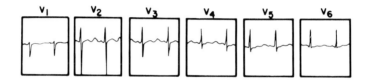

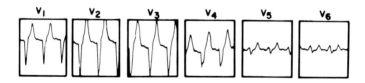

Diagnosis: Hyperkalemia.

Discussion: Severe hyperkalemia is a life-threatening condition that requires not only prompt recognition but also an understanding of its differential diagnosis to allow initiation of appropriate therapy. "Pseudo" or fictitious hyperkalemia should be the first consideration when hyperkalemic values return from the laboratory. Common causes include hemolysis, venipuncture below a tourniquet of an exercising arm, marked leukocytosis ($>$ 100,000 leukocytes/μl), and thrombocytosis ($>$ 1,000,000 platelets/μl).

Potassium redistribution, which occurs with systemic acidosis and insulin deficiency, is another cause of hyperkalemia. As pH falls, H+ ions move into the cells to be buffered and exchanged for K+, which moves into the extracellular space to maintain electrical neutrality. Insulin is an important hormone involved in the movement of K+ into cells, and its deficiency can result in hyperkalemia.

Approximately 90% of the 100 mEq daily K+ load is excreted via the kidneys, and the action of aldosterone on distal tubular secretion is a major mechanism of renal K+ elimination. Hyperkalemia usually does not develop until late in the course of chronic renal failure; serum K+ remains normal until creatinine clearance falls below 10 ml/min provided urine output remains intact. Hyperkalemia is a common accompaniment, however, of acute renal failure. In addition to low glomerular filtration rates, factors that contribute to hyperkalemia in renal insufficiency include metabolic acidosis, increased exogenous (potassium penicillin) or endogenous (rhabdomyolysis) K+ input, impaired renal tubular response to aldosterone, and various medications described below. Also, a primary K+ secretory defect of renal tubules can occur in selected disorders such as renal transplantation, systemic lupus erythematosus, sickle cell disease, and urinary tract obstruction.

Several commonly used medications may result in hyperkalemia. Potassium-sparing diuretics such as spironolactone, triamterene, and amiloride inhibit renal tubular secretion of K+, thereby potentially inducing hyperkalemia. Nonsteroidal anti-inflammatory agents inhibit renal prostaglandin biosynthesis, which results in profound renal vasoconstriction with decreased glomerular filtration and suppressed aldosterone secretion. Heparin and angiotensin-converting enzyme inhibitors,

such as captopril and enalapril, also decrease aldosterone synthesis. Digitalis intoxication may increase serum K+ by inhibiting the cellular enzyme Na+/K+-ATPase, thereby impairing cellular uptake of K+. Beta-adrenergic blocking agents may rarely inhibit catecholamine-mediated movement of K+ into cells and produce hyperkalemia.

The major clinical effects of hyperkalemia relate to the cardiovascular and peripheral neuromuscular systems and, unfortunately, often first occur without warning late in the patient's course. ECG changes of tall, thin, peaked T waves are the earliest signs and progress to prolongation of the PR interval, depression of ST segments, lengthening of the QRS interval, loss of P waves, and finally coarse ventricular fibrillation. The neuromuscular effects of hyperkalemia are weakness and paralysis due to changes in muscle cell resting membrane potential.

Treatment is determined by the severity of hyperkalemia and the extent of cardiovascular and neuromuscular symptoms. Electrocardiographic signs of hyperkalemia warrant continuous ECG monitoring and emergent therapy. The principles of therapy involve counteracting the effect of K+ on muscle cell membrane potential, redistribution of K+ from the extracellular to the intracellular space, and removal of K+ from the body.

Intravenous infusion of 10% calcium gluconate counteracts the effects of hyperkalemia on muscle cell membrane potentials within minutes, although effects may last only 30 minutes. Redistribution of K+ can be accomplished by administration of sodium bicarbonate and infusion of glucose with insulin, which lower K+ levels within 30 minutes, with effects lasting several hours. Removal of K+ from the body can be initiated with exchange resins, such as sodium polystyrene sulfonate (Kayexalate), and with hemodialysis.

The present patient was found to have a serum K+ concentration of 8.1 mEq/L, BUN of 106 mg/dl, creatinine of 5.6 mg/dl, and digoxin of 1.9 ng/dl. Contributing factors for hyperkalemia included exogenous K+ supplementation in the face of decreased K+ elimination that resulted from chronic renal failure and use of a nonsteroidal anti-inflammatory agent. Therapy included intravenous calcium chloride, dextrose with insulin, and oral Kayexalate. Hemodialysis was subsequently initiated for treatment of her renal insufficiency.

Clinical Pearls

1. Several disorders, such as renal transplantation, systemic lupus erythematosus, sickle cell disease, and urinary tract obstruction, can induce a primary K+ secretory defect of renal tubules, resulting in hyperkalemia.

2. Heparin infusions in patients with renal insufficiency can cause hyperkalemia by decreasing aldosterone synthesis.

3. Beta-adrenergic blocking agents may cause redistribution of body K+ by inhibiting catecholamine-mediated cellular influx of K+, thereby producing hyperkalemia.

REFERENCES

1. Gabow PA, Peterson LN: Disorders of potassium metabolism. In Schrier RW (ed): Renal and Electrolyte Disorders. Boston, Little, Brown and Co., 1986, pp 207–249.
2. Ponce SP, Jennings AE, Madias NE, et al: Drug-induced hyperkalemia. Medicine 64:357–370, 1985.

PATIENT 8

A 74-year-old man with oliguria following inpatient evaluation for a transient ischemic attack

A 74-year-old farmer noted transient (60 minutes) left hemiparesis. He was hospitalized for further evaluation. Medical history was unremarkable except for hypertension being treated with hydrochlorothiazide and dyrenium.

Physical Examination: Vital signs: normal. Peripheral pulses: no bruits. Neurologic: normal.

Laboratory Findings: CBC, serum electrolytes, and UA: normal. Chest radiograph: unremarkable. Head CT scan with contrast: no lesions.

Hospital Course: One day after admission, a carotid angiogram revealed diffuse, patchy atherosclerosis. On the third hospital day, he was noted to be oligoanuric. At that time, his serum creatinine had doubled from the admission value, and a UA revealed granular casts. A spot urinary Na+ concentration was 56 mEq/L.

What is the most likely cause of the patient's laboratory abnormalities?

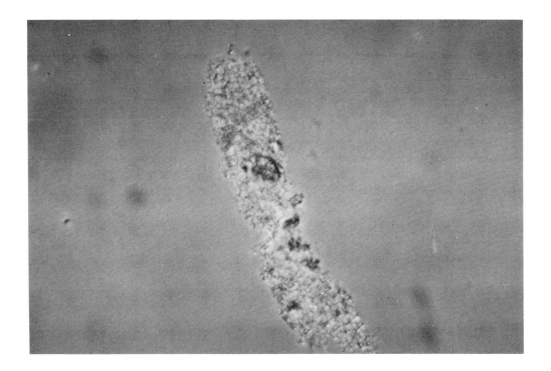

Diagnosis: Contrast-induced acute tubular necrosis.

Discussion: Recent prospective studies indicate that 2 to 5% of all patients admitted to a general medical-surgical hospital will develop acute renal failure. This incidence may be as high as 20 to 25% in critically ill patients admitted to ICUs. The development of hospital-acquired acute renal failure has major impact on patient outcome because it increases mortality rates eight-fold.

Acute renal failure classically becomes manifest by either the occurrence of oligoanuria or a rising BUN/creatinine noted in serial biochemical monitoring of seriously ill patients. It is important to recall, however, that most contemporary instances of acute renal failure are nonoliguric in nature. Thus, the presence of a good urine output (20–30 ml/hr) by no means ensures adequate renal function.

In approaching the present patient, prerenal azotemia should first be considered. This patient had been taking a diuretic and had been made NPO for several tests. Moreover, he had mild orthostatic hypotension when evaluated at the time of discovery of oliguria. Factors suggesting that he did not have prerenal azotemia included the presence of an abnormal urinary sediment and the relatively high urinary Na+ concentration. Nevertheless, intravascular volume expansion with normal saline was instituted to restore circulating blood volume and to improve renal function. Unfortunately, restoration of extracellular fluid volume did not improve his oliguria.

Next, the possibility that this patient might have postrenal azotemia (obstructive uropathy) should be considered. His advanced age and the possibility that he was treated with drugs that had anticholinergic effects could predispose him to bladder outlet obstruction. On physical examination, no evidence of bladder distention was noted, and insertion of a bladder catheter revealed only 10 ml of residual urine. A renal ultrasound examination demonstrated the presence of normal-sized kidneys without ureteral dilation. Together, these findings exclude obstructive uropathy.

After excluding pre- and post-renal causes of renal failure, it is appropriate to focus attention on the kidneys. When focusing on the kidneys, it is helpful to think in terms of renal anatomic compartments. Because this patient had an arteriogram, it is possible that his renal failure was due to atheroembolic disease. However, there was no evidence of emboli to the gut or lower extremities. There was no reason for an acute glomerular or renal interstitial inflammatory process to develop. By exclusion, acute tubular necrosis appeared to be the most likely diagnosis. The abnormal urinalysis and high urinary Na+ are compatible with this diagnosis.

Nephrotoxins cause about 25% of all cases of acute tubular necrosis. Common contemporary nephrotoxins include aminoglycoside antibiotics (which usually cause mild, nonoliguric acute renal failure), nonsteroidal anti-inflammatory agents, cisplatin, amphotericin B, pentamidine, and radiographic contrast agents. Contrast agents are usually remarkably well tolerated in most individuals. Patients with underlying renal failure, especially diabetics, however, may be especially predisposed to contrast nephrotoxicity. The mechanisms underlying the nephrotoxicity remain unknown.

In the present patient, intravascular volume depletion plus repetitive exposure to contrast likely combined to result in acute tubular necrosis. Despite volume expansion and administration of furosemide in an attempt to make him nonoliguric, his oliguric state remained and ultimately he required hemodialysis.

Clinical Pearls

1. Nephrotoxins cause 20 to 25% of contemporary cases of acute tubular necrosis.

2. Because most instances of acute renal failure are nonoliguric, the presence of a good urine output does not ensure normal renal function.

3. Radiographic contrast agents occasionally cause acute tubular necrosis, and diabetics may be especially predisposed to this complication.

REFERENCES

1. Anderson RJ: Radiocontrast and the kidneys. West J Med 142:685–686, 1985.
2. Schusterman N, Strom BL, Murray TG, et al: Risk factors and outcome of hospital-acquired acute renal failure. Am J Med 83:65–72, 1987.

PATIENT 9

A 34-year-old man with chest pain after smoking free-base cocaine

A 34-year-old man presented to the emergency room with chest pain that began two days earlier while he was smoking free-base cocaine. He reported smoking 60 gm of cocaine during the 5 days before admission. He denied seizures, loss of consciousness, or use of other illicit drug or toxins.

Physical Examination: Temperature 98.6°; pulse 80; respirations 16; blood pressure 112/74. General: muscular male in no acute distress. Chest: normal. Cardiac: normal. Extremities: no weakness, edema, or tenderness.

Laboratory Findings: Electrolytes normal; creatinine 1.5 mg/dl; Ca^{2+} 9.9 mg/dl, phosphorus 2.8 mg/dl; LDH 167 IU/L (upper limit 175), SGOT 64 IU/L (upper limit 35); creatine kinase (CK) levels obtained at 12-hour intervals: 2556, 2049, and 1509 IU/L (upper limit 165) with all skeletal muscle (MM) isoenzyme. UA: normal. Chest radiograph: normal. ECG: inversion of T waves in leads II, III, and AVF.

What diagnostic concern is suggested by the patient's presentation?

Diagnosis: Rhabdomyolysis secondary to cocaine use.

Discussion: Since the mid-1980s when cocaine abuse began to burgeon in the United States, a growing literature has described many life-threatening consequences attached to its use. These predominantly include disorders of the cardiovascular system (arrhythmias, severe hypertension, and coronary artery spasm with myocardial infarction) and central nervous system (hyperpyrexia, agitation and delirium, and intractable seizures). Recently, rhabdomyolysis has been added to the list of complications of cocaine intoxication. The mechanisms whereby cocaine causes rhabdomyolysis are unknown; however, cocaine can result in seizures and vasoconstriction of several vascular beds, suggesting that muscle ischemia may play a role.

Rhabdomyolysis is an acute syndrome resulting from skeletal muscle injury with release of muscle contents into the serum. The substances released include K+, phosphorus, organic acids, enzymes, and myoglobin. The true incidence of rhabdomyolysis is unknown; the diagnosis requires a high clinical suspicion in many cases and is probably frequently missed. Although many disorders have been reported to cause rhabdomyolysis, the three most common etiologic factors are alcohol abuse, muscle compression, and generalized seizures. Multiple factors are present in the majority of patients.

Elevations of the skeletal muscle (MM) isoenzyme of creatine kinase and myoglobin are diagnostic of muscle injury and rhabdomyolysis. Other routine blood chemistry tests are insensitive indicators, although the presence of hyperkalemia, hyperphosphatemia, hyperuricemia, hypocalcemia, and an elevated anion gap should alert the clinician to the presence of muscle tissue necrosis. Hyperkalemia, hyperphosphatemia, and hyperuricemia result from the release of muscle content into the serum, whereas hypocalcemia may be due to deposition of calcium phosphate salts in the injured or necrotic muscle. Myoglobinuria detected by the orthotolidine reagent on the urine dipstick has been considered a hallmark of rhabdomyolysis; however, Gabow and colleagues found that myoglobinuria was present using this method in only 50% of patients.

The diagnosis of rhabdomyolysis should be suspected in the presence of: (1) high-risk settings such as alcohol abuse, drug abuse including cocaine, and muscle compression; (2) edema of muscle groups; (3) orthotolidine-positive urine without red cells; and (4) unexplained elevations of SGOT, LDH, K+, uric acid, and phosphorus. Whenever rhabdomyolysis is suspected, a creatine kinase level must be determined to confirm the diagnosis.

Acute renal failure may occur during the course of rhabdomyolysis. In a recent study, 13 of 39 patients with rhabdomyolysis due to cocaine intoxication developed acute renal failure. The pathogenesis of rhabdomyolysis-induced acute renal failure is unclear. Postulated mechanisms include direct tubular toxic effects of myoglobin or ferrihemate, tubular obstruction by myoglobin or uric acid crystals, and renal ischemia due to volume depletion and release of vasoconstrictive mediators. Animal models have stressed the importance of dehydration and acidic urine in the development of renal failure in association with rhabdomyolysis. The degree of elevation of serum creatine kinase, K+, and phosphorus along with the presence of dehydration or sepsis may be factors predictive of renal failure in rhabdomyolysis. Rarely, hypercalcemia complicates the course of patients with acute renal failure due to rhabdomyolysis and may occur from the release of calcium deposited in damaged muscles.

No controlled studies addressing the treatment of rhabdomyolysis in man have been performed. Animal studies, however, strongly suggest that increasing urine flow rate and raising urine pH above 6.0 are beneficial. Ron and colleagues have reported that the induction of an alkaline solute diuresis ($>$ 300 ml/hr) prevented azotemia or renal failure in seven patients with rhabdomyolysis from extensive crush injuries. In the clinical setting, the production of an alkaline urine can be difficult. Moreover, administration of sodium bicarbonate may lead to alkalemia with increased tissue deposition of calcium phosphate, hypocalcemia, and the development of tetany. When faced with a patient with rhabdomyolysis, we favor a forced diuresis with adequate volume replacement to ensure a urine flow rate above 100 ml/hr as long as the urine remains dipstick positive. Furosemide may be needed to maintain increased urine flow. Aggressive volume administration to patients with rhabdomyolysis mandates careful serum electrolyte monitoring and serial assessment to ensure the absence of muscle swelling with neurovascular entrapment. If acute renal failure develops, dialysis may be necessary.

The present patient was admitted to the CCU because of possible myocardial ischemia. The diagnosis of rhabdomyolysis was made after return of the elevated CK and isoenzyme levels. The patient was vigorously hydrated and did not develop azotemia. The chest pain resolved without treatment, and the patient was discharged on the third hospital day.

Clinical Pearls

1. Rhabdomyolysis can occur after cocaine intoxication, with more than 30% of such patients developing acute renal failure.

2. Rhabdomyolysis occurs in many settings but is most commonly associated with alcohol abuse, muscle compression, and seizures.

3. Up to 50% of patients with rhabdomyolysis will not have myoglobinuria detected by the urine dipstick orthotolidine reagent method.

REFERENCES

1. Gabow PA, Kaehny WD, Kelleher SP: The spectrum of rhabdomyolysis. Medicine 61:141–152, 1982.
2. Ward MM: Factors predictive of acute renal failure in rhabdomyolysis. Arch Intern Med 148:1553–1557, 1988.
3. Ron D, Taitelman U, Michaelson M, et al: Prevention of acute renal failure in traumatic rhabdomyolysis. Arch Intern Med 144:277–280, 1984.
4. Roth D, Alarcon FJ, Fernandez JA, et al: Acute rhabdomyolysis associated with cocaine intoxication. N Engl J Med 317:673–677, 1988.

PATIENT 10

A 76-year-old man with 40% total body surface area burns, renal insufficiency, and volume overload

A 76-year-old man had been hospitalized for 30 days with 40% total body surface area burns and resultant ARDS requiring mechanical ventilation. He had received total parenteral nutrition and multiple antibiotics because of persistent fever. One day earlier, he underwent skin grafting in the operating room and subsequently developed bleeding and hypotension requiring transfusion with 33 units of packed red blood cells and institution of multiple vasopressor agents.

Physical Examination: Temperature 98.2°; pulse 120; respirations 24 (mechanical ventilation); blood pressure 90/60 on a norepinephrine infusion. Weight: increased 20 kg from admission. Skin: burns in various stages of healing involving head, neck, upper chest, back, and arms. Diffuse anasarca was present.

Laboratory Findings: Platelets: decreased. Na^+ 136 mEq/L, K^+ 3.8 mEq/L, Cl^- 98 mEq/L, HCO_3^- 30 mEq/L. BUN 64 mg/dl, creatinine 2.0 mg/dl. Urine output: 140 to 250 ml/hr on a furosemide infusion. ABG (100% O_2): pH 7.49, PCO_2 37 mm Hg, PO_2 66 mm Hg. Liver function tests: all elevated. Management was initiated employing the extracorporeal circuit depicted below.

What management technique was employed? What are the benefits of this procedure?

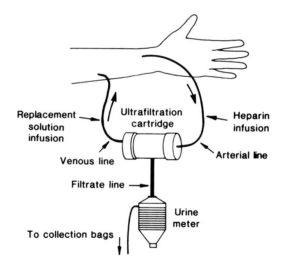

Answer: Continuous arteriovenous hemofiltration (CAVH) for the management of severe volume overload and anasarca in multiple organ failure.

Discussion: Critically ill patients commonly require multiple infusions of parenteral crystalloids and blood products, vasoactive drugs, antibiotics, and total parenteral nutrition which necessitate the infusion of large volumes of fluid. Resultant volume overload with or without renal failure can impede the normal excretion of nitrogenous waste products, solutes, and water. Several methods exist for the removal of excess solutes and water in this clinical situation and include diuretics, peritoneal dialysis, hemodialysis, isolated ultrafiltration, continuous arteriovenous hemofiltration (CAVH), and continuous arteriovenous hemodialysis (CAV-HD).

Hemodialysis, which is commonly employed in the volume-overloaded, critically ill patient, alters the solute and water composition of blood by exposing it to a dialysate solution across a semipermeable membrane or artificial kidney. Solutes pass through the membrane by diffusion or ultrafiltration (convection). The quantity of solute and water removal can be adjusted by controlling the pressures in the blood and dialysate compartments. Hemodialysis requires access to the vascular space, which in the acute setting is usually obtained by insertion of a flexible, double-lumen dialysis catheter into the subclavian, internal jugular, or femoral vein. Once placed, these catheters are ready for immediate use.

Common indications for hemodialysis in the ICU include symptomatic uremia (BUN > 100 mg/dl and/or creatinine > 10 mg/dl), fluid overload, hyperkalemia, and metabolic acidosis unresponsive to medical therapy. Hypotension, a common complication associated with hemodialysis, results from the high blood flows required (200–250 ml/min) and possibly from the vascular effects of acetate, the base commonly used in dialysis fluid. These factors often limit the use of this technique in critically ill patients who may be hemodynamically unstable. Other common complications of hemodialysis include bleeding (some anticoagulation is usually required to prevent clotting of the blood in the dialyzer) and hypoxemia (due to white cell and platelet sequestration in the pulmonary vascular bed and to alveolar hypoventilation).

Isolated ultrafiltration is another method for removing excess fluid and can be performed by modifying the usual hemodialysis apparatus. This technique does not change the composition of solutes in the blood and is, therefore, most useful in patients in volume overload without renal failure. Although isolated ultrafiltration is tolerated better than hemodialysis, excessive ultrafiltration rates can result in hypotension.

CAVH is an extracorporeal process that utilizes the patient's arterial to venous hydrostatic pressure gradient to generate and remove ultrafiltrate. A filter containing a membrane highly permeable to water is used for filtration. When blood pressure falls, the ultrafiltration rate slows, thereby decreasing the risk of hemodynamic instability. Low blood flow rates (20 to 50 ml/min) can result in high ultrafiltration rates (300 to 500 ml/hr) and removal of excess fluids. Solute removal also occurs via the process of convection: in patients who produce < 10 g/day of urea nitrogen, the BUN can be maintained at < 90 mg/dl with an exchange volume of 10 to 12 L in 24 hours. In catabolic patients, CAVH can be used to remove excess fluids and allow use of hyperalimentation to promote anabolism and reduce urea nitrogen production.

Arterial and venous access for CAVH is usually obtained using the femoral artery and vein. Catheters can routinely be left in place for weeks, and routine changing of catheters should be avoided to reduce complications. Complications of CAVH include vascular compromise, infection, and hemorrhage associated with anticoagulation of the extracorporeal circuit.

If additional solute removal is necessary, CAVH combined with hemodialysis can be performed. The circuit is similar to CAVH but dialysate is infused into one of the ports of the ultrafiltration cartridge. The replacement fluid now becomes dialysis solution and the ultrafiltration cartridge becomes a dialyzer. Ultrafiltration rates with CAV-HD can be quite low.

The present patient was treated with CAVH. In the face of hypotension requiring vasopressor agents, an ultrafiltrate of 300 ml/hr was obtained. The patient expired the next day.

Clinical Pearls

1. Hemodialysis-associated hypotension results from requisite high blood flow rates (200 to 250 ml/min) through the membrane and possibly from the vascular effects of acetate, the base commonly used in dialysis fluid.

2. CAVH can provide fluid removal along with varying degrees of solute removal without hemodynamic instability.

3. Ultrafiltration rates in CAVH decrease as blood pressure falls, thereby limiting the risks of hemodynamic instability.

REFERENCES

1. Alfred HJ, Cohen AJ: Use of dialytic procedures in the intensive care unit. In Rippe JM, Irwin RS, Alpert JS et al (eds): Intensive Care Medicine. Boston, Little, Brown and Co., 1985, pp 562–582.
2. Maguire WC, Anderson RJ: Continuous arteriovenous hemofiltration in the intensive care unit. J Crit Care 1:54–56, 1986.
3. Howard RL, Anderson RJ: Continuous arteriovenous hemofiltration and multiple organ failure. J Crit Care 3:161–162, 1988.

CHAPTER 4

Infectious Disease

Jan V. Hirschmann, M.D.

PATIENT 1

A 68-year-old man with weight loss, malaise, and bloody stools for 6 months and fever and congestive heart failure for 3 weeks

A 68-year-old previously healthy man had weight loss, malaise, and occasional bloody stools for 6 months, and fever, anorexia, and weakness for 2 weeks. During the week prior to admission he developed increasing exertional dyspnea and orthopnea.

Physical Examination: Temperature 102°; pulse 120; respirations 25; blood pressure 90/60. Skin: cool, clammy. Chest: bibasilar crackles. Cardiac: soft heart sounds, grade III/VI short, diastolic, medium-pitched decrescendo murmur along left sternal border. Rectal: stool positive for occult blood.

Laboratory Findings: Hct 26%; WBC 12,500/μl with 85% PMNs. ABG (room air): pH 7.48, PCO_2 30 mm Hg, PO_2 56 mm Hg. Chest radiograph: moderate cardiomegaly, pulmonary venous engorgement; interstitial edema; Kerley B lines. ECG: normal. Two-dimensional echocardiogram: large vegetation on aortic valve.

What is the most likely organism causing the endocarditis?

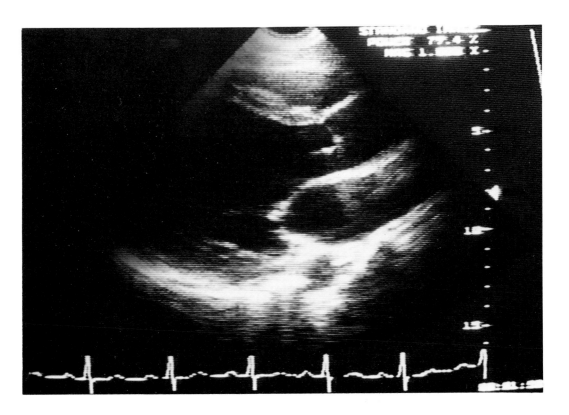

Diagnosis: Aortic valve endocarditis *(Streptococcus bovis).*

Discussion: Approximately two-thirds of patients with endocarditis have previously recognized valvular disease. In patients with aortic involvement the cause may be congenital (especially a bicuspid valve), rheumatic, or degenerative (calcific aortic valves in the elderly). Overall, about 60% of infective endocarditis is due to streptococci and 20% to staphylococci. Five to 10% of patients have negative blood cultures because of previous antibiotic therapy, fastidious organisms that are difficult to grow, or microbes that require special diagnostic techniques, such as the agent causing Q fever *(Coxiella burnetii).* When drug addiction is the predisposing factor to valve infection, *Staphylococcus aureus* is the major organism; in patients with prosthetic valves, the most common causes are *Staphylococcus epidermidis* and streptococci. In endocarditis involving native valves the aortic is the most frequently affected, followed by the mitral; in drug addicts the tricuspid valve predominates.

The most important diagnostic test in endocarditis is the blood culture; three sets should be obtained from separate venipuncture sites. More specimens are usually unnecessary, because when any of multiple samples grow the responsible organism, one or both of the first two cultures are positive in 98% of patients with native valve endocarditis and in 93% with prosthetic valve endocarditis. Timing of the cultures is generally unimportant because the bacteremia is continuous. The intensity of the bacteremia is low, however, with most cultures containing < 30 bacteria/ml of blood, illustrating the importance of withdrawing relatively large volumes (at least 10 ml) with each venipuncture.

Although echocardiography cannot provide definitive proof of the disease, it may help to confirm the diagnosis of endocarditis by demonstrating abnormalities consistent with vegetations in 40 to 80% of patients. False-negative studies can occur because the vegetations are too small to be detected, preexisting valve disease obscures them, valve destruction is pathologically more prominent than vegetations, or the valves are poorly visualized. The frequency of false-positive examinations is unknown, but they can occur with nonbacterial endocarditis (as in lupus erythematosus or cancer), myxomatous valve degeneration, calcification, or other valve thickening. Vegetations from previous infective endocarditis can persist for months to years, confounding the diagnosis of recurrent valvular infection in those with prior episodes.

Streptococcus bovis, the infecting organism in the present patient, has special diagnostic significance. Although present in the fecal flora of about 10 to 15% of healthy people and approximately equivalent numbers of those with most forms of gastrointestinal disease, its prevalence in patients with colonic carcinoma is about 60%. Among patients with *S. bovis* bacteremia, whether or not endocarditis is present, the prevalence of colonic neoplasm (carcinoma or adenoma) is about 75% and a few more have upper intestinal malignancies. These findings suggest that all patients with *S. bovis* bacteremia, even without gastrointestinal symptoms, should undergo a complete examination of the alimentary tract.

The present patient required emergent valve replacement because of severe heart failure and hypotension. Following convalescence, colonoscopy revealed an adenocarcinoma of the transverse colon that was subsequently resected. There was no evidence of local or distant metastases.

Clinical Pearls

1. Although the echocardiographic size of vegetations correlates with the severity of endocarditis, the risk of embolization from large vegetations does not appear greater than the risk from smaller lesions.

2. Because valve replacement during active endocarditis has a surprisingly low incidence (6%) of subsequent prosthetic valve infection with the same organism, urgent surgery should not be delayed, even if the patient has received relatively little antibiotic therapy.

REFERENCES
1. Bayliss R, Clarke C, Oakley CM, et al: The microbiology and pathogenesis of infective endocarditis. Br Heart J 50:513–519, 1983.
2. Klein RS, Catalono MT, Edberg SC, et al: *Streptococcus bovis* septicemia and carcinoma of the colon. Ann Intern Med 91:560–562, 1979.
3. Aronson MD, Bor DH: Blood cultures. Ann Intern Med 106:246–253, 1987.

PATIENT 2

A 50-year-old alcoholic with cirrhosis, ascites, and abdominal pain

A 50-year-old man with biopsy-proved alcoholic cirrhosis developed diffuse abdominal pain 12 hours before admission.

Physical Examination: Temperature 98°; pulse 130; blood pressure 80/40. Skin: cold, wet. Abdomen: tense ascites with moderate, diffuse tenderness.

Laboratory Findings: WBC 10,800/μl, 85% PMNs, 10% bands. Ascitic fluid obtained by paracentesis: WBC 4000/μl, 90% PMNs, protein 2.8 gm/dl, glucose 80 mg/dl. Gram stain shown below.

What is the most likely diagnosis? What treatment would you recommend?

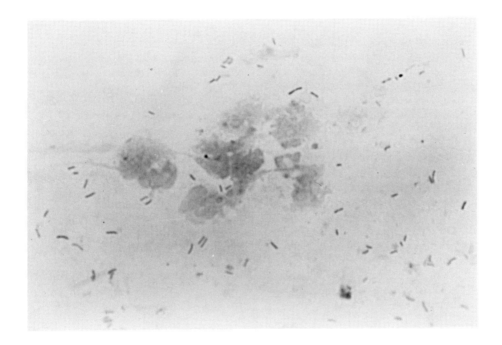

Diagnosis: Spontaneous bacterial peritonitis (*E. coli*).

Discussion: Spontaneous bacterial peritonitis may occur in patients with ascites from any cause, including various hepatic diseases, cardiac failure, the nephrotic syndrome, malignancy, or systemic lupus erythematosus; however, the most common underlying etiology by far is alcoholic cirrhosis. The infecting organism is *E. coli* in about 50% of cases, Klebsiella species in 10%, other aerobic gram-negative bacilli in 10%, streptococci (including pneumococci and enterococci) in 25%, and anaerobic or microaerophilic bacteria in only 5%. The relatively high oxygen tension in ascitic fluid may explain the rarity of anaerobes. In spontaneous bacterial peritonitis, a single species is usually isolated from ascitic fluid or blood cultures, but about 10% are polymicrobial infections.

The pathogenesis is usually uncertain, although in some cases the organisms obviously reach the periotoneum by hematogenous spread from a distant site (e.g., pneumococcal pneumonia). How gram-negative bacilli travel from the gut to the ascitic fluid, however, is unclear. Bacteria present in the bowel lumen may enter the portal vein, which provides venous drainage from the intestines to the liver, and exit into the peritoneal cavity because of high intravascular pressure. Alternatively, these organisms may travel by lymphatic or venous channels that bypass the liver, enter the systemic circulation, and reach the peritoneum via a hematogenous route. It is possible that transmural migration of bowel bacteria may occur through edematous intestinal walls due to venous congestion from the portal hypertension, or, occasionally, microbes present on the skin may enter the abdominal cavity through disruptions of the cutaneous barrier by trauma, including paracentesis.

Common clinical findings are fever (present in 50 to 80% of patients), diminished bowel sounds, abdominal tenderness, and worsening hepatic encephalopathy. Hypotension and hypothermia occur in a minority of patients. Sometimes, bacteria grow from routine cultures of ascitic fluid in asymptomatic patients. Early peritonitis may be present, but in many cases such bacterial colonization probably resolves spontaneously without causing symptoms.

Usual laboratory abnormalities include increased liver enzymes, elevated bilirubin, decreased albumin, prolonged prothrombin time, leukocytosis, anemia, and increased creatinine and urea nitrogen. The ascitic fluid usually has a total protein less than 1 gm/dl and a glucose close to the serum value. The Gram stain reveals organisms in about 30 to 40%. This low yield is not surprising because the bacterial concentration necessary for a Gram stain to be positive is about 10^5 organisms/ml, and the median concentration in spontaneous bacterial peritonitis is about 1 organism/ml. In those with a negative stain, the best indicator of infection is an absolute neutrophil count of $> 250/\mu l$, and this value warrants prompt antimicrobial therapy pending culture results. The ascitic fluid pH decreases and the lactate increases in spontaneous bacterial peritonitis, but these measurements do not add to the diagnostic accuracy of the absolute neutrophil count alone. Immediate inoculation of 10 ml of ascitic fluid into a blood culture bottle following paracentesis provides a higher microbiologic yield than routine culture techniques. Because bacteremia occurs in about 40% of patients, blood cultures are also indicated. Until these studies reveal the identity and antimicrobial susceptibility of the infecting organism, a reasonable antibiotic regimen is ampicillin plus an aminoglycoside, which provides good coverage for both aerobic gram-negative bacilli and streptococci, including enterococci.

Fever and abdominal pain in patients with ascites are sometimes caused by bowel perforation. Clues strongly suggestive of a ruptured viscus rather than spontaneous bacterial peritonitis are free air on abdominal radiographs and an ascitic fluid with WBC $> 10,000/\mu l$ and polymicrobial growth, including anaerobes, on culture. Almost all patients with intestinal perforation, but very few with spontaneous bacterial peritonitis, will have at least two of the following three values in peritoneal fluid: total protein > 1 gm/dl, glucose < 50 mg/dl, and LDH > 225 IU/L.

The present patient grew *E. coli* from both ascitic fluid and blood cultures and responded well to a 10-day course of ampicillin, to which the organism was sensitive. Unfortunately, he died a few days later from uncontrollable gastrointestinal hemorrhage from esophageal varices.

Clinical Pearls

1. Bedside inoculation of 10 ml of ascitic fluid into a blood culture bottle immediately following paracentesis results in an increased frequency of positive cultures and faster growth than conventional microbiologic techniques.

2. The hospital mortality rate for patients with spontaneous bacterial peritonitis is about 70%, but most die from complications of their hepatic disease rather than from the infection.

REFERENCES

1. Wilcox CM, Dismukes WE: Spontaneous bacterial peritonitis. Medicine 66:447–456, 1987.
2. Runyon BA, Canawati HN, Akriviadis EA: Optimization of ascitic fluid culture technique. Gastroenterology 95:1351–1358, 1988.
3. Runyon BA: Spontaneous bacterial peritonitis: An explosion of information. Hepatology 8:171–175, 1988.

PATIENT 3

A 54-year-old man with nausea, vomiting, and weakness

A 54-year-old, previously healthy man developed nausea, vomiting, and abdominal cramps about 18 hours after eating some home-canned green beans. A few hours later he noticed blurred vision followed by dry mouth, diplopia, difficulty in swallowing, arm weakness, and increasing dyspnea.

Physical Examination: Temperature 98°; pulse 70; respirations 35; blood pressure 100/70. Neurologic: alert, dysarthric speech, fixed and dilated pupils, diminished extraocular movements, ptosis, decreased gag reflex, symmetric facial muscle weakness, severe upper extremity weakness, mild lower extremity weakness, deep tendon reflexes diffusely diminished symmetrically but sensation intact.

Laboratory Findings: Hct 45%; WBC 8500/μl. Chest radiograph: normal. ABG (room air): pH 7.30, PCO_2 50 mm Hg, PO_2 58 mm Hg.

What is the most likely diagnosis?

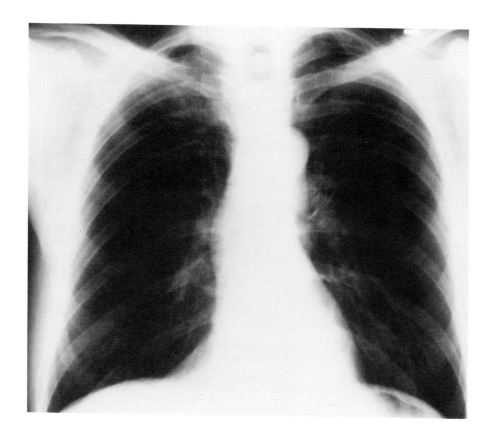

Diagnosis: Type A botulism.

Discussion: Clostridium botulinum is an anaerobic gram-positive bacillus that produces heat-resistant spores and is widely distributed in nature in soil and water. When the spores germinate and *C. botulinum* multiplies, the organism produces a heat-labile toxin that causes paralysis by inhibiting acetylcholine release at peripheral nerve endings. Most cases occur from eating improperly home-canned foods, especially vegetables, but other sources include commercially processed foods and restaurant-prepared meals. Occasionally, botulism develops from wounds contaminated with the organism. Rarely, ingested spores colonize the intestinal tract and then produce toxin; described mainly in infants, this form of botulism may also occur in adults with gastrointestinal disease. Parenteral drug abuse is a risk factor for botulism, usually from contamination of injection sites with *C. botulinum.*

There are seven types of *C. botulinum,* identified by antigenically distinct toxins elaborated, but types A, B, and E cause most human disease. *C. botulinum* type E resides in water, and most cases of botulism due to this bacterium occur from ingestion of home-processed fish or meat from marine animals. Spores of *C. botulinum* can withstand boiling for several hours but are destroyed by 30 minutes of moist heat at 120°C. The toxin is destroyed by boiling for 10 minutes or temperatures of 80°C for 30 minutes.

Symptoms of botulism usually begin about 18 to 36 hours after ingestion of the toxin, but the incubation period can range from a few hours to several days, with a short interval generally betokening severe disease. The initial symptoms are often of gastrointestinal origin—abdominal cramps, nausea, vomiting, and diarrhea. Common early neurologic symptoms include dysphagia, dry mouth, diplopia, dysarthria, and blurred vision. Subsequently, muscles of the trunk and extremities become weak and respiratory insufficiency may develop. Pupils may be normal or dilated and fixed. Deep tendon reflexes may be diminished but remain symmetric, as are the other neurologic abnormalities. Mentation is normal, sensory changes are absent, mucous membranes are often dry, and the cerebrospinal fluid examination is normal.

The differential diagnosis includes Guillain-Barré syndrome, tick paralysis, belladonna poisoning, and poliomyelitis. In Guillain-Barré syndrome, sensory abnormalities usually occur, and the protein concentration in the cerebrospinal fluid is typically increased. In most cases, the paralysis is ascending and progresses superiorly, unlike in botulism, where it is descending. A descending pattern occurs in about 1 to 4% of patients with Guillain-Barré syndrome, and the Miller-Fisher variant includes ophthalmoplegia and ataxia. In these disorders nerve conduction studies, normal in botulism, demonstrate evidence of demyelination. Tick paralysis is an ascending paralysis with loss of deep tendon reflexes that occurs mostly in small children from the bite of certain female ticks, which apparently excrete a toxin in their saliva. Progression of disease requires persistent attachment of the tick, which is commonly found in the head or neck of the victim. In belladonna poisoning, hallucinosis is characteristic. In poliomyelitis, fever and cerebrospinal fluid pleocytosis occur.

The diagnosis of botulism can be confirmed by the finding of toxin in the patient's serum or stool or in incriminated food. On electromyography (EMG), repetitive nerve stimuli at low amplitude cause decreased muscle contraction, but at high amplitude an incremental response occurs. This pattern is seen in Eaton-Lambert syndrome as well; the two disorders, however, have different clinical features.

An antitoxin for botulism is available, and, if given promptly, may slow or halt progression of the disease. Otherwise, treatment is supportive, including intubation and mechanical ventilation for respiratory insufficiency. Mortality is less than 10%, and most patients recover without neurologic sequelae, although protracted exertional dyspnea and fatigue are common.

The present patient's serum and stool contained type A botulism toxin, as did the canned string beans. The patient required endotracheal intubation and mechanical ventilation for progressive hypercapnia. He was weaned from the ventilator several weeks later when respiratory muscle strength had improved.

Clinical Pearls

1. The following features distinguish botulism from Guillain-Barré syndrome: the absence of numbness or paresthesias; a descending rather than ascending progression of paralysis, affecting facial muscles first; and a normal cerebrospinal fluid protein.

2. Botulism is a rare complication of contaminated wounds, with symptoms occurring about 10 days after the injury.

3. Intravenous drug abuse is a risk factor for botulism.

REFERENCES

1. MacDonald KL, Cohen ML, Blake PA: The changing epidemiology of adult botulism in the United States. Am J Epidemiol 124:794–799, 1986.
2. Hughes JM, Blumenthal JR, Merson MH, et al: Clinical features of Types A and B food-borne botulism. Ann Intern Med 95:442–445, 1981.

PATIENT 4

A 34-year-old man with headache, fever, and confusion 3 months after closed head trauma

A 34-year-old man lost consciousness after driving his automobile into a telephone pole while inebriated. When seen in the emergency room, he had minor scalp lacerations and evidence of a basilar skull fracture on computed tomography of the head. He awakened an hour later and was discharged the following day. Three months later he had abrupt onset of a severe headache, stiff neck, fever and mild confusion.

Physical Examination: Temperature 103°. Neurologic: oriented to place and person but not time; stiff neck; positive Kernig's sign.

Laboratory Findings: WBC 16,000/μl, 90% PMNs. Lumbar puncture: opening pressure 230 mm H_2O, WBC 1200/μl with 98% PMNs, protein 300 mg/dl, glucose 20 mg/dl. Gram stain: gram-positive diplococci. Head CT: pneumocephalus in the left frontal area (below).

What is the diagnosis?

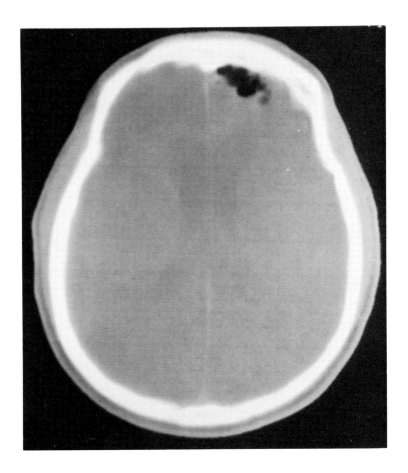

Diagnosis: Posttraumatic dural fistula complicated by meningitis (*Streptococcus pneumoniae*).

Discussion: Blunt cranial trauma can fracture the base of the skull and disrupt the dura, arachnoid, and contiguous soft tissues. The rent in the dura can create a fistula between the subarachnoid space and the nasal cavity, paranasal sinuses, or ear, permitting organisms in those locations to enter the meninges to cause bacterial meningitis. The frontal fossa in the area of the fragile cribriform plate is the most common site of fistulas, but frontal and ethmoid sinuses are also frequently involved, and multiple fistulas can occur. When the fistulas are large, cerebrospinal fluid (CSF) rhinorrhea may develop. Fractures in the temporal bone in the middle cranial fossa may produce CSF otorrhea. If the leak is small or the laceration is occluded by clot or tissue, the fistula may be unrecognized clinically.

Cerebrospinal fluid leakage, intracranial air on roentgenographic examination, and bacterial meningitis are the major manifestations of dural fistulas. The meningitis usually occurs within 1 month of the injury but may be delayed for years. If the dural fistula is undetected, multiple episodes of meningitis may occur. The most common etiology is *Streptococcus pneumoniae* (pneumococcus), responsible for about 65% of cases. Other causes include nonpneumococcal streptococci, *Hemophilus influenzae*, meningococcus, and *Staphylococcus aureus*. Enteric gram-negative bacilli are very uncommon, usually causing infection only in hospitalized patients who have received antibiotics.

Because most dural fistulas close spontaneously within 2 weeks, surgical repair is usually reserved for protracted CSF leakage, substantial pneumocephalus, or delayed presentation, where spontaneous closure is rare. If CT of the head does not demonstrate the site of the fistula, subarachnoid injection of radiolabeled albumin may localize the defect if radioactive material leaks onto cotton pledgets placed in various locations in the nasal cavity. Repair is made at craniotomy by suturing dural lacerations or covering the defect with grafts of fat, muscle, or fascia.

The present patient responded promptly to penicillin therapy and then underwent repair of the dural fistula.

Clinical Pearls

1. Cerebrospinal fluid leaks occur in approximately 10–15% of patients with known basilar skull fractures and usually appear within days of the injury. Intracranial air (pneumocephalus), definitive evidence of a dural fistula, may never be present or may become evident only weeks after the trauma.

2. Meningitis occurs in 2 to 10% of patients with recognized basilar skull fractures and in 10 to 30% of those with known CSF leaks.

3. Prophylactic antibiotics given to patients with basilar skull fractures or CSF leaks do not prevent meningitis; bacterial meningitis that does occur may be due to an organism more virulent than *S. pneumoniae* because the nasopharyngeal flora may be altered.

REFERENCES
1. Hirschmann JV: Bacterial meningitis following closed cranial trauma. In Sande MA, Smith AL, Root RK (eds): Bacterial Meningitis. New York, Churchill-Livingstone, 1985, pp 95–103.
2. Hyslop NE, Montgomery WW: Diagnosis and management of meningitis associated with cerebrospinal fluid leaks. In Remington JS, Swartz MN (eds): Current Clinical Topics in Infectious Diseases 3. New York, McGraw-Hill, 1982, pp 254–285.

PATIENT 5

A 40 year-old-woman with sore throat, fever, and dyspnea

A previously healthy 40-year-old woman had sore throat, fever, chills, painful swallowing, and dyspnea of 10 hours' duration.

Physical Examination: Temperature 103°; respirations 24. ENT: muffled voice; saliva drooling from lips. Neck: edematous erythema over anterior neck. Chest: crackles at left base and diffuse wheezing, best heard as stridor over neck.

Laboratory Findings: WBC 25,000/μl, 60% PMNs, 30% bands. Chest radiograph: left lower lobe pneumonia. Xeroradiogram of neck (below). Sputum Gram stain: many PMNs, numerous gram-negative pleomorphic coccobacilli.

What is the diagnosis? What treatment would you recommend?

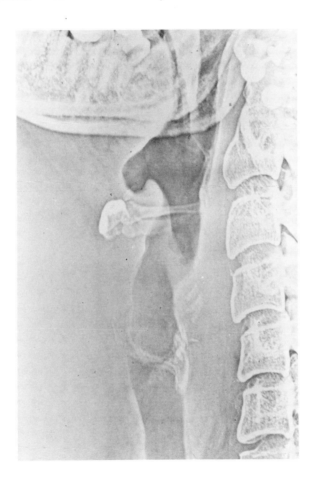

Diagnosis: Hemophilus influenzae pneumonia and epiglottitis (supraglottitis).

Discussion: Acute epiglottitis or, more accurately, supraglottitis occurs in both males and females in about equal frequency at all ages from childhood through adult life. Sore throat and dysphagia are almost always present in adults, and drooling of saliva may occur as patients try to avoid swallowing, which may be extremely painful. Other findings include a muffled voice, respiratory difficulty, and stridor. Most patients are febrile, and occasionally cellulitis appears over the anterior neck. Usually there is a leukocytosis with increased neutrophils and band forms. Chest radiographs are typically normal, but a concomitant pneumonia is sometimes present.

Oral examination, including indirect laryngoscopy, the simplest and most accurate diagnostic procedure, characteristically reveals edema and erythema of the uvula, base of the tongue, vallecula, epiglottis, and aryepiglottic folds. The false and true vocal cords are unaffected, and the oropharynx is inflamed in a minority of patients.

Lateral neck radiographs usually correlate well with the physical examination but are occasionally interpreted as normal. The most common findings, as in the present patient, are enlargement of the epiglottis and other supraglottic soft tissue edema. Blood cultures, positive in about 20–35% of cases, most commonly grow *H. influenzae*. Occasional isolates include *Streptococcus pneumoniae* and *H. parainfluenzae*. In bacteremic patients pharyngeal cultures correlate poorly with blood cultures, illustrating that the former are unreliable in defining the cause of supraglottitis. The microbial etiology in patients with negative blood cultures is unknown, but *H. influenzae* is probably the cause in many, perhaps most, cases.

Treatment should include antibiotic therapy effective against *H. influenzae* and pneumococcus. Many patients receive corticosteroids to reduce inflammatory edema of the airways, but their efficacy is unknown. Patients with progressive respiratory distress should undergo tracheal intubation or emergency tracheotomy. Because of a larger, more rigid larynx and perhaps a less marked inflammatory response, adults have a much lower incidence of airway obstruction and the need for tracheal intubation than children. All patients require close observation, however, because unexpected, abrupt deterioration can occur.

The present patient suffered a respiratory arrest shortly after her radiographic studies and underwent emergency tracheotomy. Following treatment with ampicillin and corticosteroids, she recovered rapidly.

Clinical Pearls

1. Acute supraglottitis should be suspected when sore throat is accompanied by respiratory distress, dyspnea, stridor, or very painful swallowing.

2. In suspected acute supraglottitis in adults, indirect laryngoscopy is safe and represents the simplest and most accurate diagnostic procedure.

3. Blood cultures, positive in 20 to 35% of cases, are the only valid method for establishing the microbial etiology of supraglottitis. Throat or nasopharyngeal cultures are unreliable and often misleading.

REFERENCES
1. Mayo-Smith MF, Hirsch PJ, Wodzinski SF, et al: Acute epiglottitis in adults. N Engl J Med 314:1133–1139, 1987.
2. Shapiro J, Eavey RD, Baker AS: Adult supraglottitis. JAMA 259:363–367, 1988.
3. Shih L, Hawkins DB, Stanley RB: Acute epiglottitis in adults. Ann Otol Rhinol Laryngeol 97:527–529, 1988.

PATIENT 6

A 25-year-old woman with diabetic ketoacidosis, facial swelling, and abrupt unilateral blindness

A 25-year-old woman with insulin-dependent diabetes mellitus developed fever, facial swelling, and abrupt blindness in the left eye. She had noted increased urine output, nausea, and high blood glucose values on home testing.

Physical Examination: Temperature 103°; respirations 40 and deep; blood pressure 100/70. Eyes: absent vision in left eye. Skin: marked facial edema and erythema. ENT: palatal ulcer and black eschar in left nasal turbinate. Neurologic: minimal confusion, otherwise normal.

Laboratory Findings: WBC 16,000/μl; serum glucose 1100 mg/dl; Na+ 130 mEq/L, K+ 3.1 mEq/L, Cl$^-$ 90 mEq/L, HCO$_3^-$ 10 mEq/L. ABG (room air): pH 7.06, PCO$_2$ 15 mm Hg, PO$_2$ 110 mm Hg. Turbinate biopsy (Gomori's methenamine silver stain): shown below.

What is the diagnosis?

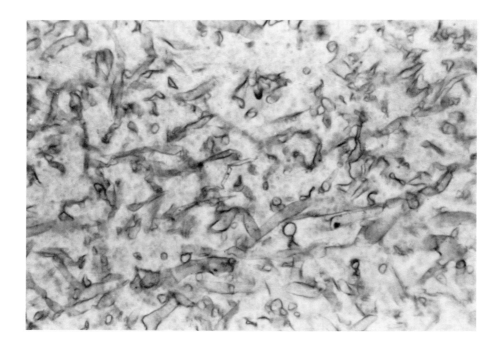

Diagnosis: Diabetic ketoacidosis with rhinocerebral mucormycosis.

Discussion: The methenamine silver stain of the turbinate biopsy demonstrated wide, thick-walled, nonseptate hyphae that branch at right angles, consistent with the organisms responsible for mucormycosis. The cultures were negative.

Mucormycosis refers to a fungal infection caused by a group of ubiquitous organisms, the most important genera being Rhizopus, Mucor, and Absidia, which grow in the soil or in decaying vegetation. Most infections in humans have occurred in those with poorly controlled diabetes mellitus, often during or after diabetic ketoacidosis, in those with immunodeficiency from underlying diseases such as leukemia, or in those receiving immunosuppressive therapy with corticosteroids or cytotoxic agents. The most common forms are rhinocerebral and pulmonary, but the infection may involve the alimentary tract, skin, and other sites, or be disseminated widely. The rhinocerebral type, seen primarily in diabetics, usually begins in the nasal mucosa or palate and extends to adjacent paranasal sinuses, retro-orbital space, and sometimes to the brain. Facial or ocular pain is a common initial symptom that is often associated with fever and facial or orbital cellulitis. Because the organism has a tendency to invade blood vessels, causing thrombotic occlusion and tissue necrosis, black eschars commonly develop on the palate or nasal mucosa, and black, necrotic, purulent material may drain from the eye. Visual loss, proptosis, and decreased ocular movement indicate involvement of the cranial muscles and nerves by fungal invasion of these structures or the cavernous sinus. Carotid artery occlusion may occur, producing seizures, hemiparesis, or other signs of brain infarction.

The diagnosis is best established by histologic examination and culture of tissue biopsies taken from involved structures. Cultures are sometimes inexplicably negative, even when the tissue demonstrates fungi. Treatment usually requires intravenous amphotericin B and surgical debridement of the necrotic tissue. The mortality rate is high, but recent reports suggest that many patients can survive with appropriate therapy.

The present patient survived the infection after therapy with amphotericin B and surgical debridement, but her unilateral blindness was permanent.

Clinical Pearls

1. Facial or orbital pain in a patient with diabetes mellitus or immunosuppression should suggest the possibility of mucormycosis, especially if accompanied by fever, facial or orbital cellulitis, or black nasal discharge.

2. The diagnosis is best established by direct examination and culture of infected tissue obtained by scraping or biopsy. Exudates, discharges, and swabs have lower yields.

3. The organisms appear as broad, nonseptate hyphae with right-angled branching, which differ from Aspergillus species, whose narrower, septate hyphae branch at acute angles.

REFERENCES
1. Lehrer RI, Howard DH, Sypherd PS, et al: Mucormycosis. Ann Intern Med 93:93–108, 1980.
2. Parfrey NG: Improved diagnosis and prognosis of mucormycosis: A clinicopathologic study of 33 cases. Medicine 65:113–123, 1986.

PATIENT 7

A 74-year-old man with fever and left upper quadrant mass

A 74-year-old man with dementia was hospitalized with fever and progressive confusion for 4 days. He had a history of recurrent urinary tract infections and stones.

Physical Examination: Temperature 103.4°; pulse 130; respirations 18; blood pressure 90/70; Abdomen: large left upper quadrant mass thought to be splenic enlargement.

Laboratory Findings: Hct 32%; WBC 18,600/µl, 80% PMNs, 15% bands. UA: 4+ WBC; BUN 60 mg/dl, creatinine 2.2 mg/dl. Blood and urine cultures: *Proteus mirabilis.* Abdominal CT scan shown below.

What is the diagnosis?

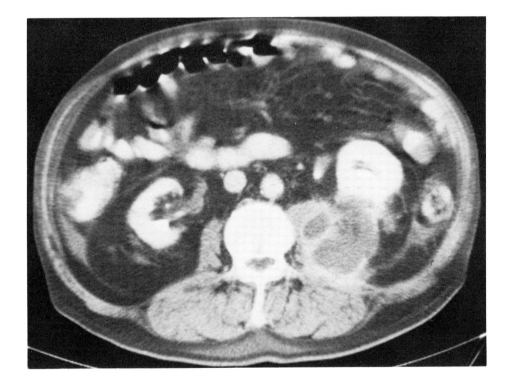

Diagnosis: Perinephric abscess with bacteremia and muscle involvement.

Discussion: A perinephric abscess lies in the perinephric space between the renal capsule and Gerota's fascia, an area that normally contains fat. Most perinephric abscesses occur when infection extends from the kidney, where the source may be a renal abscess or pyelonephritis, often associated with urinary tract obstruction from stones, malignancy, or other causes. Occasionally, suppuration may extend from contiguous infections in the liver, gallbladder, pancreas, appendix, colon, or bone. Because the site of origin is usually the urinary tract, enteric gram-negative rods are the most common cause. In about 10–15% of cases, more than one organism is isolated from the abscess. When *Staphylococcus aureus* is responsible, hematogenous spread to the renal cortex from another site, such as the skin, causes an abscess (renal carbuncle) that ruptures into the perinephric space.

The duration of symptoms may be brief or protracted, with the most common being fever, chills, flank or abdominal pain, nausea, and vomiting. Voiding complaints such as dysuria, frequency, or urgency are present in a minority of patients. On examination, most patients are febrile and have flank or abdominal tenderness; about 25 to 35% have a palpable mass. Leukocytosis or a left shift occurs in most. Urinalysis reveals pyuria in about 60% of patients. Blood cultures are positive in about 30 to 40% and urine cultures in 50 to 80%.

The excretory urogram and ultrasound demonstrate the abscess in about 60 to 70% of cases, but computed tomography is the most valuable diagnostic technique, nearly always delineating the abscess and accurately defining any local complications.

The treatment of perinephric abscesses requires antimicrobial therapy plus drainage of the abscess, either by surgery or percutaneous catheter. Surgery is indicated when concomitant problems such as obstructing stones or ruptured abdominal viscera require treatment.

The present patient had surgical drainage of the perinephric and psoas muscle abscesses but died from postoperative complications.

Clinical Pearls

1. A perinephric abscess should be considered when a patient with recurrent urinary tract infections or obstruction develops fever and abdominal or flank pain, especially if a mass is palpable or if the patient remains febrile after 5 days of appropriate antibiotic therapy.

2. Although an excretory urogram or renal ultrasound demonstrates the abscess in most cases, computed tomography is the most reliable diagnostic technique.

REFERENCES
1. Edelstein H, McCabe RE: Perinephric abscess. Medicine 67:118–131, 1988.
2. Sheinfeld J, Erturk E, Spatano RF, et al: Perinephric abscess: Current concepts. J Urol 137:191–194, 1987.

PATIENT 8

A 77-year-old man with retinal lesions and respiratory failure

A 77-year-old black man with dementia had increasing anorexia, weakness, lethargy, and dyspnea for 1 week. No other history was available.

Physical Examination: Temperature 96°; respirations 32; blood pressure 140/70. Funduscopic examination: multiple yellow-white lesions (1/4 disc diameter) visible mostly within 2 disc diameters of the optic nerve. Genitalia: a mobile, 1-cm, firm mass on right testis.

Laboratory Findings: Hct 38%; WBC 5400/μl with normal differential. UA: 25 WBC/hpf. ABG (room air): pH 7.33, PCO_2 18 mm Hg, PO_2 60 mm Hg. Chest radiograph: shown below.

Hospital Course: Over the next 2 days, he developed progressive hypoxemia requiring intubation and mechanical ventilation.

What is the diagnosis?

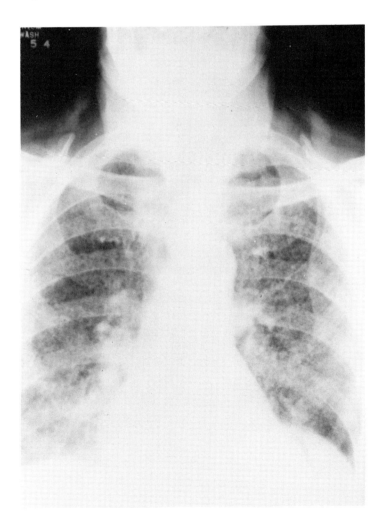

Diagnosis: Miliary tuberculosis with choroidal tubercles and hypoxemic respiratory failure.

Discussion: The present patient's chest radiograph showed a miliary pattern. His sputum contained acid-fast bacilli on smear and grew *Mycobacterium tuberculosis.* Miliary tuberculosis is the presence in many organs of numerous tuberculous granulomas of approximately equal age and size, each resembling millet (Latin: *milium*) seeds, which are about 2 mm in diameter. These lesions are derived from the discharge of large numbers of tubercle bacilli into the bloodstream from an established focus of infection. In developed countries, most cases occur in adults from recrudescence of old lesions in the lung or elsewhere, although few patients have previously had recognized tuberculous disease. Predisposing factors include alcoholism, malignancy, and impaired cell-mediated immunity from corticosteroid or cytotoxic therapy or from serious underlying disease. Pregnancy, where dilated vessels may permit hematogenous spread from a latent genital focus, is also a predisposing condition. Blacks are more likely than whites to develop miliary tuberculosis.

The predominant symptoms usually have an insidious onset and include weakness, fatigue, anorexia, weight loss, and fever. Cough and dyspnea are common but the physical examination of the chest is frequently normal, even with extensive radiographic involvement. Choroidal tubercles, seen on funduscopic examination, are present in a small number of patients and appear as rounded yellow, gray, or white lesions with ill-defined margins.

The chest radiograph, which initially may be normal, eventually demonstrates a miliary pattern in most patients. A mild anemia is common. Hyponatremia may occur from inappropriate secretion of antidiuretic hormone or, rarely, from adrenal insufficiency. Tuberculin skin tests are usually negative. Sputum smears are positive in approximately 20 to 30% and cultures in about 60% of patients. Definitive diagnosis often requires tissue biopsy, with the highest yield from lung or liver. Bone marrow biopsies, less commonly positive, have their greatest yield of revealing granulomas or demonstrating the organism on stain or culture when patients have anemia, leukopenia, monocytosis, or a combination of these findings.

Treatment should include effective antituberculous agents, such as isoniazid, rifampin, pyrazinamide, and streptomycin, although the choice and number of drugs used depend upon the clinical circumstances and history of previous therapy. Systemic corticosteroids may be useful in reducing toxic symptoms in severely ill patients. Close monitoring of the respiratory status is imperative and prompt institution of support necessary if respiratory failure ensues.

The present patient died of progressive hypoxemic respiratory failure. The autopsy demonstrated miliary tuberculosis affecting lungs, liver, spleen, urinary tract, and eyes. The lesions seen on funduscopic examination were confirmed to be granulomas containing acid-fast bacilli.

Clinical Pearls

1. In patients with miliary tuberculosis, the initial chest radiographs may be negative in up to 30% of cases; repeat roentgenograms every few days are recommended when miliary tuberculosis is suspected.

2. Miliary tuberculosis may cause the adult respiratory distress syndrome, often accompanied by disseminated intravascular coagulation, and should be considered in the differential diagnosis of these two disorders.

REFERENCES
1. Slavin RE, Walsh TJ, Pollack AD: Late generalized tuberculosis. Medicine 59:352–366, 1980.
2. Murray HW, Tuazon CV, Kirmani N, et al: The adult respiratory distress syndrome associated with miliary tuberculosis. Chest 73:37–43, 1978.

PATIENT 9

A 24-year-old woman with headache, stiff neck, and fever for 12 hours

A previously healthy 24-year-old woman was brought to the hospital by her husband, who stated that she had a severe headache, fever, and stiff neck for 12 hours and increasing somnolence and confusion over the preceding 3 hours.

Physical Examination: Temperature 104°; pulse 120; respirations 16; blood pressure 90/60. Neurologic: nuchal rigidity; somnolence and disorientation to time and place. Skin: multiple petechiae and ecchymoses on trunk, arms, and legs (below). ENT: normal tympanic membranes.

Laboratory Findings: WBC 18,500/μl, 83% PMNs, 17% bands. Lumbar puncture: opening pressure 250 mm H_2O; WBC 1580/μl, 95% PMNs; protein 230 mg/dl; glucose 10 mg/dl. Gram stain: gram-negative diplococci. CSF and blood cultures: positive for the same organism.

What is the diagnosis?

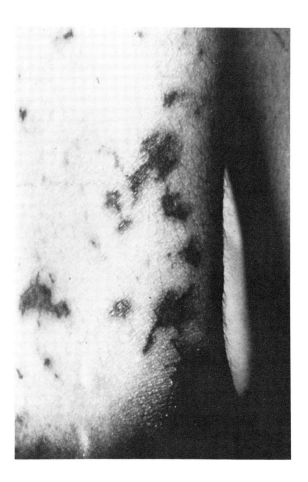

Diagnosis: Meningococcemia and meningococcal meningitis.

Discussion: Neisseria meningitidis (meningococcus) is a gram-negative diplococcus that is ordinarily present in the upper respiratory tract of 2 to 10% of the normal population. Humans are the only reservoir, and transmission of organism occurs via airborne droplets, saliva, or perhaps by inanimate objects contaminated by secretions of a carrier. Protection against invasive disease from the 13 serogroups of *N. meningitidis* depends upon certain components of serum complement and group-specific antibodies.

Meningococci enter the bloodstream from the upper respiratory tract to cause bacteremia alone (meningococcemia) or infection of distant sites such as meninges, pericardium, or joints. Often, symptoms of an upper respiratory infection, such as rhinorrhea, stuffy nose, and sore throat, precede the abrupt onset of fever, chills, malaise, weakness, arthralgias, and headache. Whether these symptoms represent a viral infection that predisposes to meningococcal disease or whether these are early manifestations of the bacterial infection is unclear. When meningitis develops, stiff neck, confusion, and even coma may occur, and hypotension is frequent. About half the patients with meningococcal meningitis have cutaneous lesions, which initially are macules that blanch on pressure. Later, they become petechial or purpuric and are most frequent on the lower extremities, trunk, and areas subjected to pressure, such as the belt line. They usually range in size from 1 to 15 mm in diameter and commonly increase in number over several hours to become generalized, but the face, palms, and soles are usually spared. They may transform into hemorrhagic bullae or large ecchymoses that can progress to cutaneous gangrene.

Blood cultures are positive in approximately one-third of patients with meningococcal meningitis but in nearly all those with cutaneous lesions. Leukocytosis is usual, and laboratory evidence of disseminated intravascular coagulation is common. Lumbar puncture typically reveals an elevated opening pressure, and the fluid will demonstrate a leukocyte count of $> 1000/\mu l$ with more than 90% PMNs, an increased protein, and a low glucose. Without previous antibiotic therapy, the Gram stain discloses the organism in 90% of patients.

Intravenous penicillin is the drug of choice; chloramphenicol is an alternative. The mortality rate for meningococcal meningitis is about 5%.

The present patient recovered promptly after receiving intravenous penicillin.

Clinical Pearls

1. Colonization of the upper airway with *N. meningitidis* may last for days to months, but disease, if it occurs, usually develops shortly after the person first acquires the organism.

2. At greatest risk for invasive disease are those without previous exposure to meningococci, especially those under 5 years of age and military recruits during the first weeks of service, when they are likely to encounter unfamiliar meningococcal types. Patients with complement deficiency are also especially susceptible, sometimes to recurrent episodes.

3. Household contacts of patients with meningococcal disease have a risk of infection 500 to 800 times greater than the general population and should receive chemoprophylaxis with rifampin. Hospital personnel caring for these patients, however, are not predisposed unless they have had intimate exposure (e.g., mouth-to-mouth resuscitation).

4. In meningococcemia, the rash usually spares the face, palms, and soles, in contrast to Rocky Mountain spotted fever.

REFERENCES
1. DeVoe IW: The meningococcus and mechanisms of pathogenicity. Microbiol Rev 46:162–190, 1982.
2. Peltola H: Meningococcal disease: Still with us. Rev Infect Dis 5:71–91, 1983.

PATIENT 10

A 74-year-old man with fever, purulent sputum, and dyspnea 3 days after colonic resection for adenocarcinoma

A 74-year-old man underwent an uncomplicated colonic resection of an adenocarcinoma of the transverse colon. Three days later he developed fever, cough, purulent sputum production, and dyspnea.

Physical Examination: Temperature 102.8°; pulse 130; respirations 28. Chest: dullness to percussion and bronchial breath sounds in right lower lobe.

Laboratory Findings: WBC 14,600/μl, 50% neutrophils, 32% bands. Sputum Gram stain: numerous PMNs and plump gram-negative bacilli with accentuated bipolar staining (below). Chest radiograph: dense right lower lung field infiltrates and patchy infiltrates in left lower lung field.

What is the most likely cause of the pulmonary infiltrates? What treatment would you recommend?

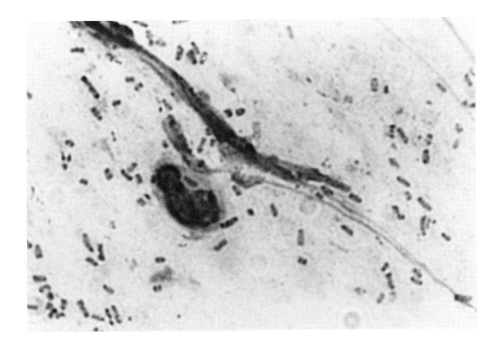

Diagnosis: Nosocomial pneumonia (*Klebsiella pneumoniae*).

Discussion: Nearly 1% of hospitalized patients develop pneumonia, which has a 20 to 50% mortality rate. Surgical patients are at highest risk, with operation on the thorax or mid or upper abdomen conferring the greatest risk, especially if the operation is lengthy. The presence of an endotracheal tube and sedation from analgesics or other medications increase the chance of aspiration. Clearance of bacteria by coughing or local host defenses is impaired because of atelectasis and decreased lung expansion due to such factors as abdominal or thoracic pain, pleural or intraabdominal fluid, and increased intestinal gas from ileus. Among those on the medical service, important predisposing factors include mechanical ventilation, corticosteroid therapy or other immunosuppressive medications, and COPD.

The predominant organisms causing nosocomial pneumonia are aerobic gram-negative bacilli, including *E. coli*, Klebsiella, Proteus, and *P. aeruginosa*. Other common causes include *Staph. aureus, Strep. pneumoniae*, and anaerobes.

Occasional nosocomial pneumonias result from hematogenous transport of organisms from a distant site of infection or from inhalation of airborne bacteria present in contaminated respiratory therapy equipment. Most, however, occur from aspiration of oropharyngeal contents. While aerobic gram-negative bacilli are rarely present in the oropharynx of normal hosts or outpatients with various illnesses, they commonly colonize the upper respiratory tract of those admitted to the hospital. The frequency and rapidity of colonization are greater in more seriously ill patients, such as those with coma, hypotension, endotracheal intubation, tracheostomy, acidosis, and azotemia. Previous antibiotic therapy is a contributory factor, and decreased gastric acidity from antacids or histamine type 2 blockers, such as cimetidine, may also increase the risk, presumably because of retrograde colonization of the pharynx from the stomach. Apparently some of these factors change the ability of gram-negative bacilli to adhere to the epithelial cells of the upper airway, which are ordinarily resistant to these organisms.

The usual clinical findings of nosocomial pneumonia are a new or progressive pulmonary infiltrate, fever, purulent sputum production, and leukocytosis. The diagnosis may be difficult because some of these findings may be absent and some noninfectious diseases can cause a clinically similar illness. The most useful tests in defining the etiology of a pneumonia are a Gram stain and culture of the sputum. The Gram stain usually helps to delineate the likely etiology before the culture confirms the specific identity of the organism. Blood cultures are positive in only 5 to 10% of patients with nosocomial pneumonia. When the patient fails to produce sputum or the results of examination are equivocal, the clinician may either initiate empirical antimicrobial therapy or obtain specimens by other means, such as percutaneous needle aspiration, transtracheal aspiration, or fiberoptic bronchoscopy. These invasive diagnostic techniques are usually reserved for patients who have not responded to empirical antibiotic therapy or for immunosuppressed hosts potentially infected with unusual pathogens.

There are several options for empirical therapy of nosocomial pneumonias if the sputum Gram stain reveals gram-negative bacilli; most experts advise using two agents, including an aminoglycoside. Many combine gentamicin, tobramycin, or amikacin with an antipseudomonal penicillin such as ticarcillin or with a third-generation cephalosporin such as cefoperazone or ceftazidime. The choice depends on the susceptibility of the hospital's predominant bacteria, the patient's condition and the physician's preference. If gram-positive cocci are the predominant organism, an antistaphylococcal penicillin such as oxacillin or a first-generation cephalosporin such as cefazolin is a good choice, unless methicillin-resistant staphylococci are common, in which case vancomycin should be used, pending culture and sensitivity results.

The present patient responded slowly to therapy with gentamicin and cephapirin; he was discharged 3 weeks after surgery.

Clinical Pearls

1. Although *Streptococcus pneumoniae* commonly causes community-acquired pneumonias, it is also frequent in nosocomial cases, being responsible for as many as 30% in some series.

2. Because patients with endotracheal tubes repeatedly aspirate oral flora whether or not the cuff is inflated, intubation is a predisposing, rather than protecting, factor in nosocomial pneumonias.

REFERENCES
1. Hessen MT, Kaye D: Nosocomial pneumonia. Crit Care Clin 4:245–257, 1988.
2. Toews GB: Nosocomial pneumonia. Am J Med Sci 291:355–367, 1986.

CHAPTER 5

Gastroenterology

William M. Lee, M.D.

PATIENT 1

A 29-year-old man with an acute abdomen one day after cadaveric renal transplant

A 29-year-old man on chronic hemodialysis for end-stage renal disease secondary to nephrotic syndrome was admitted for renal transplantation.

Physical Examination: Vital signs: normal. Chest: clear. Abdomen: benign.

Laboratory Findings: Hct 18%; WBC 6,000/μl; Na+ 134 mEq/L, K+ 6.3 mEq/L, HCO_3^- 18 mEq/L, Cl$^-$ 101 mEq/L; BUN 87 mg/dl, creatinine 14.3 mg/dl.

Hospital Course: The patient received a preoperative enema of sodium polystyrene sulfonate (Kayexalate) in sorbitol to control his hyperkalemia and underwent cadaveric transplantation on the evening of admission. Postoperative K+ level was 7.0 mEq/L and a second Kayexalate enema was administered. The following morning he had diffuse abdominal pain and distention and was febrile to 102°. Abdomen: tympanitic with absent bowel sounds and guarding in all quadrants. Rectal exam: small amounts of heme-positive material. Laboratory findings: WBC 32,000/μl, 88% PMNs, 9% bands; Na+ 133 mEq/L, K+ 7.9 mEq/L, Cl$^-$ 102 mEq/L, HCO_3^- 11 mEq/L. Abdominal flat plate (below): dilated loops of small and large bowel; thin meniscus of air in wall of transverse colon (white arrow); air in distribution of portal vein (black arrow).

What is your major diagnostic consideration?

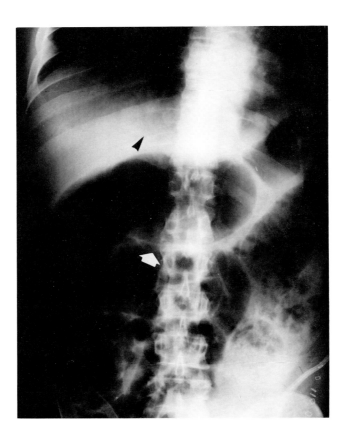

Diagnosis: Ischemic infarction of the transverse colon.

Discussion: Ischemic necrosis of the colon and/ or small intestine occurs in 1% of all renal transplant recipients and carries a 70% mortality. Surgery is necessary to remove the necrotic segment(s), and loss of the renal graft is a frequent complication due to necessary lowering of immunosuppression during the postoperative period. Atherosclerotic changes do not appear to be the main cause of this ischemic damage. The distribution of the colonic necrosis is usually patchy and, therefore, not in the characteristic "watershed" (splenic flexure or sigmoid) regions associated with conventional mesenteric arterial ischemia of the elderly.

A variety of other problems may affect the colon in transplant patients. These include diverticular perforation with abscess, intestinal pseudo-obstruction, and enterocolitis due to cytomegalovirus. The fulminant presentation in the present patient, occurring in the immediate postoperative period, suggested ischemic necrosis as the most likely diagnosis, particularly when coupled with the finding of portal venous air. Portal venous air indicates ischemic necrosis of intestine and is generally a poor prognostic sign. Air in the portal vein can be confused with air in the biliary tree, a more common and generally benign condition. Evidence in favor of portal venous as opposed to biliary tract air includes: (1) the lack of previous biliary tract surgery, which ordinarily is necessary to allow duodenal air to ascend into the biliary tree; and (2) the tendency of portal venous air to be more peripheral as opposed to biliary tract air, which is generally in a more central (pruned tree) distribution.

Several factors have been implicated in causing ischemic necrosis in transplant patients. Hypotension during the surgery may cause ischemic damage, as well as the blood volume changes associated with dialysis. Immunosuppressive agents (such as azathioprine), irradiation, vascular compromise, anemia, and uremia have also been suggested as contributing factors.

Recently, an association between intestinal necrosis and Kayexalate/sorbitol enemas has been reported. Affected patients are uremic, have undergone recent transplant operations, and have received Kayexalate and sorbitol enemas just prior to the onset of colonic infarction. Four of the five reported patients died. In experimental studies, colonic infarction occurred in rats after instillation of sorbitol and Kayexalate or sorbitol alone, but not with Kayexalate alone or saline. Sorbitol appears to be the agent that predisposes to the ischemic bowel damage. The use of sorbitol in Kayexalate enemas is unnecessary because this combination induces a cathartic effect only with oral administration. Alternate vehicles for rectal administration of Kayexalate, such as dextrose and water, appear to be equally effective and possibly safer.

The present patient's abdominal radiograph, which demonstrated air within the wall of the colon as well as portal venous air, signaled the severity of his catastrophic postoperative complication. The presence of portal venous air attests to ischemic intestinal necrosis and mandates laparotomy, which was performed the same afternoon. At operation, a necrotic transverse colon was resected, with placement of a proximal colostomy and mucous fistula. Two days later, a second exploration was necessary for resection of the splenic flexure of the colon, which also had become necrotic from ischemia. Histologic sections showed patchy through-and-through necrosis, with amorphous "crystals" of Kayexalate in the adjacent lumen. Following acute tubular necrosis and slow gastrointestinal bleeding from the damaged colon, the patient's condition slowly improved.

Clinical Pearls

1. Colonic infarction is a common complication in patients with end-stage renal disease.

2. Kayexalate/sorbitol enemas may induce colonic infarction in the early postoperative period following renal transplant despite normal graft function.

3. Radiographic evidence of portal venous air mandates surgical exploration for ischemic necrosis of the small or large bowel.

4. Efforts to avoid colonic infarction in transplant patients include careful attention to fluid balance and potassium levels, prevention of extremely low hematocrits, and avoidance of sorbitol when Kayexalate is administered per rectum.

REFERENCES

1. Perloff LJ, Chon H, Petella FJ, et al: Acute colitis in renal allograft recipients. Ann Surg 183:77–83, 1976.
2. Komorowski RA, Cohen EB, Kaufmann HM, et al: Gastrointestinal complications in renal transplant patients. Am J Clin Pathol 86:161–167, 1986.
3. Lillemoe KD, Romolo JL, Hamilton SR, et al: Intestinal necrosis due to sodium polystyrene (Kayexalate) in sorbitol enemas: Clinical and experimental support for the hypothesis. Surgery 101:266–272, 1987.
4. Julien PJ, Goldberg HI, Margulis AR, et al: Gastrointestinal complications following renal transplantation. Radiology 117:37–43, 1975.

PATIENT 2

A 67-year-old retarded woman with watery diarrhea and shock

A 67-year-old retarded woman from a nursing home was admitted for diarrhea and hypotension. She had received long-term therapy with pyridostigmine and prednisone for underlying myasthenia gravis. Three weeks earlier, she was treated successfully with 5 days of intravenous cefotetan followed by oral ampicillin for the most recent of many episodes of aspiration pneumonia. Improved well-being lasted 2 weeks, when she required admission for fever, tachypnea, tachycardia, and watery diarrhea that progressed over 2 days.

Physical Examination: Temperature 99.3°; pulse 132; respirations 58; blood pressure 90/70. Neck: supple. Chest: scattered rhonchi. Heart: regular tachycardia without murmurs or gallops. Abdomen: softly distended; nontender with bowel sounds. Extremities: normal.

Laboratory Findings: Hct 36%; WBC 13,300/μl, PMNs 73%, bands 18%; BUN 37 mg/dl, creatinine 1.0 mg/dl. UA: 5–10 WBC/hpf. ABG (room air): pH 7.41, PCO_2 27 mm Hg, PO_2 55 mm Hg. Chest radiograph: normal.

Hospital Course: The patient stabilized with rehydration, and received intravenous cefotetan and ampicillin for presumed sepsis. Two days later, the patient deteriorated with worsening abdominal distention and absent bowel sounds. Laboratory findings: WBC 7,100/μl, PMNs 24%, bands 62%, platelets 25,000/μl, prothrombin time 19.4 sec. The transverse colon was 11.4 cm in diameter on a flat plate of the abdomen and the patient underwent colonoscopy for mucosal visualization (below) and decompression. Antibiotics were changed to cefotaxime, vancomycin, and amikacin. She expired the following day.

What was the probable diagnosis that caused the patient's initial problems and eventual downhill course? How would you have managed the patient?

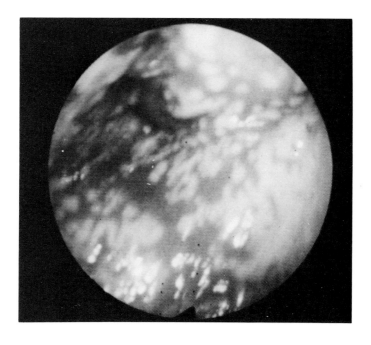

Diagnosis: Diffuse, severe pseudomembranous colitis caused by antibiotics.

Discussion: Occult antibiotic-associated colitis (AAC) due to *Clostridium difficile* has emerged as a major new threat to the elderly patient. This condition, originally known as pseudomembranous colitis, was poorly understood until the late 1970s when its association with *C. difficile* was recognized. New culture techniques and methods for identification of potent bacterial cytotoxins allowed the identification of this fastidious pathogen in patients with the disorder. Subsequently, AAC has become a commonly diagnosed condition.

Affected patients usually present in the clinical setting of previous antibiotic use, particularly ampicillin, clindamycin, or the cephalosporins. Recently, however, an association with antiviral and anticytotoxic therapy has also been documented. The diagnosis is frequently missed because diarrhea may not be a prominent feature of the disease. Furthermore, diarrhea may not begin for several days to as long as 6 weeks after antibiotic treatment has been discontinued. When present, diarrhea may be misinterpreted as a manifestation of dementia or bowel incontinence of the elderly. Prompt recognition is important because the mortality of AAC in elderly or debilitated patients approaches 20%.

Diagnosis is assisted by considering that every patient with diarrhea in the ICU is at risk for this ubiquitous and treatable condition. When suspected, stool samples should be sent for *C. difficile* culture and toxin assay, and the patient should undergo urgent sigmoidoscopy. *C. difficile* cultures must be specifically requested because the organism requires a special media. Stool examinations for white cells are usually positive but nonspecific.

Sigmoidoscopy in moderate and severe instances identifies characteristic pseudomembranes; milder degrees of AAC may not cause classic pseudomembrane formation or these lesions may be limited to the right colon above the reach of the sigmoidoscope. The pseudomembranes usually appear as white or light yellow glistening plaques 3 to 10 mm in diameter throughout the colon. A full colonoscopy is not often necessary, although it may be performed for decompression if severe dilatation is present (colon diameter > 10 cm at any point on flat plate).

In most instances of severe AAC, both culture and toxin assay results will identify *C. difficile*. Treatment should be started, however, even if only one of the tests is positive. Similarly, treatment should be initiated if pseudomembranes are observed at sigmoidoscopy before results of stool studies are known. Oral vancomycin or metronidazole are standard treatment; intravenous regimens are not required because the organism does not invade beyond the gut wall. Fulminant AAC, however, may result in dissolution of the bowel wall barrier, causing septicemia with fecal flora similar to other conditions associated with toxic megacolon. Antiperistaltic drugs are contraindicated in this condition, as are barium enemas.

Recently, treatment with oral fluoroquinolones has been suggested as effective therapy, particularly if these agents are required for an underlying condition (such as osteomyelitis). Relapses of AAC have occurred in patients not rechallenged with antibiotics because *C. difficile* is capable of reactivating from latent spores. Retreatment is required in up to 20% of patients recovering from AAC, and posttreatment surveillance has been recommended by some authors. Rapid improvement can be expected in most instances, but persistent symptoms and worsening may occur in the face of appropriate therapy in the elderly or immunosuppressed patient.

The present patient was not immediately considered to have AAC and was unfortunately treated with cefotetan and ampicillin, drugs that had initiated the colitis. The condition was recognized and confirmed by the typical mucosal features at colonoscopy. Unfortunately, proper therapy was initiated only after the patient had deteriorated to toxic megacolon and probable sepsis.

Clinical Pearls

1. Suspect *Clostridium difficile* colitis in any patient who presents with even mild diarrhea after a course of antibiotics.

2. Systemic illness with toxic megacolon and septicemia from fecal flora can result from antibiotic-associated colitis.

3. Proper diagnosis requires urgent sigmoidoscopy and stool examination for *C. difficile*.

4. Ampicillin and cephalosporins are the most common antibiotics associated with the condition.

REFERENCES

1. McFarland LV, Stamm WE: Review of *Clostridium difficile*-associated diseases. Am J Infect Control 14:99–109, 1986.
2. Bartlett JG: Treatment of *Clostridium difficile* colitis. Gastroenterology 85:1191–1195, 1985.
3. Van Ness MM, Cattau EL: Fulminant colitis complicating antibiotic-associated pseudomembranous colitis. Am J Gastroenterol 82:374–377, 1987.

PATIENT 3

A 41-year-old man with profound hypotension following a transhepatic cholangiogram

A 41-year-old man with a history of excessive alcohol intake was admitted for evaluation of a dilated common bile duct. One year earlier, an evaluation for weight loss detected pancreatic calcifications and a slightly dilated bile duct. Since then, he had abstained from alcohol but continued to lose 40 pounds. A recent CT scan demonstrated a common bile duct of 1.9 cm (normal < 0.7). After an outpatient endoscopic retrograde cholangiogram in which the common bile duct could not be cannulated, the patient was admitted for a transhepatic cholangiogram.

Physical Examination: Vital signs: normal. Thin male. Eyes: mild scleral icterus. Abdomen: soft, nontender.

Laboratory Findings: Hct 40%; WBC 8,000/μl; bilirubin 2.8 mg/dl.

Hospital Course: When the transhepatic cholangiogram needle entered the bile ducts, the patient became hypotensive and diaphoretic with rigors. A drainage catheter was rapidly inserted, and the remainder of the study was aborted. Despite rapid infusion of intravenous fluids, the patient's blood pressure became unobtainable. After transfer to the ICU, the patient remained alert despite a blood pressure of 60/40 by Doppler and a temperature of 104°. Abdomen: soft with diminished bowel sounds; minimal RUQ tenderness. Repeat laboratory findings: Hct 43%, WBC 43,000/μl, platelets 76,000/μl; BUN 12 mg/dl; prothrombin time 18.6 sec.

What is the likely diagnosis?

Diagnosis: Gram-negative septicemia with shock secondary to cholangitis. The endoscopic retrograde cholangiogram (ERCP) contaminated the biliary tree that was chronically obstructed from chronic pancreatitis, and the subsequent percutaneous cholangiogram induced the bacteremia.

Discussion: The sudden onset of rigors and hypotension in a patient undergoing any procedure that entails manipulation of an obstructed biliary tract signals bacteremia from cholangitis. Even in the absence of jaundice, partial biliary tract obstruction renders the patient susceptible to cholangitis due to stasis of bile with contamination of the biliary tree.

When common duct stones are the cause of biliary obstruction, cholangitis occurs frequently and sometimes in subtle forms. Fever is often low-grade, and altered mental status may be the only abnormal finding, especially in elderly patients. Abdominal pain or jaundice are not always present. Cholangitis is a less frequent complication of biliary stasis if the obstruction occurs at the level of the head of the pancreas either from tumor or chronic pancreatic scarring.

Gram-negative organisms predominate in cholangitis and include *E. coli,* Klebsiella sp., Pseudomonas sp., and Bacteroides sp. When patients with biliary obstruction and potential cholangitis undergo diagnostic manipulation of biliary ducts, they should receive prophylactic broad-spectrum antibiotics before and for a short period after the procedure. In the present patient, physicians had incorrectly omitted antibiotics before the percutaneous cholangiogram because the patient's obstruction had been longstanding (and presumably sterile), and the ERCP on the previous day had been unsuccessful in entering the ducts. The possibility of ductal contamination, however, from manipulation of the ampulla with the multiple cannulation attempts mandates systemic antibiotics.

Once cannulation is attempted, drainage of the biliary tree must be accomplished rapidly in addition to use of prophylactic antibiotics to avoid development of cholangitis. In the present patient, drainage was temporarily accomplished with a percutaneous catheter. Further biliary manipulation to establish drainage into the duodenum was deferred because of the rapid deterioration in the patient's status.

The patient progressed to sepsis shock with acute respiratory distress syndrome and renal failure requiring dialysis. Blood and bile cultures were positive for *E. coli,* Citrobacter and *S. faecalis.* Full recovery from sepsis occurred after 2 weeks of intravenous antibiotics and a period of mechanical ventilation and hemodialysis. An internal common duct stent was placed endoscopically 5 weeks after the patient's initial episode of sepsis, and he was discharged on pancreatic enzyme replacement to return later for surgical decompression of the biliary obstruction.

Clinical Pearls

1. Prophylactic antibiotics should always be given before and after endoscopic biliary studies when obstruction is suspected, regardless of whether ductal cannulation is successful.

2. Every patient with biliary obstruction, even without jaundice, should be considered at risk for cholangitis.

3. Once biliary obstruction is identified, drainage must be established by endoscopic, percutaneous, or surgical means.

4. Gram-negative aerobic and anaerobic organisms predominate in the biliary tree.

REFERENCES

1. Cotton PB: Endoscopic management of bile duct stones (apples and oranges). Gut 25:587–597, 1984.
2. Leese T, Neoptolemos JP, Baker AR, et al: Management of acute cholangitis and the impact of endoscopic sphincterotomy. Br J Surg 73:988–992, 1986.

PATIENT 4

A 32-year-old man with nausea, vomiting, jaundice, and a prothrombin time of 32 seconds

A 32-year-old man was admitted for nausea and vomiting. Two days earlier the patient drank three quarts of beer and developed a severe headache that persisted through the night. The next day he began vomiting and went to another hospital's ER where he appeared diaphoretic, tachycardic, and acutely ill; he was discharged with the diagnosis of alcoholic gastritis. Twenty-four hours later, he was admitted with persistent symptoms. He denied recent abdominal pain and did not have a history of pancreatitis or ulcer disease.

Physical Examination: Temperature 100.6°; pulse 120; respirations 24; blood pressure 140/70. Eyes: scleral icterus. Fundi: normal. Neck: supple. Chest: clear. Cardiac: regular tachycardia, no gallop. Abdomen: liver percussed to 5 cm; no spleen tip; no ascites. Extremities: questionable asterixis. Neurologic: lethargic; responsive to specific questions but no spontaneous speech.

Laboratory Findings: Hct 46%; WBC 13,200/μl; glucose 56 mg/dl, creatinine 3.5 mg/dl. UA: SG 1.028 protein 1+, 3–5 PMNs/hpf. Serial liver function tests: shown below.

What clinical condition explains the patient's presentation and course?

Liver function studies

Tests	Day 1	Day 2	Day 3	Day 4
Bilirubin (nl < 1.3 mg/dl)	6.2	2.3	1.2	
AST (nl < 26 IU/L)	14,800	5,340	332	
ALT (nl < 26/L)	9,560	3,255	912	
LDH (nl < 135 IU/L)	12,852	9,394	1,085	25
Alk phosphatase (nl < 170 IU/L)	128	62	113	
PT (nl < 12.4 sec)	32	20	17	14
PTT (nl < 31.2 sec)	65	70	32	32

nl = normal

Diagnosis: Alcohol/acetaminophen-induced hepatic necrosis (alcohol-acetaminophen syndrome).

Discussion: The patient's presentation was typical of alcohol-acetaminophen syndrome—a recently described syndrome comprising acute, fulminant hepatic necrosis secondary to sublethal does of acetaminophen in the setting of an alcoholic binge or chronic excessive alcohol intake. On further questioning, the patient disclosed that he had taken through the night 10 to 12 500-mg acetaminophen tablets for his headache 2 days before admission. Only careful questioning prompted by the suggestive findings of hepatic necrosis brought out this additional information, since the patient had not considered this degree of medication ingestion notable. As is true with most affected patients, he had not taken the acetaminophen as a suicide attempt but rather to treat a bothersome headache.

Peculiar to the alcohol-acetaminophen syndrome are the extremely high serum transaminase levels. If an acetaminophen history is lacking, this profound transaminasemia is a major clue to the diagnosis; transaminase levels rarely exceed 6,000 IU/L in other conditions, even including massive hepatic necrosis due to viral hepatitis or acetaminophen overdose. Levels as high as 31,000 IU/L have been reported with the alcohol-acetaminophen combination.

Differential diagnosis in this setting includes fulminant viral hepatitis or an episode of hypotension with resultant ischemic hepatic injury. The pathogenesis of alcohol/acetaminophen-induced hepatic necrosis is unclear; it is presumed that alcohol potentiates the toxicity of the acetaminophen, either by induction of the cytochrome P-450 system or by alterations in glucuronidation or in glutathione metabolism. Treatment is supportive, with attention to hypoglycemia, hypokalemia, and replacement of clotting factors if bleeding occurs. Early treatment with N-acetylcysteine or with cimetidine might be helpful but, to date, clinical trials of these agents have not been reported.

Peculiar to patients with alcohol-acetaminophen-induced hepatic necrosis is their rapid improvement, and relatively low mortality ($< 20\%$), given the apparent severity of the liver injury. The present patient's liver function test abnormalities resolved in only 3 days to near normal values, a typical result in this syndrome. No long-term sequelae have been reported.

Clinical Pearls

1. Rapid onset of hepatic necrosis in an alcoholic with extraordinarily elevated transaminase levels is typical of the alcohol-acetaminophen syndrome. Typically, a history of ingestion of large doses of acetaminophen for pain relief is obtained.

2. The initial clue to severe hepatic necrosis in any patient is the presence of altered mental status and jaundice. The jaundice may be minimal in the early stages of severe disease. Confirmation is provided by the presence of a prolonged prothrombin time.

3. A carefully obtained history is necessary to elicit the details of analgesic abuse. Intensive questioning plus screening of plasma for toxic drugs, including acetaminophen, should be undertaken in any lethargic alcoholic.

REFERENCES

1. Lesser PB, Vietti MW, Clark WD: Lethal enhancement of therapeutic doses of Tylenol by alcohol. Dig Dis Sci 31:103–105, 1986.
2. Seeff LD, Cuccherini BA, Zimmerman HJ, et al: Acetaminophen hepatotoxicity in alcoholics: A therapeutic misadventure. Ann Intern Med 104:399–404, 1986.

PATIENT 5

A 21-year-old primigravida with fever, leukocytosis, and marked transaminase elevations

A 21-year-old primigravida without previous illness was hospitalized at 33 weeks of gestation with a temperature of 103°, nausea, vomiting, and right upper quadrant abdominal pain. There were no findings or history to suggest preeclampsia. An exploratory laparotomy for presumed appendicitis was unrevealing. Fever continued, and on the sixth hospital day the patient was noted to be jaundiced. While undergoing an abdominal CT scan the next morning, she had a generalized seizure and was transferred to the ICU after undergoing tracheal intubation.

Physical Examination: Temperature 103°; pulse 110; respirations 30; blood pressure 140/88. Jaundiced, lethargic female with an oral endotracheal tube. Chest: clear. Cardiac: normal except for tachycardia. Abdomen: possible ascites, 33-week gravida uterus; normal fetal movements. Neurologic: postictal.

Laboratory Findings: Hct 31%; WBC 24,000/μl, platelets 98,000/μl; AST 3019 IU/L, ALT 1450 IU/L, alkaline phosphatase 451 IU/L, total bilirubin 10.9 mg/dl; prothrombin time 23.5 sec, fibrinogen 76 mg/dl (normal 145–348 mg/dl), fibrin split products > 40 μg/ml (normal < 10 μg/ml). Abdominal CT scan: diffuse mottling of liver with several large low-density areas, particularly in left lobe of liver (below left). Radionuclide liver scan: decreased uptake left liver lobe (below right).

What are the principal diagnostic considerations? What immediate treatment is indicated?

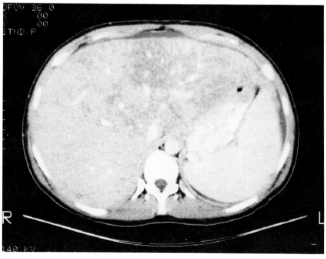
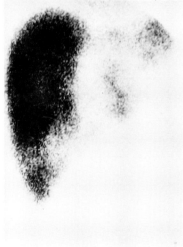

Diagnosis: Hepatic infarction associated with eclampsia. Treatment consisted of delivery of the fetus.

Discussion: Although viral hepatitis is the most common cause of jaundice in pregnant women, a constellation of liver diseases appear exclusively in pregnancy, usually in the third trimester and often in association with preeclampsia or eclampsia. These conditions include acute fatty liver of pregnancy (AFLP), the HELLP syndrome (hemolysis elevated liver function tests and low platelets), hepatic rupture, and hepatic infarction. Although the pathogenesis of these disorders is unclear and several may coexist in the same patient, each has its own unique clinical signature.

Typically, the patient with AFLP presents with hypoglycemia in late pregnancy associated with coma, prolonged prothrombin time, and increased total bilirubin with very modest increases in transaminases. Liver biopsy reveals microvesicular fat, which is also the predominant feature in Reye's syndrome and in certain hepatotoxic drug reactions. The problem in AFLP relates more to hepatocyte dysfunction than necrosis. Milder instances occur more commonly than previously suspected. In its fully developed form, AFLP is fatal in more than 80% of cases.

The HELLP syndrome is considered to be limited to patients with eclampsia. The notable features are marked thrombocytopenia and intravascular hemolysis. Transaminase levels are not markedly increased, and jaundice is not severe. The clinical picture resembles disseminated intravascular coagulation of sepsis but occurs in the setting of hypertension and proteinuria.

Hepatic infarction, as occurred in the present patient, typically is heralded by high fever, signs of eclampsia, right upper quadrant pain, and extreme transaminase elevation. This is the only one of the pregnancy-associated liver diseases to be characterized by high transaminase levels. Similarly, fever is more common in hepatic infarction and may continue for several weeks post partum. Liver-spleen scan or CT scan of the abdomen may show large mottled areas of decreased attenuation. This finding may not be easy to distinguish from fatty infiltration by imaging techniques. Liver biopsy discloses periportal areas of infarction with acute and chronic inflammatory cell infiltration.

By contrast, hepatic rupture often presents with the sudden onset of acute abdominal pain associated with bloody paracentesis fluid in a patient near term. This form of hepatic hemorrhage is often fatal. Treatment with hepatic arterial embolization can be performed, but surgery is often necessary. Rupture may be caused by hepatic infarction in close proximity to Glisson's capsule with subsequent arterial leakage through the injured capsule.

Treatment of these conditions requires, as in any patient with fulminant hepatic failure, attention to electrolyte disturbance, blood glucose levels, and intravascular volume. The presence of bleeding from any source mandates replacement of clotting factors, although asymptomatic elevation of coagulation studies are usually not treated. Intubation may be performed electively if coma develops to prevent aspiration and unexpected respiratory arrest. Cerebral edema is associated with AFLP and is best managed by mannitol infusion; there is no role for corticosteroids. In each of these pregnancy-related conditions, delivery of the infant is considered helpful in reversing the underlying process. Because hypoglycemia and coagulation abnormalities compromise infant survival, delivery may be lifesaving for the infant as well. Mortality from these conditions is high (50 to 80%), and infant mortality is even higher.

The present patient made a slow recovery after cesarean section, remaining febrile for almost a month. No other source of infection was identified. A liver biopsy after 28 hospital days showed intense periportal infarction with a dense infiltrate of mononuclear cells surrounding each infarct. She went on to full recovery.

Clinical Pearls

1. AFLP, HELLP, hepatic rupture, and hepatic infarction are high in the differential of catastrophic conditions in the third trimester of pregnancy.

2. Extremely elevated transaminase levels accompanied by fever and coagulopathy are associated with hepatic infarction, and are generally not present in AFLP or HELLP.

3. Delivery of the fetus is mandated by any of these clinical conditions.

4. Relatively rapid improvement occurs post partum in most instances but, with hepatic infarction, the resolution of the fever and biopsy findings may take several weeks.

REFERENCES

1. Rolfes DB, Ishak KG: Liver disease in toxemia of pregnancy. Am J Gastroenterol 81:1138–1144, 1986.
2. Riely CA, Latham PA, Romero R: Acute fatty liver of pregnancy. Ann Intern Med 106:703–706, 1987.
3. Weinstein L: Pre-eclampsia/eclampsia with hemolysis, elevated liver enzymes and thrombocytopenia. Obstet Gynecol 66:657–660, 1985.
4. Mokotoff R, Weiss LS, Brandon LH, et al: Liver rupture complicating toxemia of pregnancy. Arch Intern Med 119:375–380, 1967.
5. Riely CA: Case studies in jaundice of pregnancy. Semin Liv Dis 8:191–199, 1988.

PATIENT 6

A 67-year-old woman with massive upper gastrointestinal hemorrhage

A 67-year-old woman was admitted to an outlying hospital because of melena. Initial nasogastric tube suction returned a small amount of "coffee ground" material and bright red blood. The admission hematocrit was 39%. An esophagogastroduodenoscopy did not reveal esophageal varices or ulcerations of the stomach or duodenum. The next day, the patient became syncopal after vomiting 300 ml of "coffee grounds" and passing a large volume of dark blood with clots per rectum. She improved after infusion of saline and 3 units of packed RBCs, and was transferred for colonoscopy. Further questioning revealed a history of a gastric ulcer several years earlier. The patient denied recent medications except for occasional aspirin.

Physical Examination: Temperature 98.8°; pulse 112; respiration 18; blood pressure 96/60. Pale, anxious woman. Skin and mucosa: normal. Cardiac: regular tachycardia. Abdomen: soft, nontender, no liver or spleen palpable. Extremities: cool, clammy. Rectal: black to maroon stool; 4+ positive on Hemoccult.

Laboratory Findings: Hct 32%, WBC 12,400/μl, PT 11.6 sec, PTT 31.0 sec. Electrolytes and BUN: normal. Abdominal radiograph: normal.

What should be the next diagnostic procedure? What is the diagnosis?

Diagnosis: Repeat gastroscopy demonstrated a small duodenal erosion with a visible artery in its base (Dieulafoy's anomaly).

Discussion: This patient's presentation may initially appear confusing because the volume of blood retrieved from the stomach was less than expected in view of the brisk gastrointestinal bleeding that was evidenced by the patient's syncope and melenic stools. This combination of clinical features, however, suggests a bleeding duodenal ulcer, because the pylorus may prevent reflux into the stomach, allowing the bulk of blood to be rapidly transported through the colon. Despite maroon stools and a "negative" upper endoscopy, the "coffee ground" and bloody NG aspirate gave evidence of an upper tract lesion that required further investigation before considering a lower source of bleeding. The initial approach, therefore, was to repeat the upper gastrointestinal endoscopy.

Most instances of gastrointestinal bleeding stop spontaneously when the patient reaches the hospital. The initial management of bleeding episodes, therefore, is resuscitation and stabilization. A brief observation period of 1 to 2 hours allows restoration of hemodynamic equilibrium and gives the physician a chance to gauge the rate of bleeding. If the patient cannot be stabilized (less than 5% of cases), emergency upper endoscopy should be performed in anticipation of surgery or endoscopic therapy.

Brisk or recurrent gastrointestinal bleeding is almost always due to an arterial source or to esophageal varices. Arterial sources in the upper gastrointestinal tract include duodenal or gastric ulcers, Mallory-Weiss esophageal tears, and an interesting lesion termed Dieulafoy's anomaly. Dieulafoy's anomaly causes massive arterial hemorrhage either in the gastric fundus, where it was originally described, or in the antrum or duodenum. Little evidence of an ulcer is found in association with this lesion; histopathologic examination demonstrates aberrant arteries rising close to the mucosal surface where they are subject to injury from unclear causes.

Management of upper gastrointestinal bleeding from Dieulafoy's anomaly includes either endoscopic injection of alcohol, electrocautery, or application of heat via an endoscopic probe.

Although extensive experience is not yet available with injection therapy for bleeding gastric lesions, the initial results appear favorable and alcohol injections are coming into general use in the ICU setting, particularly in patients who represent poor risk for emergency surgery. If no bleeding is present at endoscopy, the lesion is usually observed. Active bleeding or a fresh clot on the lesion warrants injection or electrocautery therapy. A "visible vessel" within a Dieulafoy's anomaly is also an indication for endoscopic therapy in that this finding has a 50% chance of rebleeding during the hospitalization. Although long-term studies have not been reported, the initial results with these newer forms of therapy are remarkably good, with greater than 90% success in controlling hemorrhage in the high-risk visible vessel or rebleeding subgroup.

If the patient with upper gastrointestinal hemorrhage stabilizes in the first 2 hours, then elective endoscopy can be performed on the next hospital day. Failure to visualize a bleeding site at initial endoscopy should not deter subsequent endoscopy if the source of bleeding remains unknown. Reasons for not detecting lesions during early endoscopies relate to the emergent nature of the procedure and the conditions operative at the time. Absence of technical help, inadequate equipment support, and nonideal patient positioning all contribute in the emergency situation to a suboptimal endoscopic study.

Because of evidence that bleeding in the present patient came from the upper tract, a repeat upper endoscopy was performed. At endoscopy, there was a large blood clot in the gastric fundus. The duodenal bulb was not deformed but two shallow erosions were present, one of which had an artery protruding from its base. With gentle manipulation, it began actively pumping blood. Via an endoscopic catheter, several 0.1 to 0.2 ml aliquots of 100% alcohol were injected around the periphery of the erosions, and the bleeding stopped. The patient was placed on sucralfate and ranitidine and had no further bleeding over the next 6 months.

Clinical Pearls

1. Any evidence of upper gastrointestinal bleeding is a reliable indicator of an upper tract lesion, even if the specific bleeding site cannot be identified immediately.

2. Brisk or recurrent gastrointestinal bleeding indicates an arterial site, usually in the duodenum. Varices or a Mallory-Weiss esophageal tear is also possible. Brisk bleeding warrants emergent endoscopy for diagnosis and therapy.

3. Dieulafoy's anomaly as a cause of upper gastrointestinal bleeding may be overlooked because it is small and inapparent unless bleeding is occurring during endoscopy.

REFERENCES

1. Fleischer D: Etiology and prevalence of severe persistent upper gastrointestinal bleeding. Gastroenterology 84:538–543, 1983.
2. Rossi NP, Green EW, Pike JD: Massive bleeding of the upper gastrointestinal tract due to Dieulafoy's erosion. Arch Surg 97:797–800, 1968.
3. McClave SA, Goldschmid S, Cunningham JT, et al: Dieulafoy's cirsoid aneurysm of the duodenum. Dig Dis Sci 33:801–805, 1988.

PATIENT 7

A 68-year-old man with epigastric pain and severe hyperamylasemia

A 68-year-old retired carpenter developed the sudden onset of severe epigastric pain radiating to his back on the evening before admission. The patient denied previous episodes of pain, did not drink alcohol, and had no previous history of gastrointestinal illnesses or recent abdominal trauma. After 4 hours, nausea and vomiting ensued and he was brought to the emergency room.

Physical Examination: Temperature 100.6°; pulse 116; respiration 20; blood pressure 134/80. Writhing in pain. Skin: normal without icterus. Chest: normal. Cardiac: normal. Abdomen: exquisite tenderness in the midline and right upper quadrant; absent bowel sounds; no involuntary guarding. Extremities: diaphoretic, pulses full.

Laboratory Findings: Hct 34.3%; WBC 14,500/μl; total bilirubin 2.3 mg/dl, alkaline phosphatase 232 IU/L (normal < 115), serum amylase 7,800 IU/L (normal < 150). UA: SG 1.025, protein 1+, 3–8 WBC/hpf. ABG (room air): pH 7.45, PCO_2 32 mm Hg, PO_2 58 mm Hg. Ultrasonogram of gallbladder: common bile duct measures 1.4 cm, one stone in gallbladder, pancreatic head not visualized. ERCP: shown below.

What are the diagnosis and appropriate treatment in this setting?

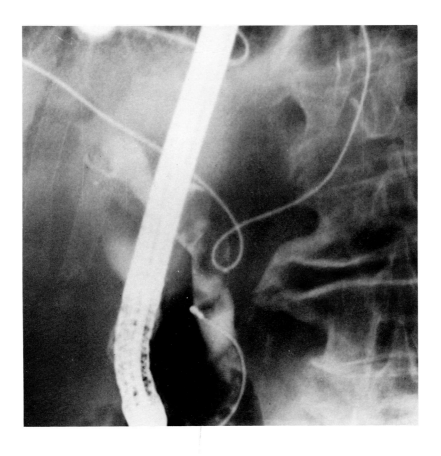

Diagnosis: Gallstone pancreatitis with suspected retained common bile duct stone.

Discussion: Gallstone disease is second only to alcohol as a cause of pancreatitis. Alcoholic pancreatitis may cause marked pain, nausea, and vomiting but usually is not as severe in terms of elevation of the serum amylase or ominous clinical sequelae as gallstone pancreatitis.

Almost one-half of patients with pancreatitis have gallstones. Passage of the gallstones through the common bile duct (CBD) appears to be the proximate cause of the pancreatitis in that virtually all patients have gallstones in their stools in the first days following an attack. The pathogenesis of pancreatitis results from the anatomically common path of the distal CBD and the main pancreatic duct, the duct of Wirsung. When the stone lodges in the ampulla, obstruction of the common channel results in sufficient back pressure in the pancreatic duct to cause disruption of cells, release of enzymes, and a chain reaction that results in severe pancreatitis.

Clinical features suggesting gallstone pancreatitis are absence of an alcohol history, marked elevations in serum amylase, and presence of gallstones. Patients are typically female (71%) and elderly, with a peak incidence in the eighth decade of life. Convincing support for the diagnosis is provided by the finding of a dilated CBD at ultrasonography and an elevated alkaline phosphatase or bilirubin level.

Prognosis can be determined by presence of these 11 criteria:

Criteria on admission	Criteria over first 48 hrs
Age > 55 yrs	Hct drop $> 10\%$
WBC $> 16,000/\mu l$	BUN increase > 5 mg/dl
Glucose > 200 mg/dl	$PO_2 < 60$ mm Hg
LDH > 350 IU/L	$Ca^{2+} < 8.0$ mg/dl
AST > 250 IU/L	Base deficit > 4 mEq/L
	Fluid retention > 6L

No. of criteria present	Mortality	Risk of major complication
< 3	1%	Zero
3–4	15%	40%
5–6	40%	90%
7–8	100%	

Evaluation of these patients by ultrasound seldom demonstrates CBD stones; the main indication for the procedure is to detect ductal dilatation and/or the presence of stones in the gallbladder. Even the presence of gallbladder stones without ductal dilatation should raise the suspicion of gallstone pancreatitis sufficiently to warrant endoscopic retrograde cholangiopancreatography (ERCP) to diagnose (and remove) a common duct stone. Evidence of dilatation of the CBD is even more supportive of the diagnosis.

The presence of CBD dilatation, pancreatitis, and increased alkaline phosphatase and/or bilirubin all provide conclusive evidence of the need for stone removal, either surgically or via endoscopic sphincterotomy. Although controversial, recent studies indicate that acute ERCP during acute pancreatitis is safe and efficacious if endoscopic sphincterotomy and stone removal are available, and may be the procedure of choice.

Conventional treatment consists of ICU support with adequate fluid replacement and maintenance of hematocrit and Ca^{2+} levels. Nasogastric suction is generally used but NPO without nasogastric suction may be equally effective. Antibiotics in the absence of proven infection are not recommended. Dreaded complications include adult respiratory distress syndrome, pancreatic abscess, uncontrolled hypotension, and gastrointestinal bleeding.

While some stones will have been passed by the time of the study, recent evidence suggests that early intervention to remove CBD stones results in improved morbidity and mortality from this otherwise highly lethal condition. In the present patient, ERCP done the same morning revealed stones in the common duct, which were removed by duodenoscopic sphincterotomy. The patient improved rapidly, with normalization of the amylase level in 48 hours.

Clinical Pearls

1. Abdominal pain and very high amylase levels in an elderly nondrinker strongly suggest gallstone pancreatitis.

2. Confirmatory evidence is provided in most instances by ultrasonogram; however, ERCP is a more definitive test for determination of the presence of CBD stones.

3. Early removal of CBD stones appears to decrease the high morbidity and mortality.

REFERENCES

1. Ranson JHC: Acute pancreatitis: Surgical management. In Go VLW, Brady FP, DiMagno EP, et al (eds): The Exocrine Pancreas. New York, Raven Press, 1986, pp 503–512.
2. Safrany L, Cotton PB: A preliminary report: Urgent duodenoscopic sphincterotomy for acute gallstone pancreatitis. Surgery 89:424–428, 1981.
3. Neoptolemos JP, London NJ, James D, et al: Controlled trial of urgent endoscopic retrograde cholangiopancreatography and endoscopic sphincterotomy versus conservative treatment of acute pancreatitis due to gallstones. Lancet 2:979–983, 1988.

PATIENT 8

A 67-year-old man with end-stage renal disease and maroon stools of 2 days' duration

A 67-year-old retired farmer developed renal failure 5 years earlier as a result of hypertension, and was placed on hemodialysis. He did well with a baseline hematocrit of 23% until during a recent hemodialysis when he complained of weakness, and a hematocrit was noted to be 17%. He improved after 1 unit of blood but noted maroon stools a week later. There was no history of alcohol, aspirin, or nonsteroidal anti-inflammatory drug ingestion.

Physical Examination: Temperature 98.8°; pulse 112; respiration 16; blood pressure 110/60 (103/65 standing). Pale, elderly man in no acute distress. Chest, cardiac, and abdomen: normal. Rectal: maroon, nonmelenic stools; 4+ Hemoccult positive.

Laboratory Findings: Hct 12%; MCV 78, platelets 275,000/μl, PT 12.3 sec; BUN 89 mg/dl, creatinine 6.7 mg/dl. Chest radiograph: cardiomegaly. ECG: left ventricular hypertrophy; minor ST depression in anterolateral leads. Colonoscopy: mucosal findings shown below.

What is the most likely diagnosis? What is your diagnostic approach?

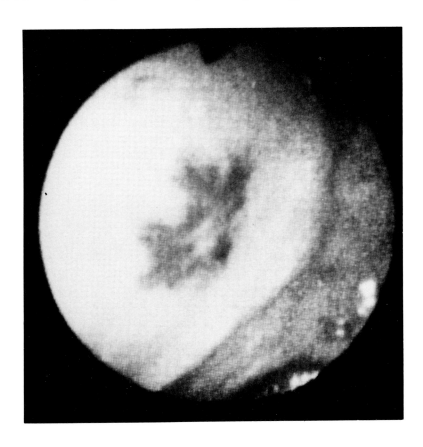

Diagnosis: Colonic bleeding secondary to arteriovenous malformations (AVMs) associated with renal failure.

Discussion: Lower gastrointestinal bleeding is a common diagnostic dilemma in the elderly. Common causes include diverticulosis, ischemic colitis, inflammatory bowel disease, and colon cancer. As in the diagnosis of upper tract bleeding, the pace of bleeding is an important diagnostic clue. Because diverticulosis results from an arterial source, bleeding is usually brisk with associated postural changes. Bleeding usually stops spontaneously, and it is often difficult to demonstrate the bleeding site by arteriographic means or by radionuclide imaging studies. Ischemic bowel will usually be associated with pain and more evidence of systemic illness and stigmata of arteriosclerotic disease elsewhere. Ulcerative proctitis can begin in later years and usually is diagnosed by flexible sigmoidoscopy, with the pace of bleeding being relatively slow. Likewise, colon cancer seldom engenders hemorrhage requiring transfusion.

A specific problem in renal failure is the development of AVMs in the colon or upper gastrointestinal tract. The usual setting is a patient on hemodialysis for more than 1 year who develops iron deficiency or maroon stools. Of note, the pace of bleeding seldom produces hypotension or orthostasis. Although transfusion is frequently required because the baseline hematocrit is low, patients seldom need more than 1 unit of packed RBCs per day during the period of active bleeding.

Diagnostic studies for identifying the site of blood loss in the lower gastrointestinal tract are less helpful than those employed for upper tract bleeding. For example, colonoscopy during the bleeding episode is helpful in identifying the bleeding site in less than 20% of cases without colon cleansing. Blood itself in addition to fecal matter obscures the endoscopist's view. Location of the region of the colon on the basis of the farthest proximal extent of blood is also unrewarding, because blood is capable of considerable to-and-fro reflux throughout the colon.

Diverticulae are usually present on the left side of the colon; however, a few right-sided diverticulae are enough to confound the clinician completely. Isotopically tagged red blood cells or serum technecium scans occasionally are of help but can be confusing unless the pace of bleeding is greater than 1 to 3 ml/min. Similarly, arteriography requires that bleeding be present at the actual time of injection and that the pace be at least 3 ml/min.

AVMs of the type associated with renal failure or valvular heart disease, particularly aortic stenosis, are clearly acquired, multiple, and often diffuse. They are not well visualized by arteriography and their demonstration by bleeding scans is equally unrewarding because the pace of blood loss is too slow. The best technique is to stabilize the patient with transfusion of blood products, correction of coagulopathies, and thorough cleansing of the colon. Elective colonoscopy can then be performed and the lesions identified.

Electrocautery therapy can be remarkably successful in ablating arteriovenous malformations; unfortunately, there are frequently too many (hundreds!) to approach in this fashion. If the lesions are strictly limited to the right colon, a hemicolectomy might be performed. A recent form of therapy applicable to upper and lower tract bleeding in renal failure is the use of estrogen-progesterone combinations (birth control pills, specifically Enovid E). Excellent results have been obtained in uncontrolled trials.

The present patient was shown to have a single large AVM in the cecum that was cauterized at colonoscopy using a bicap electrocautery probe. Radionuclide bleeding scan had been negative.

Clinical Pearls

1. Lower gastrointestinal bleeding in the elderly is primarily due to diverticulosis.
2. In the patient with renal failure or aortic valvular disease, AVMs are very common.
3. Despite the variety of radiographic studies available, elective (but not emergent) colonoscopy has the highest diagnostic yield.

REFERENCES

1. Cunningham JT: Gastric telangiectasis in chronic hemodialysis patients: A report of six cases. Gastroenterology 81:1131–1133, 1981.
2. Bronner MH, Pate MB, Cunningham JT, Marsh WH: Estrogen-progesterone therapy for bleeding gastrointestinal telangiectasis in chronic renal failure. Ann Intern Med 105:371–374, 1986.
3. Stylianos S, Forde KA, Benvenisty AI, et al: Lower gastrointestinal hemorrhage in renal transplant recipients. Arch Surg 123:739–744, 1988.

PATIENT 9

A 62-year-old man with fever and a large right pleural effusion

A 62-year-old banker was admitted with fever, right-sided thoracoabdominal pain, and dyspnea 6 weeks after an episode of acute alcoholic pancreatitis. The pain first began in the upper abdomen and then progressed to pleuritic chest pain. There was no history of cardiac or pulmonary disease and the patient stated that he had abstained from alcohol.

Physical Examination: Temperature 102°; pulse 110; respiration 28; blood pressure 134/94. Chest: right-sided dullness with diminished breath sounds. Cardiac: normal. Abdomen: normal.

Laboratory Findings: Hct 33%; WBC 12,500/μl; electrolytes normal, BUN 33 mg/dl, amylase 866 IU/L (normal < 150). ABG (room air): pH 7.43, PCO_2 32 mm Hg, PO_2 78 mm Hg. Chest radiograph: large right pleural effusion. Abdomen radiograph: pancreatic calcifications. Pleural fluid: RBC 28,500/μl, WBC 2,300/μl, protein 3.9 gm/dl, amylase 34,000 IU/L. ERP (below): pancreatic duct filled with contrast (single arrow), with fistula extending toward the right diaphragm (double arrow).

What are the likely diagnosis and appropriate approach to management?

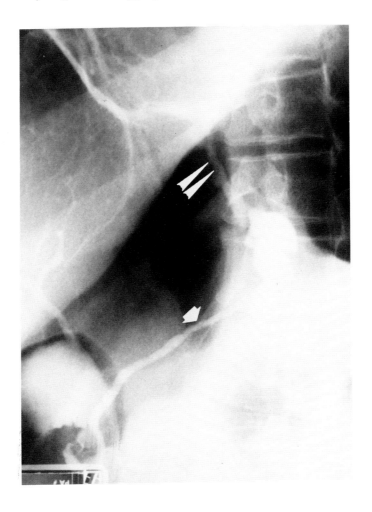

Diagnosis: Pancreaticopleural fistula.

Discussion: Pancreatic ascites and pancreaticopleural fistulae with resultant pleural effusion are two of the more interesting complications of acute or chronic pancreatitis. In both instances, the tremendous exudation of fluid results from a leakage of pancreatic ductal contents either directly into the peritoneal cavity or, in the case of the pancreaticopleural fistula, via the fistulous tract into the pleural space. Most commonly, these episodes occur at a time remote from the episode of acute pancreatitis or in the setting of chronic pancreatitis with pseudocyst formation.

It is presumed that the inflammatory process with or without pseudocyst formation results in rupture of the duct. In the case of pancreatic ascites, an anterior rupture leads to direct flow into the peritoneal cavity. The result is silent evolution of ascites, often massive and frequently confused with cirrhotic ascites. This differentiation can be made by the finding of high protein content in the fluid, but more importantly, very high amylase levels, usually in the thousands. While the fluid may become infected, it is usually sterile and the pancreatic enzymes are not activated (in contrast to the situation in acute pancreatitis where fat necrosis and phlegmon formation occur secondary to the action of the pancreatic secretions). If a posterior leak occurs, it may penetrate along the tissue planes leading to the diaphragmatic hiatus and thus enter the chest via the fistulous tract created.

The pleural fluid is sterile with a high protein content. Markedly elevated amylase levels in the fluid confirm the diagnosis. Serum amylase levels may be normal or elevated due to the absorption of the secreted amylase across serosal surfaces.

The diagnosis should be suspected in patients presenting with ascites or pleural effusions who have a history of acute or chronic pancreatitis. Consideration of the diagnosis allows testing of fluid for amylase. Endoscopic retrograde pancreatography (ERP) will in most instances show the leak and/or fistulous tract. Recently, a combination of ERP and CT scanning has been used to demonstrate the fistulous tract.

In most instances, surgical correction of the intraperitoneal leak with Roux-en-Y drainage of the leak or partial pancreatic resection is performed. Better success has been achieved with nonoperative intervention in the case of pancreaticopleural fistulae using a combination of hyperalimentation, antibiotics, and chest tube drainage. A recent addition to this regimen has been the use of the somatostatin analogue SU 4884 to diminish pancreatic secretion while the tract closes, but this form of treatment has not been subjected to controlled trials.

The present patient was found at ERP to have a pancreaticopleural fistula that required surgical repair. He recovered without further episodes of pleural effusions.

Clinical Pearls

1. Pleural effusion of rapid onset in a patient with a history of pancreatitis is due to a fistulous tract from the pancreas until proven otherwise.
2. The pleural fluid will be diagnostic in that it should have an extremely high amylase content.
3. A combination of ERP and CT scanning can demonstrate the fistulous tract; a trial of medical therapy will be successful in at least half of patients.

REFERENCES
1. Cameron JL: Chronic pancreatic ascites and pancreatic pleural effusions. Gastroenterology 74:134–140, 1978.
2. Bronner MH, Marsh WH, Stanley JH: Pancreaticopleural fistula: Demonstration by computed tomography and endoscopic retrograde cholangiopancreatography. CT 10:167–170, 1986.
3. Kimura Y, Yamamoto T, Zenda S, et al: Pancreatic pleural fistula: Demonstration by computed tomography after endoscopic retrograde pancreatography. Am J Gastroenterol 82:790–793, 1987.

PATIENT 10

A 53-year-old man with right upper quadrant pain, lethargy, and jaundice

A 53-year-old factory worker was admitted for right upper quadrant pain, lethargy, and weakness of 3 weeks' duration. The patient denied alcohol ingestion, exertional dyspnea, orthopnea, or peripheral edema.

Physical Examination: Temperature 98°; respiration 24; blood pressure 132/90. Obese, icteric male intermittently restless and confused. Neck: no venous distention. Chest: normal. Cardiac: distant heart sounds; no gallops or rubs. Abdomen: protuberant with possible ascites; no splenomegaly; liver tender with span of 10 cm in mid-clavicular line. Extremities: trace pretibial edema.

Laboratory Findings: CBC: normal, PT 14.9 sec. Na+ 132 mEq/L, K+ 3.5 mEq/L, Cl⁻ 102 mEq/L, HCO_3^- 25 mEq/L; total bilirubin 2.5 mg/dl, AST 1780 IU/L (normal < 24), alkaline phosphatase 143 IU/L (normal < 115), albumin 3.0 g/dl, serum ammonia 74 mg/dl (normal < 40). Drug screens: negative; serologic tests for hepatitis A and B: negative. Chest radiograph: cardiomegaly. Head CT: normal. Percutaneous needle liver biopsy: shown below.

What is the etiology of this patient's hepatic insufficiency?

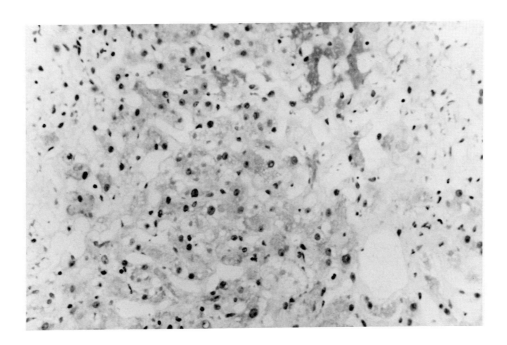

Diagnosis: Cardiomyopathy with ischemic hepatic injury causing fulminant hepatic failure.

Discussion: Severely diminished cardiac output ("forward" failure) may precipitate hepatic dysfunction that may simulate acute viral hepatitis with fulminant hepatic necrosis (FHN). The usual clinical setting is a patient who has undergone cardiac arrest with resuscitation, cardiogenic shock, ventricular or supraventricular tachyarrhythmia, or any process resulting in a low cardiac output state. The resultant ischemia to vital organs, such as the liver and kidneys, causes an acute rise in transaminases to several thousand and a parallel increase in creatinine levels.

Hepatic dysfunction from cardiac dysfunction can be separated from other causes of hepatic injury by the pattern of serum enzyme abnormalities. Transaminases rise more rapidly (up to several thousand in 24 hours) in cardiac dysfunction compared with viral hepatitis and toxic hepatic injury. Normalization of enzyme levels is equally swift (48 to 96 hours) if cardiac function is restored. Jaundice and other alterations in hepatic function due to cardiac disease may not be present and usually represent a more sustained hepatic injury.

Predominantly right-sided heart failure, as seen in tricuspid insufficiency, presents a different pattern of hepatic dysfunction. Hepatomegaly is pronounced and the liver may be pulsatile and tender to palpation. Liver function tests in these individuals demonstrate mild cholestatic changes with slightly increased bilirubin and alkaline phosphatase levels.

The combination of both "forward" and "backward" congestive failure occurs in patients with severe cardiomyopathy. The presence of both forms of cardiac failure can be detected on liver biopsy because each causes a distinctive pathologic pattern in the centrilobular zones. High right ventricular pressure causes hepatic venous congestion, whereas decreased hepatic perfusion produces centrilobular necrosis.

The *de novo* appearance of hepatic failure in a patient with clinically occult congestive heart failure is an uncommon event. As in the present patient, clinical features of hepatic dysfunction may overshadow physical signs of cardiac failure. Additionally, symptoms of fatigue, altered mental status, hepatomegaly, ascites, edema, and jaundice may be observed in either condition and may not, therefore, suggest the correct primary diagnosis. Only orthopnea, central venous distention, and auscultatory cardiac signs serve to distinguish cardiac from hepatic failure.

The present patient underwent a liver biopsy that demonstrated pathologic features of cardiac dysfunction with ischemic necrosis and centrilobular congestion (previous page). The physicians then returned to the bedside and noted previously overlooked evidence of central venous distention and a gallop rhythm. A Swan-Ganz catheter documented reduced cardiac output (1.8 L/min) and increased pulmonary artery wedge pressure (34 mm Hg). Right atrial pressure was 21 mm Hg. Echocardiogram showed a dilated cardiomyopathy with an ejection fraction of 15%. The patient's mental status improved markedly with furosemide, vasodilators, and digoxin, and laboratory values returned rapidly to normal.

Clinical Pearls

1. Altered mental status, jaundice, and elevated transaminases are seen in patients with severe congestive heart failure.

2. Striking rises and equally rapid falls in transaminase levels are typical for hepatic ischemic injury.

3. Rapid diagnosis and treatment of the underlying heart disease render further hepatic treatment unnecessary.

REFERENCES
1. Cohen JA, Kaplan MM: Left-sided heart failure presenting as hepatitis. Gastroenterology 74:583–587, 1978.
2. Kisloff B, Schaffer G: Fulminant hepatic failure secondary to congestive heart failure. Dig Dis Sci 21:895–900, 1976.
3. Kaymaklan H, Dourdourekas D, Szanto PB, et al: Congestive heart failure as a cause of fulminant hepatic failure. Am J Med 65:384–388, 1978.
4. Nouel O, Henrion J, Bernuau J, et al: Fulminant hepatic failure due to transient circulatory failure in patients with chronic heart disease. Dig Dis Sci 25:49–52, 1980.

CHAPTER 6

Hematology/Oncology

Maurie Markman, M.D.

PATIENT 1

A 65-year-old man with dyspnea and bilateral arm swelling

A 65-year-old man with a long smoking history was well until 2 weeks prior to admission when he developed the gradual onset of bilateral arm and hand swelling. He noted progressive increase in shortness of breath the day before admission.

Physical Examination: Temperature 98.8°; pulse 110; respirations 35; blood pressure 160/90. Thorax: prominent venous pattern over anterior chest. Chest: decreased breath sounds bilaterally. Cardiac: normal. Extremities: bilateral arm swelling. Neurologic: normal.

Laboratory Findings: Hct 45%; WBC 13,000/μl. Chest radiograph (below left): widened upper mediastinum. Superior venacavagram: below right.

Consider the likely diagnosis and your approach to management.

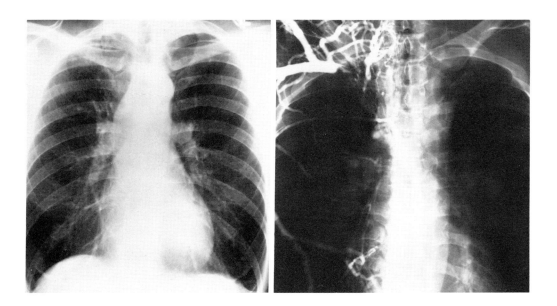

Diagnosis: Superior vena cava syndrome secondary to squamous cell carcinoma of the lung.

Discussion: Compression of the superior vena cava (SVC) by adjacent masses leads to decreased venous return from the upper extremities, head, and chest. This process (SVC syndrome) may result in a number of symptoms, including dyspnea, easy fatigability, headache, altered consciousness, and decreased visual acuity. Physical findings include cervicofacial edema, dilated veins over the chest, neck, and face, and upper extremity edema. Less common are Horner's syndrome and vocal cord paralysis. Clinical symptoms and signs will vary depending upon how rapidly the SVC is compressed and whether or not collateral circulation has become established.

More than 80% of cases of SVC syndrome are due to neoplastic invasion of the mediastinum. Three-quarters of neoplasms are lung cancer, most commonly squamous and small cell carcinomas. Approximately 10% are secondary to lymphomas (most commonly diffuse large cell type). Fewer than 15% of patients have a benign cause for the obstruction (tuberculosis, aneurysms, goiter, fibrosing mediastinitis).

Patients presenting with the SVC syndrome often do not have a previously known diagnosis of malignancy. The least invasive diagnostic technique should be selected because bleeding from high venous pressures may be excessive following incisional biopsies. Sputum cytology, bronchoscopy with brushings and washings, or biopsy of palpable lymph nodes, therefore, are the preferred procedures. Recent observations, however, suggest that more invasive procedures are tolerated with acceptable morbidity when necessary to reach a diagnosis.

It is rarely necessary to make a definitive diagnosis of SVC syndrome. The presence of appropriate clinical symptoms and a pathologically confirmed malignancy is usually sufficient to initiate treatment. If the presence of SVC obstruction is uncertain, a contrast superior venacavagram or a nuclear medicine scan can be performed.

It was previously believed that SVC syndrome should be treated as a medical emergency. While treatment should be initiated promptly, most patients may be systematically evaluated to obtain an underlying diagnosis before starting therapy. In addition, appropriate treatment planning (for example, simulation for chest radiotherapy) should be conducted prior to beginning therapy.

Treatment should be directed toward the underlying malignancy. Chemotherapy may be employed as initial treatment if the tumor is known to be responsive (lymphomas, small-cell lung cancer). Initial therapy with radiation therapy is reserved for patients with tumors poorly responsive to chemotherapy (other types of lung cancer) or of unknown histologic type. Seventy percent of patients with lung cancer and 95% of patients with lymphomas will experience improvement in the signs and symptoms of SVC syndrome following the institution of antineoplastic therapy.

Although controversial in SVC syndrome, corticosteroids may reduce edema and improve symptoms in patients presenting with dyspnea. Anticoagulation is avoided because of hemorrhagic risks from high venous pressure. Furthermore, anticoagulation does not appear to improve survival in this clinical setting.

It is important to note that signs and symptoms of cardiac involvement with cancer may closely resemble SVC syndrome. Ten to 20% of patients with metastatic malignancies will have autopsy evidence of pericardial or cardiac involvement with cancer. Approximately 10% of these patients have symptomatic evidence of cardiac dysfunction during life, which most commonly results from malignant pericardial effusion. Tumor can spread to the pericardium by direct local extension, lymphatic invasion, or hematogenously. The most common malignancies involving the pericardium are cancers of the lung and breast as well as lymphomas and melanoma.

The present patient underwent bronchoscopy, which demonstrated squamous cell carcinoma of the lung. Radiotherapy was initiated with improvement in symptoms.

Clinical Pearls

1. Over 80% of patients with SVC syndrome will be found to have a malignancy, most often lung cancer.

2. The least invasive diagnostic technique available is preferred in SVC syndrome because of the hemorrhagic risks from high venous pressure; however, patients tolerate excisional biopsies sufficiently well to warrant their use when necessary.

3. Overall, 70 to 95% of patients with SVC syndrome caused by a malignancy can be expected to improve symptomatically following the institution of antineoplastic therapy.

REFERENCES

1. Perez CA, Presant CA, Van Amburg AL III: Management of superior vena cava syndrome. Semin Oncol 5:123–134, 1978.
2. Ahmann FR: A reassessment of the clinical implications of the superior vena caval syndrome. J Clin Oncol 2:961–969, 1984.
3. Sculier JP, Feld R: Superior vena cava obstruction syndrome: Recommendations for management. Cancer Treat Rev 12:209–218, 1985.
4. Shepherd FA, Ginsberg JS, Evans WK, et al: Tetracycline sclerosis in the management of malignant pericardial effusion. J Clin Oncol 3:1678–1682, 1985.

PATIENT 2

A 25-year-old man with skin rash, liver function abnormalities, and severe diarrhea following bone marrow transplantation

A 25-year-old man with acute myelocytic leukemia received a bone marrow transplant, with his HLA-identical sister serving as the donor. Twenty days after transplant he developed a diffuse rash and severe diarrhea (> 8 liters/day).

Physical Examination: Temperature 101.0°; pulse 100; respirations 22; blood pressure 120/88. Skin: diffuse maculopapular rash. Chest: normal. Cardiac: normal. Abdomen: hyperactive bowel sounds.

Laboratory Findings: Hct 26%; WBC 700/μl, platelets 24,000/μl. Alkaline phosphatase 65 IU/L (normal 13–39), bilirubin 2.2 mg/dl, SGOT 115 IU/L (normal 7–27), LDH 190 IU/L (normal 45–90). Bone marrow at time of original diagnosis (below): diffuse infiltration with myeloblasts.

What diagnosis explains the patient's presentation?

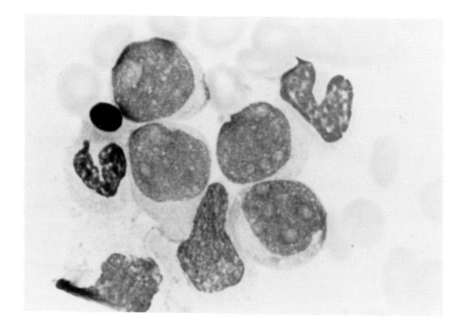

Diagnosis: Acute graft-versus-host disease (GVHD).

Discussion: GVHD is a common and frequently fatal complication of allogenic bone marrow transplantation. It occurs in acute and chronic forms and in varying degrees of severity. Incidence varies from 25 to 60% of patients receiving marrows from HLA-identical donors with unreactive mixed lymphocyte cultures. Virtually 100% of patients given a non-HLA matched bone marrow graft will develop acute GVHD.

The symptoms of acute GVHD include skin rash, hepatic dysfunction, severe diarrhea, and fever. Typically, onset of acute GVHD occurs from 20 to 100 days following the marrow transplant. The skin rash usually develops rapidly, may initially resemble a drug reaction (diffuse maculopapular), and can progress to appear indistinguishable from scalded-skin syndrome. While the rash may spontaneously resolve, it may also herald more serious symptoms. On biopsy, a lymphocytic infiltration is observed along with basilar vacuolization. Diarrhea can be voluminous and may be associated with crampy abdominal pain and severe electrolyte loss. Biopsy specimens of the rectum reveal necrosis, mucosal ulcerations, and crypt drop out. These histologic features are relatively specific and can be helpful in distinguishing acute GVHD from infectious enteritis.

Patients experiencing liver dysfunction secondary to acute GVHD have both a hepatocellular destructive (elevated SGOT) and cholestatic (elevated bilirubin) profile. Hepatic biopsy demonstrates necrosis of hepatocytes, damaged bile ducts, and a periportal lymphoid infiltration.

The etiology of acute GVHD has not been fully elucidated. Although histoincompatibility clearly plays a major role, other undefined factors contribute, because not all patients receiving allogenic marrows develop the disorder. Viral infection and radiation injury to normal cells may induce alterations in local cells leading to subsequent immunological damage.

The treatment of established acute GVHD has had limited success. Standard therapeutic regimens include high doses of immunosuppressive drugs, principally corticosteroids. Prednisone has been administered up to doses of 5 to 10 mg/kg in this clinical setting. Although improvement in symptoms of acute GVHD usually occurs, steroids in patients already severely immunocompromised and neutropenic will frequently lead to fatal opportunistic infections. Recently, investigators have begun to explore anti-T cell monoclonal antibody therapy in the treatment of acute GVHD. While results remain preliminary, impressive clinical results have been observed. Other agents used with varying degrees of success include antithymocyte globulin and cyclosporine A.

Survival following the development of acute GVHD is clearly related to the severity of the symptoms. Patients with mild or moderate disease have an overall survival comparable to patients who have not developed acute GVHD. Individuals with severe GVHD, however, have a survival of less than 20%.

Considering the poor prognosis of severe acute GVHD once established, attention has focused on the development of strategies to prevent the disease. These include the posttransplant administration of low doses of methotrexate, prednisone, antithymocyte globulin, and cyclosporine A. Other investigators have been exploring the potential of removing the immunoreactive cells responsible for GVHD in vitro before marrow transfusion.

Paradoxically, considerable evidence suggests that the total elimination of GVHD is associated with a higher incidence of relapse of leukemia compared with that in individuals who experience mild or moderate acute GVHD. These observations suggest that GVHD may have a positive influence on outcome secondary to the development of a graft versus tumor effect.

The present patient was treated with high doses of corticosteroids. Although his rash and diarrhea improved, he subsequently developed fatal Candida sepsis.

Clinical Pearls

1. Acute GVHD can initially mimic an acute drug reaction when it presents as a maculopapular drug eruption. In many cases, skin biopsy can successfully differentiate the two conditions.

2. Patients with acute myeloblastic leukemia who develop mild to moderate GVHD have a better overall prognosis than individuals who demonstrate no evidence of the disease.

3. Chronic GVHD generally follows an episode of GVHD. Manifestations include generalized erythematous rash, dry mouth, loss of dentition, hepatocellular damage and cholestasis, dysphagia, diarrhea, abdominal pain, steatorrhea, restrictive or obstructive lung disease, arthritis, arthralgia, leukopenia, anemia, and thrombocytopenia.

REFERENCES

1. Neudorf S, Filipovich A, Ramsay N, et al: Prevention and treatment of acute graft-versus-host disease. Semin Hematol 21:91–100, 1984.
2. Champlin RE, Gale RP: The early complications of bone marrow transplantation. Semin Hematol 21:101–108, 1984.
3. Wick MR, Moore SB, Gastineau DA, et al: Immunologic, clinical, and pathologic aspects of human graft-versus-host disease. Mayo Clin Proc 58:603–612, 1983.

PATIENT 3

A 26-year-old man with lymphoma and anuria

A 26-year-old man was recently diagnosed as having a diffuse poorly differentiated lymphoma. He began chemotherapy 2 days earlier and became anuric 24 hours later.

Physical Examination: Vital signs: normal. Lymph nodes: enlarged cervical nodes. Chest: clear. Abdomen: nontender; several palpable masses in the pelvis.

Laboratory Findings: Hct 25%; WBC 17,500/μl, 70% "immature" lymphocytes, platelets 450,000/μl. Na+ 135 mEq/L, K+ 6.3 mEq/L, Cl$^-$ 103 mEq/L, HCO$_3^-$ 18 mEq/L; uric acid 22 mg/dl, BUN 60 mg/dl, creatinine 3.2 mg/dl. Chest radiograph (below left): left mediastinal mass. Bone marrow (below right): malignant lymphoma cells.

What is the probable cause of the sudden anuria?

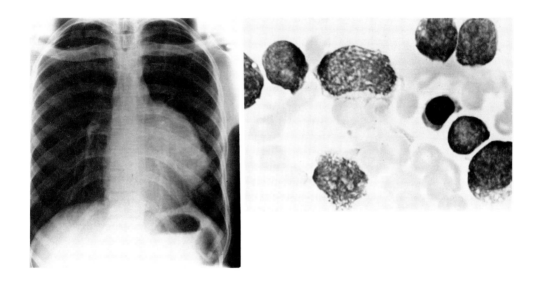

Diagnosis: Tumor lysis syndrome with resultant uric acid nephropathy.

Discussion: The tumor lysis syndrome may develop following the institution of systemic chemotherapy for rapidly growing bulky tumors for which effective treatment exists. Thus, the syndrome is most often observed in patients with acute lymphoblastic lymphomas, acute lymphocytic leukemia, Burkitt's lymphomas, and diffuse undifferentiated lymphomas. It can also be seen in patients with small-cell carcinoma of the lung and testicular carcinoma but is very uncommon in other solid tumors in that rapid responses to chemotherapy are rarely seen.

Rapid lysis of tumor leads to release of intracellular uric acid, potassium, and phosphate with resultant hyperuricemia, hypocalcemia (secondary to calcium and phosphate precipitation in the presence of an elevated serum phosphorus), hyperkalemia, and hyperphosphatemia. Renal failure may result from uric acid and/or calcium-phosphate deposition in the renal tubules. Sudden death secondary to arrhythmias caused by the rapid rise in serum potassium has been reported.

Risk factors for the development of the tumor lysis syndrome include preexisting renal dysfunction, increased lactate dehydrogenase levels (suggestive of spontaneous tumor lysis prior to the administration of chemotherapy as well as the presence of substantial tumor bulk), and high uric acid levels before treatment. The syndrome generally develops from 1 to 4 days following the initiation of therapy.

Prevention of the syndrome is far more successful than treatment once the tumor lysis becomes established. If at all possible, chemotherapy should be delayed until any serious pretreatment metabolic abnormalities have been corrected. Patients should be pretreated with allopurinol (300 mg b.i.d.) to normalize uric acid levels and prevent the formation of more uric acid following therapy. Patients should be prehydrated at a rate of 200 to 300 ml/hr with fluid continuance for at least 24 hours following the initiation of chemotherapy. The urine should be alkalinized (urine pH > 7.5) before treatment to enhance renal uric acid excretion. This is best accomplished by administering sodium bicarbonate intravenously at a dose of 100 mEq/m^2 daily. Frequent (at least twice daily) determinations of electrolytes, calcium, phosphorus, creatinine, and uric acid levels should be obtained for 48 hours following the initiation of treatment. It is important to maintain the serum uric acid level within the normal range.

Patients with severe tumor lysis syndrome may require hemodialysis to lower the serum potassium, uric acid, and phosphorus, as well as to treat fluid overload and renal insufficiency. Indications for hemodialysis include a serum K+ > 6.0 mEq/dl, serum uric acid > 10 mg/dl, serum phosphorus > 10 mg/dl, symptomatic hypocalcemia, and volume-overloaded with oliguria. Although patients with renal insufficiency can recover normal renal function, recovery may take considerable time during which both hemodialysis and other supportive measures may be required.

The present patient's serum creatinine rose to 5.6 mg/dl, but did not require hemodialysis. Renal function gradually returned to normal, and he experienced a complete response to the antineoplastic regimen.

Clinical Pearls

1. The tumor lysis syndrome is a serious but preventable complication of treatment of rapidly growing malignancies for which effective systemic chemotherapy exists.

2. If at all possible, systemic chemotherapy for such patients should be withheld for several days to correct preexisting metabolic abnormalities.

3. Alkalinization of the urine is an important measure to prevent uric acid precipitation in the renal tubules of patients at risk for developing the tumor lysis syndrome.

REFERENCES

1. Schilsky RL: Renal and metabolic toxicities of cancer chemotherapy. Semin Oncol 9:75–83, 1982.
2. Tsokos GC, Balow JE, Spiegel RJ, et al: Renal and metabolic complications of undifferentiated and lymphoblastic lymphomas. Medicine 60:218–229, 1981.
3. Vogelzang NU, Nelimark RA, Nath KA: Tumor lysis syndrome after induction chemotherapy of small cell bronchogenic carcinoma. JAMA 249:513–514, 1983.

PATIENT 4

A 47-year-old woman with acute leukemia and hemorrhagic cystitis

A 47-year-old woman with acute myelocytic leukemia presented with hematuria consisting of gross blood and clots. Five days earlier, she had begun a chemotherapy program of high-dose cytarabine and cyclophosphamide.

Physical Examination: Temperature 99.8°; pulse 90; respirations 16; blood pressure 140/75. Chest: clear. Cardiac: normal. Abdomen: normal. Pelvic: bleeding through the urethra; normal female organs.

Laboratory Findings: Hct 29%; WBC 500/μl, platelets 29,000/μl; fibrinogen 260 mg/dl (normal 150–350); PT and PTT: normal. Bone marrow (below): hypocellular with rare blast cells demonstrating Auer rods.

What are your clinical impression and management plan?

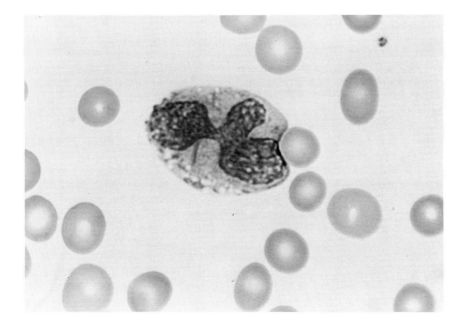

Diagnosis: Hemorrhagic cystitis secondary to cyclophosphamide.

Discussion: Cyclophosphamide, a cytotoxic alkylating agent with a wide spectrum of clinical indications, can cause bladder mucosal edema, ulcerations, and minor to severe hemorrhage. Long-term use can result in chronic bladder fibrosis.

Bladder toxicity is believed to be due to metabolites of cyclophosphamide, including chlorethyl-aziridine and acrolein, which are activated by hepatic microsomes and excreted in the urine. These metabolites concentrate in the bladder and react with the urothelium, causing damage. The incidence of hemorrhagic cystitis from cyclophosphamide administered at conventional doses is unknown because serial urinalysis is not routinely performed; patients receiving high-dose regimens, however, develop this complication in approximately 10% of courses. Pathological examination of the bladder in these patients will reveal edema and hyperemia with diffuse punctate hemorrhagic lesions.

Uncontrolled clinical observations suggest that the continuous administration of cyclophosphamide is more frequently associated with hemorrhagic cystitis than is intermittent therapy. Unfortunately, bladder toxicity may occur months after the last dose of the drug. Prevention is far more successful than treatment of established disease.

Prevention consists of providing adequate hydration following drug administration. With standard dose regimens (such as used in the treatment of breast cancer or when the drug is used chronically as an immunosuppressive agent in nonmalignant disease) oral hydration is usually satisfactory. High-dose cyclophosphamide treatment requires vigorous intravenous hydration (urine output > 200–250 ml/hr for 6 to 12 hours following drug delivery).

When hematuria is present, cyclophosphamide should be discontinued and vigorous hydration instituted or continued. Foley catheter placement is controversial, as some investigators believe the catheter may induce bladder spasm and inhibit the passage of blood clots. Continuous bladder irrigation, however, may prevent clot formation, although the pathologic process and patient's course may not be altered. If conservative measures fail, cystoscopy should be performed and bleeding sites cauterized. For severe hemorrhage the use of formalin instillations may successfully stop bleeding. Unfortunately, side effects of formalin therapy may be severe (bladder fibrosis and contraction, hydronephrosis, papillary necrosis, ureterofibrosis, intraperitoneal extravasation, and anuria). Efficacy appears to be maintained (80–90% successful in stopping bleeding with a single instillation) with acceptable toxicity using 4% or weaker solutions. When life-threatening bleeding persists, the patient may undergo bilateral ligation of the hypogastric arteries and urinary diversion, with or without cystectomy.

The present patient underwent cystoscopy with findings compatible with cyclophosphamide-induced hemorrhagic cystitis. Because of the severity of the bleeding, she received 4% instillation of formalin, which stopped the hemorrhage.

Clinical Pearls

1. Adequate hydration must be delivered both before and after administration of cyclophosphamide to prevent hemorrhagic cystitis. Although oral hydration is adequate following conventional doses of the drug, intravenous hydration is required with high-dose regimens.

2. Oral cyclophosphamide administered on a chronic basis should be taken in the morning to avoid nocturnal pooling of the drug in the bladder, which occurs with late afternoon or evening dosing.

3. The use of 4% formalin instillation to control cyclophosphamide-induced hemorrhagic cystitis appears to maintain efficacy and reduce the toxicity associated with higher formalin concentrations.

REFERENCES

1. Fair W: Urologic emergencies. In DeVita VT, Hellman S, Rosenberg SA (eds): Cancer: Principles and Practice of Oncology. Philadelphia, J.B. Lippincott, 1985, pp 1894–1905.
2. Droller MJ, Saral R, Santos G: Prevention of cyclophosphamide-induced hemorrhagic cystitis. Urology 20:256–258, 1982.
3. Shrom SH, Donaldson MH, Duckett JW Jr, et al: Formalin treatment for intractable hemorrhagic cystitis. Cancer 38:1785–1789, 1976.

PATIENT 5

A 70-year-old man with acute leukemia and shortness of breath

A 70-year-old man noted increasing fatigue over the previous 2 weeks. For the 12 hours before admission, he experienced the gradual onset of shortness of breath.

Physical Examination: Temperature 99.2°; pulse 110; respirations 28; blood pressure 150/100. Fundi: retinal vein distention. Chest: decreased breath sounds left lower lobe. Cardiac: normal. Abdomen: normal. Extremities: no calf tenderness.

Laboratory Findings: Hct 22%; WBC 120,000/μl, with 90% blast forms (below left); platelets 18,000/μl; prothrombin and partial thromboplastin times: normal. ABG (room air): pH 7.41, PO_2 39 mm Hg, PCO_2 35 mm Hg. Bone marrow (below): replacement of normal marrow with cells resembling myeloblasts.

Explain the cause of the patient's dyspnea and hypoxemia.

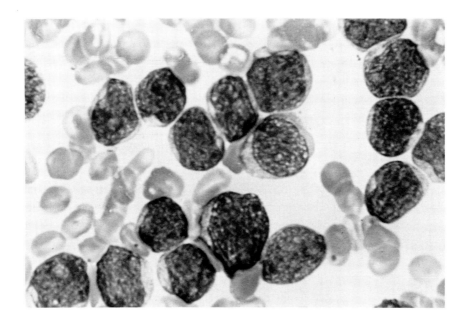

Diagnosis: Hyperleukocytic syndrome secondary to acute myeloblastic leukemia.

Discussion: The hyperleukocytic syndrome, which occurs in patients with acute myeloblastic, chronic myelocytic, and acute lymphoblastic leukemia, is characterized by signs and symptoms secondary to the high concentration of leukocytes in the blood. The process can involve multiple organs, including the lung (dyspnea, tachypnea, hypoxia), the nervous system (stupor, tinnitus, ataxia, delirium, papilledema, visual blurring, retinal vein distention, intracranial hemorrhage), and the vascular compartment (blood clots, priapism, vascular insufficiency). Sudden death has been observed, most frequently believed secondary to intracranial hemorrhage. Artifactual hypoxia is also commonly encountered because the PO_2 rapidly falls in blood samples obtained for blood gas analysis. This finding results from the extremely high metabolic rate of large concentrations of immature leukocytes.

Blood viscosity increases with extreme elevations in immature leukocyte concentration because of the limited deformability of these cells (principally blast forms) compared with that of red blood cells. Histologic studies demonstrate aggregates of blast cells and thrombi in involved organs. These aggregates are predisposed to occlusion of small vessels, particularly veins. The combination of sluggish blood flow through an organ and the high rate of metabolism of intravascular blasts lead to severe local tissue hypoxia.

Treatment of the hyperleukocytic syndrome is directed toward the rapid lowering of the white blood cell count. Uncontrolled clinical observation suggests that the combination of cytotoxic chemotherapy (cytarabine and an anthracycline in acute myeloblastic leukemia; hydroxyurea in chronic myelocytic leukemia; prednisone, vincristine, L-asparaginase in acute lymphoblastic leukemia) and leukapheresis best accomplish this goal.

Leukapheresis rapidly lowers white blood cell concentrations in the plasma, but the cells will return if effective antineoplastic therapy is not employed. Daily leukapheresis for several days may be necessary before the effects of the cytotoxic agent on leukemia cell number becomes evident. Leukapheresis has the added benefit of reducing tumor bulk and thus limiting the risk of severe tumor lysis syndrome.

With the reported success of leukapheresis in symptomatic patients with established hyperleukocytic syndrome, many oncologists recommend it prophylactically as a supplement to standard cytotoxic therapy in patients with high peripheral blood blast counts. Recommended threshold white blood counts for initiating leukapheresis in acute myeloblastic leukemia range from 50,000 to 100,000/μl.

The present patient underwent emergency leukapheresis with marked improvement in respiratory symptoms within 12 hours. Chemotherapy was begun on the second day of hospitalization and the patient ultimately experienced a complete remission.

Clinical Pearls

1. High blast concentrations in the peripheral blood cause artifactual hypoxia secondary to the increased metabolic rate of a large number of malignant cells that consume oxygen in blood samples.

2. Patients with acute myeloblastic leukemia presenting with white blood cell counts > 50,000 to 100,000/μl may benefit from leukapheresis (along with cytotoxic chemotherapy) to prevent the hyperleukocytic syndrome.

3. Transfusion to correct anemia in patients with high peripheral blast counts requires caution because resultant increased viscosity may cause the hyperleukocytic syndrome.

REFERENCES
1. Cuttner J, Holland JF, Norton L, et al: Therapeutic leukapheresis for hyperleukocytosis in acute myelocytic leukemia. Med Pediatr Oncol 11:76–78, 1983.
2. Lichtman MA, Rowe JM: Hyperleukocytic leukemias: Rheological, clinical, and therapeutic considerations. Blood 60:279–283, 1982.
3. Karp DD, Beck JR, Cornell CJ: Chronic granulocytic leukemia with respiratory distress: Efficacy of emergency leukapheresis. Arch Intern Med 141:1353–1354, 1981.

PATIENT 6

A 22-year-old woman with epistaxis and diffuse purpura

A 22-year-old woman with no history of prior serious illnesses noted the sudden onset of epistaxis and purpura on her arms, legs, and chest. She was not taking any medications.

Physical Examination: Temperature 98.8°; pulse 90; respirations 16; blood pressure 120/80. Skin: diffuse purpuric lesions on trunk and extremities. Lymph nodes: nonpalpable. Chest: clear. Cardiac: normal. Abdomen: no spleen tip.

Laboratory Findings: Hct 33%; WBC 7,500/μl, normal differential, platelets 3,000/μl. Peripheral blood: normal red and white cell morphology, marked decrease in platelet number; PT and PTT: normal. Bone marrow (below): increased number of normal-appearing megakaryocytes.

What is the prime diagnostic possibility?

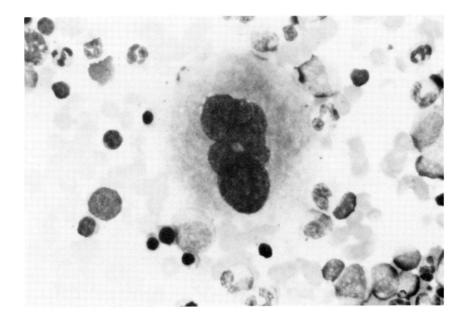

Diagnosis: Autoimmune idiopathic thrombocytopenic purpura (AITP).

Discussion: AITP is a syndrome characterized by isolated thrombocytopenia in the setting of normal platelet, leukocyte, and erythrocyte morphology. Coagulation factors are preserved, and no other systemic diseases that might be the cause of the thrombocytopenia (systemic lupus, sepsis) are apparent. Anemia, if present, is proportional to the extent of blood loss. Bone marrow examination reveals either normal or, more commonly, increased numbers of megakaryocytes. Other marrow elements are normal. In most patients, the etiology of AITP remains unknown, although viral infections are suspected in many instances.

The course of AITP may be acute or chronic, with an onset that varies from insidious to sudden. Patients with severe thrombocytopenia are at risk of spontaneous bleeding into vital organs (particularly the brain), but this risk (for unclear reasons) is usually greatest in the first few days of the illness. Fortunately, more than 80% of patients will gradually recover regardless of therapy, but symptoms can persist for greater than 6 months and occasionally the syndrome will become chronic.

Platelet counts of between 40,000 and 60,000/μl are necessary to maintain normal hemostasis. Patients with AITP and platelet counts greater than 100,000/μl, therefore, may be observed with monthly platelet counts, as the risk of serious bleeding is minimal.

Corticosteroids are the mainstay of therapy for patients with AITP. Approximately 70 to 90% of patients experience a rise in platelet number following the institution of steroid therapy. Steroids are believed to act by several mechanisms, including reducing sequestration of antibody-coated platelets in the spleen, increasing platelet production, impairing immunoglobulin synthesis, and inhibiting antibody-platelet interactions. A prednisone dose between 40 and 60 mg/day is usually employed initially in adult patients.

Platelet transfusions are of limited usefulness because transfused cells are rapidly destroyed; transfusions may be life-saving, however, in patients with serious hemorrhage or in those requiring emergency surgery. Splenectomy is advised if large doses of steroids are required beyond a 6-month period. This surgical procedure is effective in 70 to 90% of patients with AITP. Unfortunately, 10 to 15% of patients will relapse following an initial response to splenectomy. Such patients may be successfully maintained on a low dose of prednisone (10 mg or less per day). If splenectomy is unsuccessful in raising the platelet count, alternative immunosuppressive regimens may be effective (high-dose intravenous gamma globulin, danazol, azathioprine, vincristine).

Most patients with AITP have antiplatelet antibodies. When a patient responds to corticosteroids, the amount of platelet-bound immunoglobulin decreases. The antibody appears to modify the platelet surface in such a way that the reticuloendothelial system will dramatically accelerate the removal of platelets from the circulation.

The differential diagnosis of thrombocytopenia includes abnormalities in platelet production (marrow injury from drugs, radiation, alcohol, metastatic carcinoma, fibrosis), ineffective platelet production (vitamin B_{12} and folate deficiency), platelet sequestration (splenomegaly), and accelerated destruction (AITP, lymphoreticular disorders producing autoantibodies, drug-induced, fetal-maternal incompatibility, transfusion reactions, disseminated intravascular coagulation, sepsis, prosthetic cardiac valves, thrombotic thrombocytopenic purpura).

In most cases of thrombocytopenia, it is fairly easy to determine the presence of ineffective platelet production, platelet sequestration, or accelerated destruction. When the cause is unclear, a bone marrow examination will be helpful. In cases of destruction or sequestration, a normal or increased number of megakaryocytes will always be found.

Thrombotic thrombocytopenic purpura (TTP) is a serious clinical entity that may on initial presentation simulate AITP. TTP is characterized by several cardinal features, including thrombocytopenic purpura, microangiopathic hemolytic anemia, transient and fluctuating neurologic findings, fever, and renal abnormalities. The etiology of TTP remains obscure, but it is believed to be a generalized disorder of the microcirculation. Results of treatment of this previously fatal disease (60 to 80% mortality) have improved significantly since the addition of plasma infusion, plasmapheresis, and exchange transfusions to standard management. In addition to these measures, corticosteroids and antiplatelet agents are commonly employed in the treatment of TTP.

The present patient was treated with prednisone at a dose of 60 mg/day with slow tapering over several months. Bleeding stopped and the platelet count gradually rose to 120,000/μl.

Clinical Pearls

1. Platelet transfusions should only be employed in AITP when severe hemorrhage is present or there is evidence of bleeding into a vital organ (brain, lung, or heart).

2. More than 90% of patients with AITP will not have a palpable spleen. When enlarged, the spleen should not be felt > 1 cm below the left costal margin. Larger spleens suggest alternative diagnoses such as lymphoma.

3. In AITP the bone marrow will demonstrate either normal or, more commonly, increased numbers of megakaryocytes.

REFERENCES

1. Kelton JG, Gibbons S: Autoimmune platelet destruction: Idiopathic thrombocytopenic purpura. Semin Thromb Hemost 8:83–104, 1982.
2. Marcus AJ: Hemorrhagic disorders: Abnormalities of platelet and vascular function. In Wyngaarden JB, Smith LH Jr (eds): Cecil Textbook of Medicine, 18th ed. Philadelphia, W.B. Saunders Co., 1988, pp 1042–1060.

PATIENT 7

A 69-year-old woman with breast cancer, severe low back pain, and lower extremity weakness

A 69-year-old woman with known metastatic breast cancer and chronic bone pain controlled with non-narcotic analgesia noted the sudden onset of low back pain that progressed over 24 hours. She thought her legs were weaker than usual, although she was not certain if the decreased strength was due to the pain.

Physical Examination: Temperature 99.0°; pulse 88; blood pressure 160/100. Chest: clear. Thorax: no spinal tenderness to palpation; healed mastectomy scar. Cardiac: normal. Abdomen: benign. Neurologic: equivocal weakness of both legs; sensory normal; Babinski sign absent.

Laboratory Findings: Hct 34%; WBC 9,900/μl, normal differential; platelets: normal. Chest radiograph: normal. Spine radiographs: diffuse bone metastases. Bone scan (below left): multiple metastatic lesions. Myelogram: below right.

What clinical diagnosis is confirmed by the myelogram?

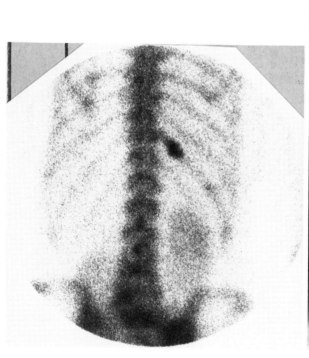 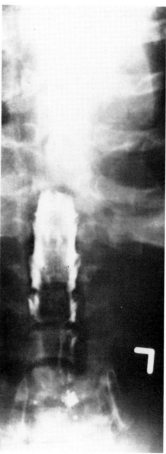

Diagnosis: Complete spinal cord block from metastatic breast cancer.

Discussion: Spinal cord involvement with cancer usually develops from vertebral body or pedicle erosion with tumor extension into the anterior epidural space. The resultant cord compression causes neurologic deficits and occurs most commonly in patients with cancers of the lung, breast, and prostate.

More than 95% of patients with epidural spinal cord compression will have preexisting back pain. The pain may precede neurologic dysfunction by hours, days, or even weeks. Unfortunately, the neurologic significance of this symptom is often overlooked because back pain from bony spinal metastases is one of the more common symptoms observed in all patients with metastatic cancer, most of whom do not progress to cord compression.

Any patient with metastatic cancer and back pain, however, should be approached with a high index of suspicion in that early diagnosis of cord compression and prompt initiation of therapy improve outcome. In one large series, 80% of patients who were ambulatory when therapy for cord compression was initiated remained ambulatory following the completion of treatment. Conversely, only 30% of patients who were not ambulatory at diagnosis regained use of their legs.

Several symptoms, signs, and radiographic features assist in determining the level of cord compression. These include the location of pain and spinal tenderness to percussion, the radicular distribution of symptoms, region of plain film abnormalities, and bone scan findings. A myelogram is indispensable, however, to precisely define the location of the compression and to determine the upper and lower limits of the block to design ports when external radiation is indicated. In addition, a myelogram may detect multiple blocks which will influence the therapeutic plan.

Recently, the magnetic resonance imaging (MRI) scan has proved valuable in the evaluation of spinal cord block secondary to metastatic cancer. This procedure has the major advantage of eliminating the need for a lumbar puncture to instill contrast material. Although the role of MRI in this clinical setting is not yet determined, early indications suggest that it may replace myelography as the diagnostic procedure of choice.

Studies indicate that external radiation therapy is equally effective compared with laminectomy in preserving neurologic function in most patients with cord compression from metastatic disease. Patients typically undergo treatment with 3000 cGy in 10 fractions over 2 weeks. The radiation portal is extended over 1 or 2 vertebral segments beyond the region documented to be involved on myelography to ensure inclusion of the entire area of tumor. The optimal initial treatment strategy for the management of patients with spinal cord compression and metastatic cancer, however, depends on several factors and must be individualized. A history of prior radiotherapy to the involved site may obviate additional radiotherapy, necessitating alternate treatment. It is even difficult to radiate a spinal region near a previously radiated area because of the risk of radiation damage to the cord. In other patients with spinal cord symptoms without a confirmed diagnosis of a malignant etiology, a laminectomy with biopsy may be indicated. Also, patients with tumor cell types known to be radioresistant, such as renal cell carcinoma, may forego radiation therapy.

Steroids are administered to all patients with documented or suspected cord compression to reduce edema. Although the optimal dose of corticosteroids is unknown, many neurologists recommend high doses of dexamethasone (100 mg IV bolus followed by 24 mg orally every 6 hours with rapid tapering) to ensure a rapid response to therapy.

The present patient received radiation therapy to the spinal lesion with improvement in pain. The leg weakness did not progress. The patient subsequently developed evidence of progressive metastatic disease in the liver.

Clinical Pearls

1. The initial symptom of spinal cord compression from malignancy is back pain. Early diagnosis of cord compression before the onset of neurologic dysfunction improves the probability of maintaining patient ambulation.

2. External radiation is equally effective as surgical decompression in preventing deterioration of neurologic function in patients with spinal cord compression secondary to metastatic tumor.

3. The MRI may replace contrast myelography as the diagnostic procedure of choice in patients with suspected spinal cord compression.

REFERENCES

1. Gilbert RW, Kim J-H, Posner JB: Epidural spinal cord compression from metastatic tumor: Diagnosis and treatment. Ann Neurol 3:40–51, 1978.
2. Greenberg HS, Kim J-H, Posner JB: Epidural spinal cord compression from metastatic tumor: Results from a new treatment protocol. Ann Neurol 8:361–366, 1980.
3. Sundaresan N, Galicich JH, Lane JM, et al: Treatment of neoplastic epidural cord compression by vertebral body resection and stabilization. J Neurosurg 63:676–684, 1985.

PATIENT 8

An 18-year-old man with severe chest and left upper quadrant pain

An 18-year-old black man presented to the emergency room with severe chest pain of 8 hours' duration. During the previous 3 hours the patient also had noted abdominal pain in the left upper quadrant.

Physical Examination: Temperature 100.8°; pulse 110; respirations 22; blood pressure 150/80. Anxious male in pain. Chest: clear. Cardiac: tachycardia; flow murmur. Abdomen: left upper quadrant tenderness; spleen not palpable; bowel sounds hypoactive.

Laboratory Findings: Hct 21%; WBC 12,000/μl, normal differential, platelets 425,000/μl. Peripheral smear: below. Chest radiograph: normal. ECG: sinus tachycardia. ABG (room air): pH 7.47, PCO_2 34 mm Hg, PO_2 85 mm Hg.

What is the cause of the patient's complaints? What other complications are associated with the underlying condition?

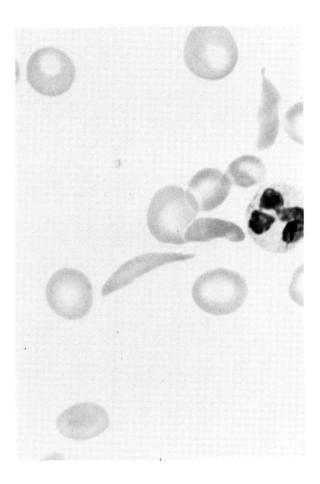

Diagnosis: Sickle cell anemia with an infarctive crisis.

Discussion: Although patients with sickle cell anemia may experience one or more of several types of crises, the infarctive crisis is by far the most common. It is caused by obstruction of small blood vessels by rigid sickled red cells which results in tissue hypoxia. Pain is the major symptom and may involve many body regions, most commonly the bones, chest, and abdomen. Splenic infarction (presenting as left upper quadrant abdominal pain) is so common that by early adulthood most patients with sickle cell anemia will have small spleens secondary to scarring. In contrast to patients with sickle cell anemia, individuals with either sickle/beta-thalassemia or hemoglobin SC disease will commonly have splenomegaly in adulthood.

Fever is frequently observed during an infarctive crisis. This may make the differential diagnosis of pain more difficult, as patients with sickle cell anemia are highly susceptible to a number of infections, including pneumococcal sepsis and salmonella osteomyelitis. Pulmonary infarctions are also common in sickle cell anemia and are difficult to differentiate from infectious processes. The acute chest syndrome in sickle cell anemia is characterized by fever, chest pain, leukocytosis, and a pulmonary infiltrate. It has been suggested that patients presenting with these clinical features and no predominant organism on Gram stain of the sputum should not receive antibiotics unless they appear seriously ill.

Treatment of an infarctive crisis is supportive in nature. The patient should be given hydration and analgesia as necessary. As multiple crises over many years are the rule rather than the exception in sickle cell anemia, narcotic analgesia should be employed only when absolutely necessary and for as short a time as possible. While the role of supplemental oxygen in infarctive crisis remains unsettled, it is unlikely to cause harm and may provide some limited benefit by improving tissue oxygenation.

Patients with sickle cell anemia may also develop an aplastic crisis, most frequently secondary to infection. Marrow reserve in these patients is limited. Folate deficiency is a common problem in individuals with sickle cell anemia and must be considered in patients with a sudden fall in hematocrit. Sequestration crisis occurs in infants, may be fatal, and is caused by the sudden and massive pooling of blood in the spleen. Finally, patients with sickle cell anemia may present with a hemolytic crisis as a result of an acceleration in the "normal" hemolytic clinical picture chronically present in patients with sickle cell anemia. Patients experiencing this complication usually have a secondary cause for hemolysis, such as concurrent G-6-PD deficiency or a transfusion reaction.

Patients with sickle cell anemia may be chronically jaundiced (secondary to chronic hemolysis) or may develop clinical difficulties associated with jaundice, including infectious hepatitis, gallstones (particularly bilirubin stones), cirrhosis, and sepsis. In addition, during an infarctive crisis, the liver may transiently increase in size.

The present patient was treated with intravenous hydration and analgesia, with resolution of the pain over several days.

Clinical Pearls

1. Patients with sickle cell anemia will undergo autosplenectomies secondary to multiple infarctive crises, such that the spleen can rarely be palpated beyond childhood.

2. The acute chest syndrome, secondary to pulmonary infarction, may mimic pulmonary infection. In the absence of further documentation of an infectious process (positive sputum Gram stain), antibiotics should be withheld. However, if the patient appears seriously ill, appropriate antibiotic coverage should be instituted until the etiology of clinical process has been established.

3. Fever frequently accompanies an infarctive crisis in sickle cell anemia in the absence of infection.

REFERENCES
1. Charache S: The treatment of sickle cell anemia. Arch Intern Med 133:698–705, 1974.
2. Maugh TS II: A new understanding of sickle cell emerges. Science 211:468–470, 1981.

PATIENT 9

A 60-year-old man with headache, epistaxis, visual disturbances, and an abnormal serum paraprotein

A 60-year-old man with no significant medical history presented with decreased vision, headaches, and epistaxis.

Physical Examination: Temperature 98.0°; pulse 80; respirations 16; blood pressure 160/95. Fundi: sausage-shaped retinal vein engorgement; retinal hemorrhage. Chest: clear. Cardiac: normal.

Laboratory Findings: Hct 30%; WBC 8,500/μl, normal differential, platelets 250,000/μl; albumin 3.2 g/dl, globulin 6.5 g/dl; serum protein electrophoresis: monoclonal paraprotein; quantitative immunoglobulin determination: IgA 2,500 mg/dl (normal: 70–312 mg/dl); serum viscosity: 6 (normal: 1.4–1.8). Bone marrow examination (below): 40% of nucleated cells are plasma cells.

What diagnosis and pathophysiologic sequelae underlie the patient's presentation?

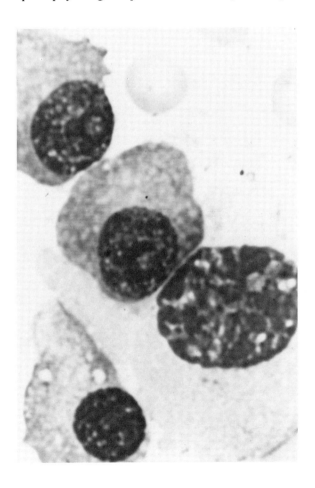

Diagnosis: IgA myeloma with hyperviscosity syndrome.

Discussion: Multiple myeloma is a malignant neoplasm that is characterized by the proliferation of plasma cells. This abnormal proliferation can ultimately lead to anemia, renal insufficiency, hypercalcemia, destructive bone lesions, a susceptibility to serious infections, and amyloidosis. In the majority (60 to 70%) of cases of multiple myeloma, an IgG paraprotein is secreted, whereas in a smaller number of cases either IgA (20%) or only immunoglobulin light chains (15%) will be found. Fewer than 1% of cases will secrete IgD or IgE or will be nonsecretors of a paraprotein.

Patients with IgA myeloma and, more commonly, individuals with an IgM paraprotein (Waldenstrom's macroglobinemia), may develop symptoms secondary to hyperviscosity of the blood and subsequent decreased blood flow to multiple organs. The IgA molecule itself is able to produce the syndrome despite its much smaller size than IgM due to polymerization of the paraprotein.

Symptoms of the hyperviscosity syndrome include headache, dizziness, seizures, epistaxis, decreased hearing, decreased mentation, congestive heart failure, and visual disturbances including blindness. Patients may be anemic and have coagulation abnormalities (secondary to the paraprotein). Blood or serum viscosity (measured relative to the viscosity of water) will be abnormal. Symptoms attributable to hyperviscosity will generally not become evident until the patient has a serum viscosity of > 4 (normal: 1.4–1.8). When the serum viscosity rises to > 6, essentially all patients will be symptomatic.

Treatment is directed at the underlying malignancy (systemic chemotherapy) and to lowering the serum viscosity by plasmapheresis. This technique can rapidly improve both the signs and symptoms of hyperviscosity, but the duration of benefit may be short, such that frequent exchanges are required. Plasmapheresis should be instituted in any patient with severe hyperviscosity (visual disturbances, impending coma, paresis, serious bleeding). As many as 6 to 8 liters of plasma may be removed by this technique over several days. As plasmapheresis will treat only the symptoms and not the underlying malignant neoplasm, chemotherapy should be initiated at the same time pheresis is begun. Chlorambucil is the most commonly used agent in this clinical setting, but more intensive chemotherapeutic regimens have been employed and are quite appropriate in a patient able to tolerate the side effects of such a treatment strategy. Pheresis can usually be discontinued when a therapeutic response is observed. Special caution is required in treating patients with hyperviscosity and anemia. Transfusion of red cells will increase the blood viscosity and may exacerbate symptoms. It is often best to transfuse such patients very slowly and in association with plasma exchange.

The present patient underwent plasmapheresis with the removal and replacement of 6 liters of plasma (over two sessions). Symptoms improved markedly following the first pheresis. Oral chlorambucil was also instituted.

Clinical Pearls

1. Waldenstrom's macroglobinemia and IgA myeloma are the two diseases most commonly associated with the development of hyperviscosity.

2. Plasma exchange with removal of the abnormal paraprotein can rapidly improve the signs and symptoms of hyperviscosity.

3. Red cell transfusions in a patient with the hyperviscosity syndrome may lead to congestive heart failure or cerebral vascular accidents secondary to a rapid rise in blood viscosity.

REFERENCES
1. McGrath MA, Penny R: Paraproteinemia: Blood hyperviscosity and clinical manifestations. J Clin Invest 58:1155–1162, 1976.
2. Waldenstrom's macroglobinemia. Lancet 2:311–312, 1985.

PATIENT 10

A 32-year-old woman with newly diagnosed acute leukemia and multiple coagulation abnormalities

A 32-year-old woman was found to have acute leukemia. At initial presentation the patient reported a 3-day history of bleeding gums, nose bleeds, and the appearance of multiple bruises on her body.

Physical Findings: Temperature 101°; pulse 110; respirations 18; blood pressure 130/80. Skin: multiple echymoses and purpuric lesions. Mouth: blood oozing from gums. Chest: clear. Cardiac: normal.

Laboratory Findings: Hct 21%; WBC 1,100/μl, 90% "immature" appearing forms (same cells as in bone marrow), platelets 12,000/μl, prothrombin time 16 sec, fibrinogen 60 mg/dl (normal 150–350), fibrin degradation products: elevated. Bone marrow (below): marked increase in promyelocytes.

What is the cause of the patient's coagulation abnormalities? What is your planned therapeutic approach?

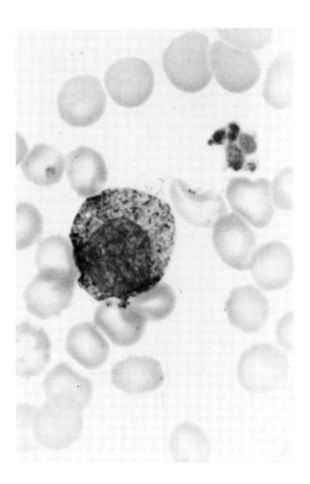

Diagnosis: Acute promyelocytic leukemia and disseminated intravascular coagulation (DIC).

Discussion: Defining a specific etiology for bleeding and multiple coagulation abnormalities in a patient with acute leukemia may be difficult. Thrombocytopenia secondary to bone marrow infiltration with leukemic cells is common, as is sepsis (with subsequent DIC) in a patient without an adequate granulocyte reserve. It is standard clinical practice to initiate empirical broad-spectrum antibiotics (to cover the most common organisms infecting this patient population) with evidence of fever in individuals presenting with very low white blood cell counts (granulocytes $< 1000/\mu l$).

A unique feature of bleeding and coagulation abnormalities in patients with acute nonlymphocytic leukemia (ANLL) is the potential for the development of DIC as a direct result of the malignancy itself. Although any subtype of ANLL may be associated with DIC, it is most commonly observed in patients with acute promyelocytic leukemia (APL). In APL the development of DIC (which at a subclinical level may be found in virtually all cases) is secondary to the release of a procoagulant found in the granules of the leukemic cells.

In past years APL had been considered to be associated with an inferior prognosis compared with other subtypes of ANLL, principally because of early deaths following diagnosis. The recognition that patients with APL present with DIC, the severity of which may initially worsen after therapy (with release of procoagulant material), and institution of appropriate treatment to manage DIC, have dramatically altered the outcome. Currently, individuals with APL can be expected to respond well if not better to antileukemic therapy compared with patients with other subtypes.

The earliest laboratory evidence of DIC is an elevation of the prothrombin time (PT) with increased fibrin degradation products (FDP). Patients will subsequently develop decreasing fibrinogen levels, a fall in platelets, and an elevated partial thromboplastin time (PTT). Treatment of DIC secondary to acute leukemia includes the rapid institution of cytotoxic chemotherapy and appropriate transfusion support. This includes the administration of platelets (despite the concern for their rapid removal in the presence of DIC) in patients with active bleeding and a markedly abnormal coagulation profile. Platelets may need to be transfused twice daily until the bleeding stops or coagulation parameters improve. It is reasonable to attempt to keep the platelet count $> 30,000$ to $40,000/\mu l$, although this goal may be difficult to attain in the face of ongoing DIC. When fibrinogen is < 70 to 80 mg/dl, it is appropriate to transfuse either fresh frozen plasma or cryoprecipitate to replace coagulation factors.

Finally, although its value has never been demonstrated in controlled clinical trials, the use of heparin in the setting of DIC in patients with acute leukemia appears to have had an overall positive influence on the course of the disease. The justification for administering this agent in the presence of bleeding or severe coagulation abnormalities is that it will inhibit the abnormal coagulation cycle responsible for the consumption of clotting factors. Heparin is delivered as a continuous infusion at low dose levels (approximately 500 units/hour). This strategy runs the serious risk of increasing bleeding. Coagulation parameters (PT, PTT, fibrinogen) must be carefully monitored to be certain they improve when heparin is administered. In general, heparin can be discontinued 5 to 7 days after institution of antineoplastic therapy, as release of procoagulant material from the leukemic blasts should have increased by this time. Invasive procedures (such as Hickman catheter placement) should be avoided if at all possible while the patient is receiving heparin. Use of heparin in DIC associated with acute leukemia is a unique clinical situation. If sepsis is suspected to be the major cause of DIC, appropriate management includes antibiotics and transfusion support, and not heparin.

The present patient was treated with heparin and platelets along with combination chemotherapy. Her coagulation profile improved and, despite a difficult course, she had a complete remission.

Clinical Pearls

1. Acute promyelocytic leukemia is associated with a unique form of DIC that is secondary to the release of procoagulant material from the leukemic blasts.

2. The administration of low-dose heparin and blood-product transfusion in patients with leukemia-induced DIC are important management strategies.

REFERENCES

1. Daly PA, Schiffer CA, Wiernick PH: Acute promyelocytic leukemia—clinical management of 15 patients. Am J Hematol 8:347–359, 1980.
2. Seifter EJ, Bell WR: Coagulation abnormalities in patients with cancer. Clin Oncol 2:657–704, 1983.

CHAPTER 7

Endocrinology

Gary P. Zaloga, M.D.

PATIENT 1

A 70-year-old woman with worsening congestive heart failure

A 70-year-old woman was admitted to the ICU for worsening congestive heart failure (CHF) and lethargy. She had been ill for 10 years with progressive dyspnea and weakness. CHF was diagnosed 5 years previously and initially responded to digoxin and furosemide. Despite recent hospitalization and maximal medical therapy, no improvement was noted. Her family reported a 30-pound weight loss over the previous few years, which was attributed to anorexia. She had been disinterested in her surroundings and herself, and was considered "senile."

Physical Examination: Temperature 99°; pulse 150; respirations 28; blood pressure 130/60. Skin: dry. Neck: multinodular, mildly enlarged thyroid gland. Chest: bibasilar rales. Cardiac: irregularly rapid heart rate; S_3; 2+ edema in lower extremities; jugular venous distention. Neurologic: lethargic, no focal findings.

Laboratory Findings: Hct 35%; WBC 7800/μl; Na+ 138 mEq/L, HCO_3^- 28 mEq/L, Ca^{2+} 9.8 mg/dl, PO_4^{-2} 3 mg/dl, glucose 110 mg/dl, albumin 3.8 g/dl; BUN 35 mg/dl; creatinine 1.3 mg/dl. ABG (O_2 2 L/min): pH 7.45, PCO_2 38 mm Hg, PO_2 78 mm Hg. Chest radiograph: cardiomegaly; interstitial infiltrates. ECG: atrial fibrillation.

Hospital Course: On the third hospital day, the patient developed fever to 103° and became unresponsive, hypotensive, and tachycardic. Gram stain tracheal aspirate: gram-positive diplococci. Chest radiograph: new right middle lobe infiltrate.

What disease processes are responsible for the patient's clinical status?

Diagnosis: Thyroid storm precipitated by pneumococcal pneumonia. CHF and atrial fibrillation worsened by untreated hyperthyroidism.

Discussion: Hyperthyroidism, a hypermetabolic disease that results from the secretion of excess thyroid hormone, may be due to Graves' disease, thyroiditis, or nodular thyroid disease. Hyperthyroidism is manifested by symptoms of excess organ function which include nervousness, anxiety, diaphoresis, heat intolerance, palpitations, dyspnea, fatigue, weight loss, and impaired cognitive function. Signs of hyperthyroidism include an enlarged thyroid gland, ophthalmopathy (i.e., lid retraction, exophthalmos), tachycardia, atrial fibrillation, muscle weakness, CHF, tremor, hyperactivity, and impaired mentation. Elderly patients frequently have "apathetic hyperthyroidism" in which signs and symptoms are limited to a few organ systems and the presentation may be only stupor or coma.

The present patient had an enlarged thyroid gland, CHF, atrial fibrillation, impaired cognitive function, weakness, apathy, and weight loss, all suggestive of hyperthyroidism. Many of these symptoms and signs, however, are nonspecific and may occur in patients with critical illness unrelated to thyroid dysfunction. Nevertheless, the findings of an enlarged thyroid gland coupled with refractory CHF and atrial fibrillation should raise the suspicion of hyperthyroidism. An elevated T4 (thyroxine) and/or T3 (tri-iodothyronine) level indicates the presence of the hyperthyroid state; a suppressed TSH level and TSH response to TRH are confirmatory. Thyroid function tests in the present patient showed: T4 14.7 μg/dl (normal 4–12), T3 210 ng/dl (normal 70–200), T3RU 39% (normal 25–35), FTI 16.1 (normal 4–12), TSH < 1.5 μU/ml (normal < 7), and TRH stimulation: flat.

Thyroid storm represents severe life-threatening hyperthyroidism and is usually associated with marked agitation and/or psychosis, impaired mentation, fever, tachycardia, and diarrhea. Untreated, it may progress to pulmonary edema, cardiovascular collapse, hepatic failure, and death. It is usually precipitated by stress (trauma, surgery, infection) in a patient with untreated or incompletely treated hyperthyroidism. With infection, it is often difficult to determine whether symptoms and signs result from the infection or from thyrotoxicosis.

Treatment of hyperthyroidism is aimed at suppressing the thyroid gland, inhibiting peripheral conversion of T4 to T3, and blocking the systemic manifestations of thyroid hormone excess. Propylthiouracil (PTU), methimazole, iodide, lithium, radioactive iodine, and thyroidectomy all can be used to limit thyroid hormone secretion. PTU not only blocks thyroid hormone synthesis but also inhibits T4 to T3 conversion. Inorganic iodide inhibits iodide organification and thyroid hormone release. Its antithyroid effect is more rapid than that of other antithyroid drugs. It may be given as potassium iodide, Lugol's solution, or ipodate. Iodide should be given after PTU or methimazole to avoid thyroidal organification of iodide. Lithium inhibits thyroid hormone synthesis and release but its use is limited by toxicity. Radioactive iodine is trapped in the thyroid gland but takes weeks to months to achieve an antithyroid effect. Since surgery may itself precipitate thyroid storm, it is preferable to render patients euthyroid with antithyroid medications prior to thyroidectomy.

Agents that inhibit T4 to T3 conversion include PTU, glucocorticoids, propranolol, and ipodate. Agents that ameliorate the systemic effects (sympathetic hyperactivity) of hyperthyroidism include propranolol, reserpine, and guanethidine. Most hyperthyroid patients can be controlled with PTU and propranolol. However, because thyroid storm has a high mortality, many prefer to treat thyroid storm or impending thyroid storm with a combination of antithyroid drugs (PTU and iodide), monodeiodination inhibitors (PTU, ipodate, and/or propranolol), and a catecholamine blocker (propranolol). Glucocorticoids are usually given until it can be verified that the patient does not have adrenal insufficiency. Supportive measures include treatment of infection or concomitant disease, hydration, fever control, nutrition, and ventilatory and cardiac support.

If left unrecognized, the present patient would most likely have died. She survived with antibiotic treatment and therapy aimed at controlling her thyrotoxicosis. Following control of hyperthyroidism, CHF an atrial fibrillation resolved, her mental function improved and weight gain ensued.

Clinical Pearls

1. The occurrence of refractory CHF and atrial fibrillation or tachycardia should suggest the possibility of hyperthyroidism.

2. The diagnosis of hyperthyroidism in the critically ill patient is difficult because many of the signs and symptoms of hyperthyroidism are nonspecific. A high index of suspicion is required.

3. The diagnosis of hyperthyroidism is made by finding an elevated T4 and/or T3 level in a patient with a compatible clinical picture. A suppressed TSH and flat TSH response to TRH are indicative of primary hyperthyroidism.

4. Treatment of thyroid storm is aimed at suppression of the thyroid gland, inhibition of T4 to T3 conversion, and use of agents that block sympathetic overactivity.

REFERENCES

1. Zaloga GP, Chernow B: Addisonian crisis, hyperthyroidism, and hypothyroidism. In Parrillo JE (ed): Current Therapy in Critical Care Medicine. Toronto, B.C. Decker, 1987, pp 300–305.
2. Studer H, Ramelli F: Simple goiter and its variants: Euthyroid and hyperthyroid multinodular goiters. Endocrinol Rev 3:40–61, 1982.
3. Robbins J: Thyroid storm. In Krieger DT, Bardin CW (eds): Current Therapy in Endocrinology and Metabolism. Toronto, B.C. Decker, 1985, pp 66–69.

PATIENT 2

A 20-year-old man with dehydration and "cardiac arrest"

A 20-year-old man was admitted to the ICU unconscious following a "cardiac arrest." He worked on an assembly line in a factory and had experienced nausea most of the day. The ambient temperature in the factory was 94°F. He vomited several times, complained of dizziness, became confused, and collapsed. CPR was begun by his fellow workers. He had a palpable blood pressure and was breathing spontaneously when the EMS arrived.

Physical Examination: Temperature 101°; pulse 130; respirations 18; blood pressure 88/40; Skin: tan; dry mucous membranes. Chest: normal. Cardiac: regular tachycardia. Neurologic: no focal findings; unresponsive to verbal commands; withdrawal to pain only.

Laboratory Findings: Hct 48%; WBC 12,000/μl, Na+ 120 mEq/L, K+ 6.7 mEq/L, Cl⁻ 82 mEq/L, HCO₃⁻ 18 mEq/L; glucose 50 mg/dl, BUN 30 mg/dl, creatinine 1.8 mg/dl, Ca²⁺ 9.6 mg/dl, PO₄⁻² 3.6 mg/dl. Urinalysis: SG 1.030, no cells. ECG: shown below.

What diagnosis is suggested by the data? What tests should be performed to confirm the diagnosis? What emergency treatment is indicated?

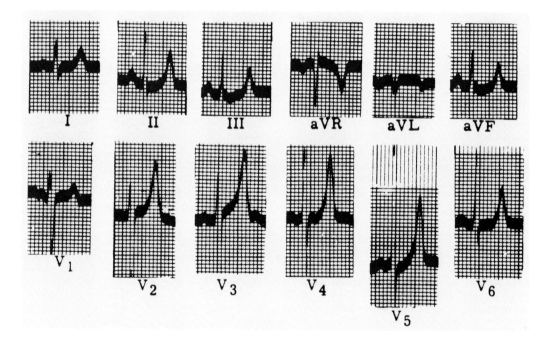

Diagnosis and Treatment: Primary adrenal insufficiency. The diagnosis is confirmed by finding a low serum cortisol, absent cortisol response to ACTH stimulation, and an elevated serum ACTH level. Emergency treatment is intravenous fluids to restore intravascular volume and administration of hydrocortisone.

Discussion: Adrenal insufficiency can result from adrenal gland failure (primary adrenal insufficiency) or from hypothalamic-pituitary gland failure (secondary adrenal insufficiency). Primary glandular failure results in loss of both aldosterone and cortisol secretion, whereas secondary glandular failure results in loss of cortisol only. Primary adrenal insufficiency results from autoimmune disease, infection (tuberculosis, CMV, meningococcus), tumor, hemorrhage into the gland, and from surgical removal of the glands. Metabolic failure of the adrenal gland may result from drugs such as aminoglutethimide and ketoconazole. Over 90–95% of adrenal tissue must be destroyed before adrenal insufficiency will occur. Secondary adrenal insufficiency results from exogenous glucocorticoid withdrawal, hypopituitarism (after surgery, irradiation, or tumor invasion), or hypothalamic failure.

Clinical features of adrenal insufficiency result from loss of glucocorticoid and/or aldosterone effects. Glucocorticoid deficiency impairs cardiovascular function and may cause hypotension and impaired pressor responses. Free water clearance is limited and may result in hyponatremia; hepatic glucose output is diminished with potential for hypoglycemia. Gastrointestinal manifestations include anorexia, nausea, and vomiting. In general, the ability to tolerate stress is impaired. Aldosterone reabsorbs sodium in the distal renal tubule in exchange for potassium and hydrogen. Loss of mineralocorticoids results in salt wasting, hypovolemia, hypotension, and ultimately shock. In addition, hyperkalemia and metabolic acidosis are common.

A serum cortisol level < 20 μg/dl in a severely stressed patient is usually sufficient to confirm the diagnosis of adrenal insufficiency. In less stressed patients, a short ACTH stimulation test may be helpful in making a definitive diagnosis. A low serum cortisol (< 20 μg/dl) 30 to 60 minutes following short ACTH stimulation indicates adrenal insufficiency; however, it does not separate primary from secondary insufficiency. The finding of an elevated plasma ACTH concentration or failure to respond to prolonged ACTH infusion indicates primary adrenal insufficiency. A low ACTH and/or a normal response to long ACTH infusion indicates secondary adrenal insufficiency. Patients who display a normal response to short ACTH stimulation do not have primary adrenal insufficiency but may still have secondary adrenal insufficiency (failure of the hypothalamic-pituitary axis to respond). A normal response to stress (critical illness, hypoglycemia) or metyrapone is required in these patients to exclude secondary adrenal insufficiency.

Treatment of adrenal insufficiency includes IV fluids, hormone replacement, and correction of the underlying disease. Intravascular volume should be replaced with normal saline; if hypoglycemia is present, 5% dextrose in saline should be given. Dexamethasone should be used for initial hormone replacement because it does not interfere with serum cortisol measurement and ACTH testing. Following adrenal testing, hydrocortisone, which has both glucocorticoid and mineralocorticoid activity, should be given (100 mg q 6–8 hours). If mineralocorticoid activity is not required, another steroid may be used (methylprednisolone, prednisone). The dosage of glucocorticoid should be tapered to maintenance levels based upon the clinical condition. It may be necessary to add fluorocortisone (a mineralocorticoid) if fluid and electrolytes become problematic.

The present patient responded to aggressive fluid resuscitation and corticosteroid administration. A serum cortisol level drawn on admission was < 20 μg/dl, and primary hypoadrenalism was subsequently diagnosed.

Clinical Pearls

1. Dehydration in a young individual should suggest adrenal insufficiency.
2. Total body tanning suggests ACTH excess.
3. The occurrence of hyponatremia and hyperkalemia indicates adrenal insufficiency until proven otherwise.
4. A normal short ACTH stimulation test does not exclude secondary adrenal insufficiency.

REFERENCES

1. Zaloga GP, Chernow B: Addisonian crisis, hyperthyroidism, and hypothyroidism. In Parrillo JE (ed): Current Therapy in Critical Care Medicine. Toronto, B.C. Decker, 1987, pp 300–305.
2. Borst GC, Michenfelder HJ, O'Brian JT: Discordant cortisol response to exogenous ACTH and insulin-induced hypoglycemia in patients with pituitary disease. N Engl J Med 306:1462–1464, 1982.
3. Nerup J: Addison's disease—clinical studies. A report of 108 cases. Acta Endocrinol 76:127–141, 1974.
4. Angeli A, Frairia R: Simultaneous diagnosis and treatment of acute adrenocortical insufficiency. Lancet 2:1217–1218, 1975.

PATIENT 3

A 69-year-old man with refractory hypotension

A 69-year-old man with chronic renal failure (not on dialysis) was admitted to the hospital for emergent surgery for a leaking abdominal aortic aneurysm. He had a history of hypertension treated with clonidine and furosemide.

Physical Examination: Temperature 97°; pulse 130; respirations 28; blood pressure 190/110. Chest: normal. Cardiac: normal heart sounds without murmurs. Abdomen: pulsatile mass; rebound tenderness in epigastric area. Extremities: bilateral femoral bruits; pulses intact and symmetric. Neurologic: oriented; no focal findings.

Laboratory Findings: Hct 30%; WBC 14,200/μl, platelets 51,000/μl, PT 13.7 sec, PTT 45 sec, Na+ 137 mEq/L, K+ 4.8 mEq/L, Cl$^-$ 97 mEq/L, HCO$_3^-$ 25 mEq/L; BUN 68 mg/dl, creatinine 6.7 mg/dl, glucose 136 mg/dl, albumin 4.2 g/dl, Ca^{2+} 9.5 mg/dl, PO$_4^{-2}$ 4.9 mg/dl, Mg^{2+} 2.7 mg/dl, bilirubin 0.6 mg/dl. CT abdomen: 8 cm abdominal aortic aneurysm.

Hospital Course: The patient was taken to surgery and a leaking abdominal aortic aneurysm was repaired. In the ICU following surgery, he developed progressive hypotension, oliguria, and an anion gap metabolic acidosis. Cardiac index was 2 L/min/m^2, and he received 7 L of normal saline and 50 g of albumin over the next several hours to maintain his P$_{CW}$ above 15 mm Hg. He received dopamine at 15 μg/kg/min, but CI and blood pressure were unresponsive. Sodium bicarbonate was given repeatedly to maintain the arterial pH above 7.25. Following the last ampule of bicarbonate, the patient developed progressive bradycardia, became asystolic, and had a cardiac arrest.

What is a likely cause for the cardiac arrest? What therapeutic maneuvers may have contributed to the cardiac arrest?

Diagnosis: The cardiac arrest resulted from acute hypocalcemia. Large quantities of Ca^{2+} free intravenous fluids, albumin, and sodium bicarbonate all contributed to the hypocalcemia.

Discussion: An ionized Ca^{2+} level at the time of the patient's arrest was 2.0 mg/dl (normal 4.1–5.1). Total serum Ca^{2+} was 4.7 mg/dl, PO_4^{-2} 7.7 mg/dl, Mg^{2+} 2.5 mg/dl, and K+ 4.3 mEq/L.

Ionized hypocalcemia develops in patients as a result of insufficient parathyroid hormone secretion, diminished synthesis of calcitriol (1,25-dihydroxy-vitamin D), or as a result of Ca^{2+} precipitation/chelation. Parathyroid gland insufficiency may result from hypoparathyroidism (autoimmune or surgical) or from severe hypomagnesemia or hypermagnesemia. This patient's serum Mg^{2+} was normal at the time of the cardiac arrest and an n-terminal parathyroid hormone level (from plasma obtained just prior to the arrest) subsequently returned at 57 pg/ml (normal 11–24). Thus, the patient's parathyroid gland responded appropriately to hypocalcemia. A calcitriol level on the same blood sample was undetectable in the face of a normal calcidiol (25-hydroxyvitamin D) level. This inappropriately low level is common in patients with renal failure because the 1-hydroxylase enzyme, which converts calcidiol to calcitriol, is located in renal tissue.

The inability to synthesize calcitriol predisposes patients with renal failure to ionized hypocalcemia. Calcium precipitation/chelation also may contribute to hypocalcemia. This patient had an elevated serum PO_4^{-2} of 7.7 mg/dl just prior to his arrest. In addition, he received albumin, which is capable of binding Ca^{2+}, and large amounts of Ca^{2+} free fluids, which can dilute the circulating Ca^{2+} level. Finally, the patient received sodium bicarbonate, which can decrease the ionized Ca^{2+} level by increasing its binding to albumin. All these factors contributed to the acute hypocalcemia and cardiac arrest in this patient.

Low total serum Ca^{2+} concentrations are common in critically ill patients and usually result from hypoalbuminemia; most will have normal ionized Ca^{2+} levels. However, some of these patients will have true ionized hypocalcemia. Adjustment of the total Ca^{2+} for alterations in albumin concentrations and/or pH cannot reliably predict the ionized Ca^{2+} value. Direct measurement is the only reliable method of determining ionized Ca^{2+} concentrations.

Ionized hypocalcemia in critically ill patients most commonly presents with cardiovascular compromise (low cardiac output, hypotension, bradycardia). Neuromuscular irritability, although less common, also may occur. These patients usually improve with intravenous Ca^{2+} therapy.

The present patient was unsuccessfully resuscitated. At autopsy, he was found to have minimal coronary artery disease and an intact aortic graft.

Clinical Pearls

1. Hypocalcemia results from parathyroid gland insufficiency, vitamin D deficiency, and Ca^{2+} precipitation/chelation.

2. Acute or chronic renal failure predisposes to hypocalcemia by impairing synthesis of calcitriol.

3. Rapid infusion of large quantities of Ca^{2+} free fluids, albumin, and sodium bicarbonate can contribute to hypocalcemia.

4. Total serum Ca^{2+} and adjustment of the total serum Ca^{2+} concentration for albumin level are poor predictors of the true ionized Ca^{2+} value.

REFERENCES

1. Zaloga GP, Chernow B: Divalent ions: Calcium, magnesium, and phosphorus. In Chernow B, Holaday JW, Zaloga GP, Zaritsky AL (eds): The Pharmacologic Approach to the Critically Ill Patient. Baltimore, Williams and Wilkins, 1988, pp 603–636.
2. Zaloga GP, Chernow B, Cook D, et al: Assessment of calcium homeostasis in the critically ill patient: Diagnostic pitfalls of the McLean Hastings Nomogram. Ann Surg 202:587–594, 1985.
3. Zaloga GP, Chernow B: Hypocalcemia in critical illness. JAMA 256:1924–1929, 1986.

PATIENT 4

A 57-year-old man with confusion

A 57-year-old previously healthy man was admitted for fever, chills, and lethargy of 1 week's duration. Review of systems was significant for urinary frequency and anorexia. He denied weight loss, cough, or dyspnea. He had a 20 pack-year history of cigarette smoking.

Physical Examination: Temperature 102°; pulse 115; respirations 20; blood pressure 135/88. Chest: clear. Cardiac: normal heart sounds; no murmurs. Abdomen: tender over left flank; no hepatosplenomegaly. Rectal: prostatic tenderness; no blood in stool. Neurologic: alert; oriented; no focal findings.

Laboratory Findings: Hct 42%; WBC 17,000/μl. Na+ 145 mEq/L, K+ 4.2 mEq/L, HCO$_3^-$ 23 mEq/L; glucose 110 mg/dl, BUN 24 mg/dl, creatinine 1.3 mg/dl, albumin 4.4 g/dl, Ca^{2+} 9.7 mg/dl, PO$_4^{-2}$ 3.6 mg/dl; Mg^{2+} 2.0 mg/dl. UA: SG 1.024, protein 2+, blood 1+, microscopic (below). Blood and urine cultures: *E. coli* sensitive to tobramycin.

Hospital Course: Management was initiated with intravenous tobramycin for a diagnosis of *E. coli* pyelonephritis, and the patient was noted to improve. On the fifth hospital day, the patient was confused and lethargic with hyperactive deep tendon reflexes. Blood pressure and temperature were normal. An ECG demonstrated many premature ventricular contractions. ABG (room air): pH 7.32, PCO$_2$ 48 mm Hg, PO$_2$ 78 mm Hg.

What metabolic abnormality is most likely responsible for the patient's clinical condition? What workup is appropriate?

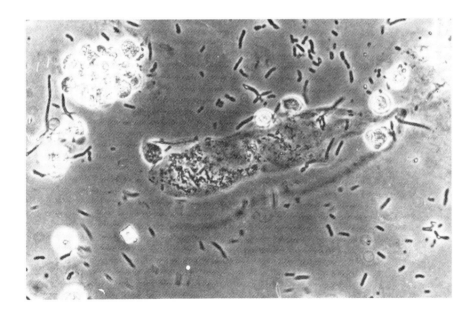

Diagnosis: Hypomagnesemia. Appropriate laboratory studies should include serum Mg^{2+}, Ca^{2+}, PO_4^{-2}, $Na+$, $K+$, glucose, BUN, and creatinine; urine collection (12 hour) for Mg^{2+} and creatinine.

Discussion: The development of a metabolic encephalopathy during treatment for an underlying disorder as occurred in the present patient warrants the exclusion of several differential diagnoses. Major clinical considerations include hypoxia and/or hypercapnia, hypoglycemia, adverse reactions to medications, and electrolyte disturbances. This patient's ABG values demonstrated mild hypercapnia without hypoxia, not severe enough to explain the encephalopathy. A blood glucose concentration was 88 mg/dl. Results of an SMA-6 were only mildly abnormal. The physicians suspected hypomagnesemia because the patient had recently received little nutrition (anorexic for over a week) and was undergoing aminoglycoside therapy. Most diets are marginal in fulfilling daily requirements for Mg^{2+}; lack of dietary intake alone can lead to Mg^{2+} deficiency. Additionally, aminoglycoside antibiotics interfere with renal conservation of Mg^{2+}, further increasing the risks for hypomagnesemia.

Hypomagnesemia is frequently associated with other electrolyte abnormalities. Hypocalcemia results from parathyroid gland suppression and peripheral resistance to vitamin D action in the setting of decreased Mg^{2+}. Parathyroid hormone levels in this patient were inappropriately low and improved with Mg^{2+} repletion. Hypokalemia can result from renal K+ wasting because the renal $Na+/K+$ exchange pump is Mg^{2+} dependent.

The most common clinical features of Mg^{2+} deficiency involve the cardiovascular and neuromuscular systems. Hypomagnesemia potentiates the action of vasoconstrictors and may lead to coronary artery spasm; arrhythmias and cardiac failure also can occur. Total muscle weakness, including the respiratory muscles, is common and may result in respiratory failure, most likely responsible for the hypercapnia in the present patient. Mg^{2+} deficiency may cause paresthesias, muscle spasms, seizures, tetany, confusion, obtundation, and coma. It is unclear whether signs and symptoms result from Mg^{2+} deficiency alone or from concomitant electrolyte disturbances.

The present patient's blood chemistry demonstrated the following results: K+ 3.0 mEq/L, total Ca^{2+} 6.2 mg/dl, ionized Ca^{2+} 3.0 mg/dl (nl 4.1–5.1), albumin 4.0 g/dl, Mg^{2+} 0.8 mg/dl (nl 2–3), PO_4^{-2} 3.7 mg/dl (nl 3.0–4.5). A 12-hour urine collection contained 30 mEq of Mg^{2+} and 80 mEq of K+, consistent with both Mg^{2+} and K+ wasting. The patient responded to Mg^{2+} supplementation with improvement in his mental status.

Clinical Pearls

1. The occurrence of hypokalemia and hypocalcemia should suggest hypomagnesemia.
2. Renal Mg^{2+} wasting is common in patients receiving aminoglycoside antibiotics.
3. Hypomagnesemic hypocalcemia results from parathyroid gland suppression and peripheral vitamin D resistance.
4. Hypomagnesemia may cause respiratory muscle weakness and respiratory failure.

REFERENCES

1. Zaloga GP, Chernow B: Divalent ions: Calcium, magnesium, and phosphorus. In Chernow B, Holaday JW, Zaloga GP, Zaritsky AL (eds): The Pharmacologic Approach to the Critically Ill Patient. Baltimore, Williams and Wilkins, 1988, pp 603–636.
2. Zaloga GP, Chernow B, Pock A, et al: Hypomagnesemia is a common complication of aminoglycoside therapy. Surg Gynecol Obstet 158:561–565, 1984.
3. Anast CS, Winnacker JL, Forte LR, et al: Impaired release of parathyroid hormone in magnesium deficiency. J Clin Endocrinol Metab 42:707–717, 1976.
4. Rude RK, Singer FR: Magnesium deficiency and excess. Ann Rev Med 32:245–259, 1981.

PATIENT 5

A 16-year-old boy unresponsive following a motor vehicle accident

A 16-year-old boy was admitted to the ICU following a motor vehicle accident. He was the driver of the car and drove off the road into a ditch. He was obtunded and responded only to pain. Medical history, obtained from his mother, was unremarkable.

Physical Examination: Temperature 97°; pulse 124; respirations spontaneous at 30; blood pressure 90/70. Skin: contusions on face and arms. Fundi: normal. Ear canals: clear. Chest: clear. Cardiac: normal. Abdomen: generalized tenderness. Extremities: full range of motion; pulses intact. Rectal: normal. Neurologic: obtunded; withdraws to pain; no focal signs.

Laboratory Findings: Hct 48%; WBC 16,000/μl. Na+ 126 mEq/L, K+ 4.3 mEq/L, Cl− 100 mEq/L, HCO_3^- 6 mEq/L, glucose 847 mg/dl, BUN 38 mg/dl, creatinine 2 mg/dl. ABG (room air): pH 7.08, PCO_2 12 mm Hg, PO_2 80 mm Hg. Urine output 100 ml/hr; UA: SG 1.036, glucose 4+, ketones 4+. ECG: sinus tachycardia.

Why is the patient obtunded?

Diagnosis: Diabetic ketoacidosis.

Discussion: Patients presenting with trauma may have many causes of obtundation or coma other than intracranial disorders. Metabolic conditions not only may result from injuries received, but also may be the underlying cause of altered consciousness leading to the traumatic event, as in the present patient. It is essential that primary metabolic abnormalities, drug overdose, and myocardial disease be excluded rapidly. Delay in treatment of these disorders by performing head CT scans and focusing on presumed intracranial events may increase morbidity and mortality.

Polyuria in a patient with hypotension following trauma suggests diabetes insipidus, diuretic use, or an osmotic diuresis from glucose, mannitol, or radiocontrast dye. The high urine SG in this patient suggested an osmotic diuresis. The elevated urine glucose and marked hyperglycemia pointed to diabetes mellitus as the cause. The marked ketosis and acidemia further indicated that the patient had diabetic ketoacidosis.

The clinical features of diabetic ketoacidosis result from hyperglycemia and ketosis. Hyperglycemia causes fluid and electrolyte losses with resultant dehydration that may result in shock. In addition, hyperglycemia interferes with organ function (especially the brain) as a result of hyperosmolality. Ketosis primarily causes problems as a result of acidosis.

Hyperglycemia and ketosis result from an imbalance between insulin and its counterregulatory hormones (glucagon, epinephrine, cortisol). Treatment is aimed at replenishing intravascular volume and electrolytes, administering insulin, and treating the underlying disease. Volume replacement reestablishes organ (liver and renal) perfusion, allowing for excretion and metabolism of glucose and ketones. In addition, volume expansion decreases counterregulatory hormone secretion. Insulin decreases hepatic glucose output and increases glucose uptake by the liver, muscle, and fat.

Total body $K+$, PO_4^{-2}, and Mg^{2+} are frequently depleted in patients with diabetic ketoacidosis and should be replaced during therapy. Total body depletion exists despite normal serum levels upon admission. Potassium is the most important electrolyte that must be replaced during treatment to avoid the possibility of life-threatening arrhythmias. Potassium decreases as a result of volume expansion, osmotic diuresis, and insulin (K+ shifts into cells). If bicarbonate is given, it also may cause an intracellular K+ shift and exacerbate hypokalemia. Acidosis is well tolerated by patients with diabetic ketoacidosis, and treatment with bicarbonate frequently leads to a rebound metabolic alkalosis, once perfusion is reestablished and insulin is given. Most authorities recommend that bicarbonate not be given unless the pH is below 7.10.

The present patient regained consciousness when the blood glucose and serum osmolality decreased towards normal. A CT of the head, performed soon after admission, was normal.

Clinical Pearls

1. Coma following head trauma may result from metabolic causes.

2. Polyuria in hypotensive patients suggests diabetes insipidus, diabetes mellitus, use of diuretics (furosemide, mannitol), or radiocontrast agents.

3. CNS dysfunction in patients with diabetic ketoacidosis correlates best with hyperosmolality.

4. Total body $K+$, PO_4^{-2}, and Mg^{2+} are usually depleted in patients with diabetic ketoacidosis despite normal serum levels on admission.

5. Acidosis in patients with diabetic ketoacidosis is usually well tolerated, and treatment with bicarbonate is frequently associated with rebound alkalosis.

REFERENCES

1. Zaloga GP, Chernow B: Insulin and oral hypoglycemics. In Chernow B, Holaday JW, Zaloga GP, Zaritsky AL (eds): The Pharmacologic Approach to the Critically Ill Patient. Baltimore, Williams and Wilkins, 1988, pp 637–658.
2. Kreisberg RA: Diabetic ketoacidosis: New concepts and trends in pathogenesis and treatment. Ann Intern Med 88:681–695, 1978.
3. Morris LR, Murphy MB, Kitabchi AE: Bicarbonate therapy in severe diabetic ketoacidosis. Ann Intern Med 105:836–840, 1986.

PATIENT 6

A 45-year-old asthmatic woman with coma

A 45-year-old woman living alone was found unresponsive in her apartment and brought to the hospital by a friend. She had a history of asthma that was usually controlled with inhaled beta-agonists. A recent asthmatic exacerbation necessitated prednisone, 40 mg daily. She had been seen 1 week earlier by her local physician who noted decreased bronchospasm at that time.

Physical Examination: Temperature 98°; pulse 112; respirations 22; blood pressure 100/80. Skin: poor turgor; dry mucous membranes; no contusions or trauma. Chest: minimal expiratory wheezes. Cardiac: rapid rate; no murmurs. Abdomen: obese. Neurologic: unresponsive to verbal stimuli; withdraws to pain, pupils equal and reactive; oculocephalic response normal; no focal abnormalities.

Laboratory Findings: Hct 48%; WBC 14,000/μl, 82% PMNs. Electrolytes: pending. ABG (room air): pH 7.45, PCO_2 34 mm Hg, PO_2 89 mm Hg. UA: SG 1.015, 4+ glucose, no protein or ketones.

What is your admitting clinical impression?

Diagnosis and Treatment: Hyperglycemic hyperosmolar nonketotic coma precipitated by glucocorticoid therapy. Treatment consists of fluid and electrolyte replacement and insulin administration. Glucocorticoids should be tapered slowly to avoid adrenal crisis.

Discussion: The major metabolic differential diagnoses that should be considered in patients presenting with coma include hypo- and hyperglycemia, drug overdose (narcotics, barbiturates), uremia, hypoxia/hypercapnia, hypo- and hypernatremia, hepatic failure, and thiamine deficiency. Hyperglycemic hyperosmolar nonketotic coma typically occurs in middle-aged or elderly non-insulin–dependent diabetics, although it occasionally may be the initial presentation of diabetes mellitus. It is frequently precipitated by comorbid conditions such as stroke, myocardial infarction, burns, trauma, surgery, infection, or intravenous hyperalimentation. Drugs that may cause the syndrome include glucocorticoids, thiazide diuretics. phenytoin, cimetidine, and propranolol.

Most patients experience polydipsia and polyuria over several days, culminating in dehydration and altered consciousness. Hyperglycemia produces an osmotic diuresis that causes volume depletion, impaired renal glucose clearance, and resultant hyperglycemia. The exact mechanism by which ketoacidosis is suppressed is unclear. Depressed CNS function may range from lethargy to coma. Transient, focal neurologic signs occur on occasion, and some patients may present with seizures. The altered sensorium parallels the hyperosmolality and requires prompt treatment. Serum osmolalities above 350 mOsm/L are usually found in patients with CNS depression.

Serum sodium concentrations are usually lowered by about 1.5 mEq/L for each 100 mg/dl increase in serum glucose above normal. When the serum sodium is not appropriately decreased, it is indicative of a relative hypernatremia and volume depletion. If insulin is given to these patients without fluid, hypotension may result as glucose (an osmotically active particle) shifts intracellularly and is followed by fluid movement, thereby depleting intravascular volume. Azotemia, hemoconcentration, and an anion gap metabolic acidosis due to lactic acid also may result from intravascular volume depletion.

Treatment is first aimed at correcting intravascular volume and reestablishing organ perfusion. Concomitant electrolyte replacement is required. Insulin is then given to treat the hyperglycemia and hyperosmolality. Cerebral and pulmonary edema may result if glucose is lowered too rapidly. The serum glucose should be lowered by no more than 100 mg/dl/hr.

The present patient presented with coma that did not appear related to trauma. The absence of focal neurologic signs suggested a metabolic/toxic encephalopathy or infection as the underlying etiology, although a CNS structural lesion could not be immediately excluded. Initial laboratory evaluation suggested hyperglycemia as the etiology; the serum glucose returned at 1600 mg/dl. A drug screen subsequently returned negative and a head CT scan was normal.

Clinical Pearls

1. Glucose abnormalities are common causes of nontraumatic coma.
2. Drugs that can precipitate hyperglycemic hyperosmolar nonketotic coma include glucocorticoids, thiazide diuretics, phenytoin, cimetidine, and propranolol.
3. Depressed sensorium correlates best with hyperosmolality; a serum osmolality > 350 mOsm/L usually is associated with depressed sensorium.
4. The serum sodium is decreased by 1.5 mEq/L for each 100 mg/dl increase in serum glucose above normal. A normal serum sodium in hyperglycemic coma suggests relative hypernatremia and volume depletion.

REFERENCES
1. Zaloga CP, Chernow B: Insulin and oral hypoglycemics. In Chernow B, Holaday JW, Zaloga GP, Zaritsky AL (eds): The Pharmacologic Approach to the Critically Ill Patient. Baltimore, Williams and Wilkins, 1988, pp 637–658.
2. Arieff AI, Carroll HJ: Nonketotic hyperosmolar coma with hyperglycemia: Clinical features, pathophysiology, renal function, acid-base balance, plasma-cerebrospinal fluid equilibria and effects of therapy in 37 cases. Medicine 51:73–94, 1972.
3. Khardori R, Soler NG: Hyperosmolar hyperglycemic nonketotic syndrome. Am J Med 77:899–904, 1984.

PATIENT 7

A 62-year-old woman with coma and hypotension

A 62-year-old woman was found unresponsive at home with a slow pulse, shallow respirations, and a low blood pressure. She was intubated by EMS, placed on oxygen, and begun on IV fluids. Her husband reported that she had been nauseated and weak over the previous week. He denied that she took any medications and stated that her appetite was diminished and her memory recently poor.

Physical Examination: Temperature 100°; pulse 56; respirations 34; blood pressure 100/76. Skin: poor turgor; no evidence of trauma. Eyes: pupils 3 mm, normal light reflex; extraocular movements intact; normal fundi. Chest: clear. Breasts: small lump in right. Cardiac: normal. Neurologic: no response to verbal stimuli; withdraws from pain; moves all extremities spontaneously; no focal signs; depressed reflexes.

Laboratory Findings: Hct 30%; WBC 12,000/μl, platelets 200,000/μl, Na+ 154 mEq/L, K+ 4.8 mEq/L, Cl$^-$ 118 mEq/L, HCO$_3^-$ 23 mEq/L, glucose 134 mg/dl, BUN 55 mg/dl, creatinine 2.0 mg/dl; Ca^{2+} 10.5 mg/dl, albumin 3.0 g/dl, PO$_4^{-2}$ 5.7 mg/dl, Mg^{2+} 1.8 mg/dl. UA: SG 1.004; dipstick and microscopic: negative. Urine drug screen: negative. ABG (room air): pH 7.47, PCO$_2$ 35 mm Hg, PO$_2$ 87 mm Hg. Head CT: normal. CSF: protein 35 mg/dl, glucose 80 mg/dl, 0 cells, Gram stain: negative.

What is the cause for the patient's unresponsiveness? What test can confirm the diagnosis?

Diagnosis: Hypercalcemia. An ionized Ca^{2+} level should be performed to confirm the diagnosis.

Discussion: The patient's presentation in coma following a prodrome of nausea, weakness, and deteriorating memory was suggestive of a toxic or metabolic encephalopathy. Although the absence of focal neurologic abnormalities supported this impression, plans were made for a head CT scan to exclude an intracranial mass or hemorrhage while laboratory studies were pending. The initial emergency evaluation considered the potential metabolic etiologies of the patient's altered sensorium. There was no history of drug ingestion, and a urine drug screen was negative. Because the patient had a low-grade fever and leukocytosis, meningitis was excluded with a lumbar puncture. Infectious encephalitis remained a diagnostic possibility; however, analysis of her admission laboratory data revealed a total serum Ca^{2+} in the upper ranges of normal despite a low serum albumin level. These findings suggested the presence of hypercalcemia; an ionized Ca^{2+} subsequently confirmed the diagnosis in that it was markedly elevated at 2.0 mM (normal 1.0–1.2).

Total serum Ca^{2+} is a poor predictor of the ionized Ca^{2+} concentration even when the effects of albumin and pH are considered. However, a Ca^{2+} in the upper normal ranges in a critically ill patient should always suggest the presence of hypercalcemia. The most common causes of hypercalcemia in a fasting patient are hyperparathyroidism and malignancy. Parathyroid hormone and 1,25-dihydroxy-vitamin D levels were measured in the present patient and found to be low, excluding hyperparathyroidism. A bone scan revealed multiple areas of increased uptake consistent with metastatic disease. A biopsy of the right breast mass noted on the admission physical examination revealed carcinoma.

The patient appeared dehydrated on admission with hypotension and poor skin turgor; paradoxically, her urine was dilute. This presentation is consistent with hypercalcemia-induced nephrogenic diabetes insipidus. The patient also had an elevated serum PO_4^{-2}, which is consistent with metastatic bone disease. Serum PO_4^{-2} is usually low or normal in patients with hyperparathyroidism.

Hypercalcemia commonly affects the neuromuscular system, causing disorientation, obtundation, coma, memory impairment, depression, psychosis, weakness, and seizures. Cardiovascular effects include hypertension, bradycardia, and arrhythmias. Calcium may also form stones within the kidney or disrupt tubular function. Anorexia, nausea, and constipation are common. Skeletal symptoms relate to direct tumor invasion (bone pain, fractures) or skeletal resorption by tumor products. The most common causes of death from hypercalcemia are renal failure, arrhythmias, and CNS effects.

The initial goal of treatment in hypercalcemia is to lower the circulating Ca^{2+} level with fluids, to increase renal Ca^{2+} excretion with diuretics, and to decrease bone resorption. Definitive treatment is directed at the underlying disease. The present patient was hydrated with normal saline, given furosemide to increase renal Ca^{2+} excretion, and treated with calcitonin to decrease bone resorption. When the ionized Ca^{2+} level continued to be elevated despite this therapy, she was treated with mithramycin to effect decreased bone resorption. Over the next few days she regained consciousness as ionized Ca^{2+} level normalized. Chemotherapy for breast cancer was instituted.

Clinical Pearls

1. Serum total Ca^{2+} is a poor predictor of the ionized Ca^{2+} concentration even when adjusted for serum albumin levels.
2. Hyperparathyroidism and malignancy are the most common causes of fasting hypercalcemia.
3. Hypercalcemia causes nephrogenic diabetes insipidus and dehydration.

REFERENCES
1. Zaloga GP, Chernow B: Divalent ions: Calcium, magnesium, and phosphorus. In Chernow B, Holaday JW, Zaloga GP, et al (eds): The Pharmacologic Approach to the Critically Ill Patient, 2nd ed. Baltimore, Williams and Wilkins, 1988, pp 603–636.
2. Zaloga GP, Chernow B, Cook D, et al: Assessment of calcium homeostasis in the critically ill patient: Diagnostic pitfalls of the McLean Hastings Nomogram. Ann Surg 202:587–594, 1985.
3. Stewart AF, Horst R, Deftos LJ, et al: Biochemical evaluation of patients with cancer-associated hypercalcemia. N Engl J Med 303:1377–1383, 1980.

PATIENT 8

A 40-year-old woman with polyuria following craniotomy

A 40-year-old woman was evaluated for chronic headaches. A head CT scan revealed a tumor in the pituitary region with suprasellar extension. She denied symptoms of endocrine deficiency, and preoperative endocrine testing demonstrated normal thyroid and adrenal function. She took no medications. Following a frontal craniotomy for removal of a craniopharyngioma, the patient developed polyuria with 150 to 200 ml of urine per hour.

Physical Examination: Temperature 97°; pulse 100; respirations 18; blood pressure 110/75 mm Hg. Chest: clear. Cardiac: normal. Neurologic: alert, oriented; no focal findings.

Laboratory Findings: Hct 42%; WBC 9,000/μl, Na+ 144 mEq/L, K+ 4.0 mEq/L, Cl− 99 mEq/L, HCO_3^- 25 mEq/L; BUN 12 mg/dl, creatinine 1.1 mg/dl, glucose 90 mg/dl. UA: SG 1.001; glucose, protein and microscopic: negative. Serum osmolality: 291 mOsm/L H_2O; urine osmolality: 80 mOsm/L H_2O. Water deprivation test: shown below.

	Urine Output (ml/hr)	Urine Osmolality (mOsm/L)	Serum Osmolality (mOsm/L)
Onset of test	200	75	292
Water deprivation	180	80	312
5U IV vasopressin	100	190	310

What is the cause of the patient's polyuria?

Diagnosis: Central diabetes insipidus.

Discussion: The concentration of solutes in the blood is usually maintained within a narrow range (285 to 290 mOsm/L), despite large fluctuations in water and solute intake. Renal free water excretion is primarily regulated by the action of antidiuretic hormone (ADH) on the collecting ducts in the kidney. ADH is synthesized in the hypothalamus and transported to and secreted by the posterior pituitary. Surgery on or close to the pituitary gland, as in the present patient, can interfere with ADH secretion and cause DI.

Polyuria has multiple causes and it is important to determine the specific etiology, so that appropriate treatment can be given. In polyuria resulting from excessive water intake, ADH secretion is suppressed in an attempt to excrete the excess fluid. These patients develop polyuria with a maximally dilute urine (< 100 mOsm/L) but do not develop hypotension. Serum sodium remains normal and results of water deprivation testing are normal.

Hypothalamic-neurohypophyseal lesions may interfere with ADH secretion and cause central diabetes insipidus (DI). These patients continue to produce dilute urine despite volume depletion, develop hypernatremia, and demonstrate an abnormal water deprivation test. They respond appropriately, however, to exogenous ADH.

Polyuria also may result from reduced renal responsiveness to ADH (nephrogenic DI). This disorder may occur secondary to adverse reactions from drugs, such as amphotericin B, lithium, and demeclocycline. Other causes include hypercalcemia, hypokalemia, primary renal disease, and renal medullary washout. These patients continue to produce dilute urine despite volume depletion, develop hypernatremia, and have an abnormal water deprivation test. They do not, however, respond appropriately to exogenous ADH. Finally, polyuria may result from diuretic agents (osmotic agents, loop diuretics). Osmotic diuresis produces concentrated urine and may result from glucose, mannitol, or radiocontrast dyes.

The standard test for evaluating patients for DI is the water deprivation test. Fluids are withheld until serum osmolality increases into the hyperosmolar range (> 310 mOsm/L), such that ADH secretion is stimulated maximally. The patient then is given 5U of aqueous vasopressin intravenously and urine and serum osmolalities are obtained hourly. Patients with normal neurohypophyseal function and patients with excess water intake achieve a urine osmolality that is greater than serum osmolality at the end of water deprivation. Urine osmolality in these patients does not increase more than 5% after vasopressin injection. Patients with complete central DI have a urine osmolality less than serum osmolality following water deprivation and their urine osmolality increases more than 50% after vasopressin. In patients with partial central DI, urine osmolality can increase above serum osmolality following water deprivation but it also increases more than 9% after vasopressin. In contrast, patients with nephrogenic DI have a urine osmolality less than serum osmolality after water deprivation and it fails to increase above serum osmolality with vasopressin.

In the present patient, the lack of an increase in urine osmolality following water deprivation and the significant increase (138%) in urine osmolality after vasopressin indicate the presence of central DI. Although the urine remained hypotonic, it represented a significant increase in urine osmolality. Urine osmolality may not reach higher levels due to renal medullary washout from polyuria.

Central DI is most effectively treated with DDAVP (1-desamino-8-D-arginine-vasopressin), intravenously or intranasally. This agent has little vasopressor activity, unlike arginine vasopressin.

Clinical Pearls

1. Postoperative polyuria may result from DI, excess water intake during surgery, or osmotic and loop diuretics.
2. Polyuria from osmotic agents produces concentrated urine.
3. Normal postoperative diuresis alone does not cause hypotension or hypernatremia, and there is a normal response to water deprivation.
4. Amphotericin B, lithium, hypercalcemia, and hypokalemia may cause nephrogenic DI.

REFERENCES

1. Chernow B, Wiley SC, Zaloga GP: Critical care endocrinology. In Shoemaker WC, et al (eds): Textbook of Critical Care, 2nd ed. Philadelphia, W.B. Saunders, 1989, pp 736–766.
2. Balestrieri FJ, Chernow B, Rainey TG: Postcraniotomy diabetes insipidus. Crit Care Med 10:108–110, 1982.
3. Miller M, Dalakos T, Moses AM, et al: Recognition of partial defects in antidiuretic hormone secretion. Ann Intern Med 73:721–729, 1970.

CHAPTER 8

Neurology

Jerome E. Kurent, M.D.

PATIENT 1

A 53-year-old woman with recurrent, generalized tonic-clonic seizures

A 53-year-old woman with a previously well-controlled seizure disorder developed recurrent, generalized tonic-clonic seizures. She had been taking phenytoin, 300 mg daily, with recent serum levels ranging from 15 to 20 μg/ml.

Physical Examination: Temperature 100.8°; pulse 110; respirations 28; blood pressure 150/96. Neurologic: cranial nerves II to XII intact; no focal motor findings; Babinski sign present bilaterally; unresponsive with frequent generalized tonic-clonic seizures lasting 2 to 5 minutes.

Laboratory Findings: Hct 34%; WBC 11,300; Na+ 141 mEq/L, Ca^{2+} 9.1 mg/dl, Mg^{2+} 2 mg/dl; BUN, creatinine, and glucose: normal. Toxin screen: negative. Serum phenytoin level: 0 μg/ml. Head CT: cortical atrophy with mildly enlarged ventricles. Chest radiograph: normal. ECG: normal. Lumbar puncture: normal opening pressure, RBC 1/μl, WBC 8/μl (mononuclears), protein 60 mg/dl, glucose 74 mg/dl, negative stains and cultures, India ink negative, cryptococcal antigen negative.

*Hospital Course:*The patient was intubated and mechanically ventilated. She was treated with IV diazepam 10 mg and IV phenytoin 1200 mg at 50 mg/min. She was subsequently given 1000 mg of IV phenobarbital for continued intermittent seizures. Major motor activity subsided, but the patient remained unresponsive 24 hours later. Serum phenytoin level: 22 μg/ml; phenobarbital level: 34 μg/ml.

What is the most likely explanation for the patient's failure to regain consciousness by 24 hours?

Diagnosis: Refractory status epilepticus with electrical status. Coma due to toxic levels of phenobarbital.

Discussion: Many patients who present in status epilepticus have a known seizure disorder and have stopped taking their anticonvulsant medications. In the acute management of such patients, therefore, anticonvulsants should be urgently administered on the assumption that drug levels are low or absent. Serum levels should be determined as soon as possible, however, for diagnosis and assistance with seizure control.

Provision of a patent airway and adequate oxygenation is the initial step in management of status epilepticus. Emergency drugs include IV diazepam, phenytoin, and barbiturates for seizure control and a bolus of 50% glucose with thiamine for the possibilities of hypoglycemia with incipient Wernicke-Korsakoff syndrome. Indicated blood studies include routine chemistries with calcium and magnesium, CBC, serum anticonvulsant levels, and toxicology screens. The administration of 5 to 10 mg of IV diazepam in the adult usually will suppress seizure activity. The control may be short-lived, however, requiring definitive anticonvulsant therapy with IV phenytoin at a rate not exceeding 50 mg/min and blood pressure and ECG monitoring. If seizure activity continues, phenobarbital should be given. If hypotension occurs, phenobarbital can be held temporarily until the blood pressure returns to baseline. Patients with status receiving aggressive barbiturate therapy should be intubated in anticipation of respiratory depression.

If refractory status epilepticus continues after initial treatment, other therapeutic alternatives should be considered. Additional IV barbiturates may be given, placing the patient in barbiturate coma. Some authorities recommend inducing coma with IV pentobarbital in preference to phenobarbital because of its shorter half-life.

Major motor activity usually will subside during barbiturate coma. Rarely, general anesthesia may be necessary. Even though control of clinical major motor activity is accomplished, the patient may still be in electrical status as demonstrated by EEG. Electrical status represents an unacceptable metabolic stress to neurons and can result in irreversible neuronal damage. Despite the absence of motor expression of seizure activity, these patients require aggressive anticonvulsant therapy.

Patients developing new onset seizures within the first 7 days of head injury (posttraumatic seizures) and after 7 days (delayed posttraumatic) represent a special situation. Up to 30% of patients will develop intractable seizures that are drug-resistant. Fortunately, most instances of posttraumatic seizures do not persist, although anti-seizure medications should be continued for 2 years. Delayed posttraumatic seizure disorders are more likely to become chronic. Risk factors after trauma for seizures include posttraumatic amnesia > 24 hours, dural tear, depressed skull fracture, and focal neurologic signs. Patients presenting with two or more of these clinical features should receive prophylactic anti-seizure medications.

In the present patient, an EEG after therapeutic blood levels were reached showed frequent generalized bursts of spike and slow wave activity. Additional IV phenobarbital under EEG monitoring resolved this abnormal pattern, although the patient remained in coma with a serum phenobarbital level of 47 μg/ml. The patient regained consciousness several days later when the serum phenobarbital concentration decreased to 22 μg/ml. Additional history from family members indicated that the patient had stopped taking her phenytoin "a few days ago" because of viral gastroenteritis.

Clinical Pearls

1. Electrical status epilepticus can exist in the absence of major motor clinical seizure activity and represents unacceptable metabolic stress on cerebral neurons. Prompt, aggressive therapy, such as barbiturate coma, is indicated in electrical status.

2. Refractory status epilepticus associated with recently acquired structural brain lesions, such as stroke or hematoma, may be especially difficult to treat and may necessitate barbiturate coma.

3. Patients with status epilepticus may demonstrate minimal CSF pleiocytosis and protein elevation, which require the exclusion of other causes before attributing them to status epilepticus.

REFERENCES

1. Amit R, Goitein KJ, Mathot I, et al: Prolonged electro-cerebral silent barbiturate coma in intractable seizure disorders. Epilepsia 29:63–66, 1988.
2. Fishman BA: Cerebrospinal Fluid Findings in Diseases of the Nervous System. Philadelphia, W.B. Saunders, 1980.
3. Rashkin MC, Youngs C, Penovich P: Pentobarbital treatment of refractory status epilepticus. Neurology 37:500–507, 1987.

PATIENT 2

A 47-year-old man with new-onset seizures and obtundation

A 47-year-old man with a history of chronic alcohol abuse was admitted following the new onset of recurrent tonic-clonic seizures. He reportedly had not drunk alcohol during the previous 4 months. There was no history of recent head trauma.

Physical Examination: Temperature 98.4°; pulse 90; respirations 26; blood pressure 140/90. Eyes: pupils equal and reactive; fundi normal. HEENT: normal. Neurologic: unresponsive to painful stimuli; corneal and gag reflexes present bilaterally; deep tendon reflexes symmetric: no focal findings.

Laboratory Findings: Hct 42%; WBC 11,300/μl, 81% PMNs, 0 bands. Na+ 139 mEq/L, Ca^{2+} 8.9 mg/dl, Mg^{2+} 2.5 mg/dl; BUN 8 mg/dl, creatinine 0.7 mg/dl, glucose 116 mg/dl. Liver function tests: normal. RPR: negative. Chest radiograph: cardiomegaly with normal lung fields. ECG: normal. Head CT scan with contrast: moderate cortical atrophy. Lumbar puncture: opening pressure 140 mm H_2O, 3 mononuclear cells/μl, protein 50 g/dl, glucose 66 mg/dl. Gram and AFB stain negative; India ink preparation negative.

Hospital Course: The patient was given IV thiamine and phenytoin with prompt resolution of seizure activity. Mental status improved slowly, although he remained confused for several days after his last seizure despite therapeutic serum phenytoin levels.

Based on the CSF findings, has chronic CNS infection been excluded?

Diagnosis: Cryptococcal meningitis.

Discussion: *Cryptococcus neoformans* is an important cause of chronic meningitis. Although negative in this patient, the preliminary diagnosis is often made by a positive India ink preparation performed on CSF (below).

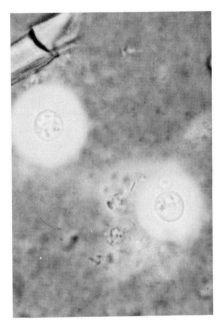

A more sensitive diagnostic test, however, is Latex agglutination for cryptococcal antigen. This test may be positive before CSF pleiocytosis occurs and even when India ink and CSF cultures are negative. The presence of cryptococcus is confirmed by growth on Sabouraud's or chocolate agar culture medium; identification usually requires 4 to 7 days.

Classic forms of cryptococcal infection include pneumonia and disseminated disease in addition to meningitis. Patients without underlying immunocompromise may develop cryptococcal pneumonia that may simulate bacterial pneumonia or pulmonary infarction with hemoptysis, fever, and pleuritic chest pain. In previously normal hosts, the natural history of cryptococcal pneumonia is spontaneous recovery and chemotherapy is, therefore, not required. Immunocompromised hosts, however, usually rapidly develop meningitis and require amphotericin B therapy. Disseminated disease is particularly common in AIDS patients and may not respond to therapy or may recur when therapy is discontinued. Although cryptococcal meningitis is usually associated with defective T-cell immunity, some studies indicate that up to 50% of patients will not have any clinically detectable underlying disease.

Patients with cryptococcal meningitis may present with headaches often associated with impaired mental status, nausea, vomiting, and neck stiffness. Less commonly, visual complaints such as diplopia or photophobia, papilledema, and seizures may occur. As in the present patient, cryptococcal meningitis may not be suspected early in the clinical course. If untreated, cryptococcal meningitis is fatal.

Typical CSF findings in cryptococcal meningitis include elevated protein and low glucose concentrations and a mononuclear pleiocytosis. The India ink preparation is positive in approximately 60% of patients. In the present patient, the relatively benign nature of the preliminary CSF findings emphasizes the importance of obtaining cryptococcal antigen and sending CSF for culture either to establish or exclude the diagnosis of cryptococcal meningitis. Recurrent cryptococcal meningitis may occur in patients who appear to have been treated successfully with appropriate antifungal therapy.

Cryptococcal meningitis is treated with combination therapy that includes amphotericin B and flucytosine for 6 weeks. This regimen is effective but associated with frequent adverse reactions that include renal insufficiency and bone marrow suppression.

The present patient was treated with IV amphotericin B and flucytosine. One week later, the patient's mental status improved. Following completion of therapy, reexamination of the CSF was negative for cryptococcal antigen as well as for growth of cryptococcus.

Clinical Pearls

1. Any patient with altered mental status of uncertain etiology should be evaluated for cryptococcal meningitis with India ink staining, Latex agglutination for cryptococcal antigen, and culture of the CSF.

2. Although commonly associated with defective cell-mediated immunity, many patients with cryptococcal meningitis have no apparent underlying disease.

3. Cryptococcal meningitis may recur after a long period of apparent cure.

REFERENCES

1. DeWytt CN, Dickson PL, Holt GW: Cryptococcal meningitis: A review of 32 years experience. J Neurol Sci 53:283–292, 1982.
2. Diamond RD, Bennett JE: Prognosis factor in cryptococcal meningitis: A study of 111 cases. Ann Intern Med 80:176–181, 1974.
3. Sabetta JR, Andriole VT: Cryptococcal infection of the central nervous system. Med Clin North Am 69:333–344, 1985.

PATIENT 3

A 23-year-old woman with slowly progressive respiratory failure

A 23-year-old woman developed progressive dyspnea several days following an upper respiratory tract infection. She was intubated in a community hospital and transferred for further care. Four years earlier myasthenia gravis had been diagnosed, and the patient was started on a medical regimen with which she was noncompliant.

Physical Examination: Temperature 100.2°; pulse 96; respirations 20; blood pressure 100/70. Chest: diffuse rhonchi. Neurologic: awake and alert; mild bilateral ptosis; bilateral facial weakness; proximal upper and lower motor strength 4/5; distal motor strength 5/5; deep tendon reflexes 2+; Babinski sign absent, sensory examination normal.

Laboratory Findings: Hct 39%; WBC 8,400/μl. Electrolytes, BUN, and glucose: normal. Serum assay for anti-acetylcholine receptor antibody: 4.8 (normal < 0.5). FVC: 700 ml. ABG (ventilator FiO_2 0.5): pH 7.44, PCO_2 35 mm Hg, PO_2 140 mm Hg. Chest radiography: no acute infiltrates. Sputum: normal flora.

Hospital Course: The patient was given IV edrophonium and saline in a double-blind fashion with subjective and objective improvement in muscle strength only after edrophonium. She was treated with prednisone, 100 mg q.d., without improvement after one week.

What further therapeutic option should be considered?

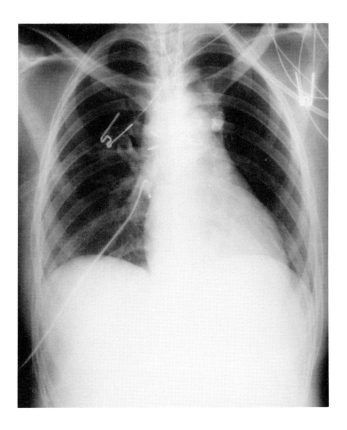

Diagnosis: Myasthenia gravis with respiratory failure. Additional therapy includes plasma exchange.

Discussion: Myasthenia gravis, an acquired autoimmune disease, is characterized by exercise-induced muscle fatigue that resolves after rest. The pathogenesis results from antibody destruction of muscle acetylcholine receptor sites, making acetylcholine binding ineffectual. Circulating acetylcholine receptor antibodies are found in 80 to 90% of patients, although there is no absolute correlation between acetylcholine receptor antibody titer and clinical severity of disease. The peak incidence is in the third decade in females and the sixth and seventh decades in males, with the disease being slightly more common in females. The diagnosis is confirmed by response to anticholinesterase drugs.

Patients with myasthenia gravis require intensive ICU management during myasthenic or cholinergic crises and following thymectomy. A myasthenic crisis frequently is exacerbated by infection but can also occur without apparent cause. Despite increased doses of anticholinesterase drugs, respiratory failure can ensue, requiring intubation and mechanical ventilation. In general, a progressive decrease in forced vital capacity is noted; when the FVC decreases to less than 15 ml/kg, respiratory support is usually necessary. It is recommended that the decision for intubation be made before the development of hypercapnia to avoid an emergent procedure. Potential neuromuscular blocking drugs, such as morphine, aminoglycoside antibiotics, procainamide, quinidine, and tetracycline, should be avoided in impending myasthenic crisis.

Anticholinesterase drugs administered at toxic levels can cause cholinergic crisis, resulting in respiratory failure. The nicotinic action of the anticholinesterase drugs paradoxically produces profound, generalized weakness and bronchoconstriction, and the muscarinic effects produce excess respiratory secretions. Anticholinesterase therapy should be withheld and ventilatory support maintained until the patient stabilizes.

Plasma exchange has been documented to be effective adjunctive therapy in patients with severe myasthenia gravis. Plasmapheresis can provide transient clinical improvement in patients with impending or actual respiratory failure. It may also avoid a crisis in those with severe muscle weakness and may be beneficial in preparing the patient for thymectomy. Plasma exchange can be implemented without interfering with the respiratory care of the patient in crisis. Muscle strength usually improves within 48 hours following the first plasmapheresis. Progressive improvement generally follows subsequent exchanges.

Plasma exchange can be performed at the bedside with an antecubital or femoral vein utilized for vascular access and a smaller vein for return of packed red cells, albumin, potassium and magnesium. Fifty milliliters of plasma/kg body weight is removed and replaced, providing an exchange of 60 to 70% of the total plasma volume. The risk of hepatitis and AIDS is avoided by using albumin rather than pooled plasma as the replacement fluid. Plasma exchange in myasthenia gravis is not used as the primary therapeutic modality. Improvement following plasma exchange appears to be limited to a period no longer than 12 weeks.

The present patient was treated with plasma exchange and was able to be weaned from mechanical ventilation over the next 7 days. She was maintained on pyridostigmine, and prednisone was tapered.

Clinical Pearls

1. Patients with myasthenia gravis requiring ICU care include those in myasthenic or cholinergic crisis and those in the postoperative period following thymectomy. Mechanical ventilation has dramatically reduced the morbidity and mortality of the condition.

2. When the FVC gradually decreases to less than 15 ml/kg body weight, intubation and mechanical ventilation are usually necessary.

3. Plasma exchange has been shown to be an effective adjunct in the management of patients with severe myasthenia gravis. It has been successful in avoiding mechanical ventilation and preventing long-term mechanical ventilation. Improvement in muscle strength generally is seen within 48 hours of the first plasma exchange, with subsequent improvement with further exchanges.

REFERENCES

1. Engel AG: Myasthenia gravis and myasthenic syndrome. Ann Neurol 16:519–534, 1984.
2. Olarte MR, Schoenfeldt RS, Penn AS, et al: The effect of plasmapheresis in myasthenia gravis 1978–1980. Ann NY Acad Sci 377:725–728, 1981.
3. Perlo VP: Treatment of the critically ill patient with myasthenia. In Ropper AH, Kennedy SF (eds): Neurological and Neurosurgical Intensive Care, 2nd ed. Rockville, MD, Aspen Publishers, Inc., 1988.

PATIENT 4

A 52-year-old man with hypertension, headache, and lethargy

A 52-year-old man with chronic hypertension presented with a 2-day history of dull headache and progressive lethargy. His family initially thought that he had "the flu."

Physical Examination: Temperature 98.8°; pulse 86; respirations 20; blood pressure 164/100. The patient was lethargic but oriented with dysarthric speech. Neck: supple. Eyes: pupils meiotic with anisocoria (right 1 mm smaller than left); reactive to light and accommodation; fundi normal except for a-v nicking. Neurologic: extraocular movements normal; minimal right upper and lower facial weakness; fine motor coordination impaired; rapid alternating movements mildly dysrhythmic (right > left); appendicular and gait ataxia. Sensory examination: normal.

Laboratory Findings: Hct 42%, WBC 11,200/μl. Technetium brain scan: interpreted as normal at referring hospital. Lumbar puncture (from outlying hospital): normal opening pressure; trace xanthochromia; 13 RBC/μl, 3 WBC/μl (mononuclears), Gram stain, AFB stain and India ink preparation: negative. EEG: mild diffuse theta slowing.

Hospital Course: Following transfer, the patient had a head CT scan (below). Posterior fossa angiography was normal. Over the first 24 hours following admission, the patient became more difficult to arouse.

What is the most likely diagnosis, and what is the most appropriate management?

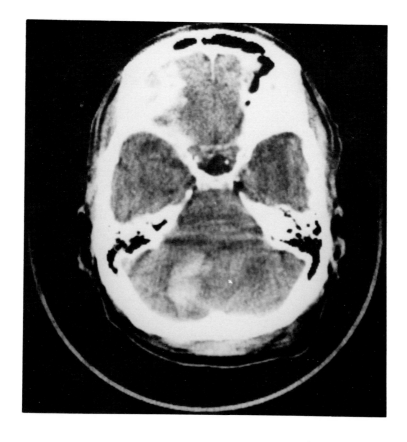

Diagnosis: Hypertensive cerebellar hemorrhage.

Discussion: Chronic hypertension causes numerous vascular disorders in end organs, but none is more lethal or dramatic in onset as hypertensive intracerebral hemorrhage. Despite a decrease in incidence of stroke in the general population, brain hemorrhage continues to contribute to morbidity and mortality in 60,000 persons in the United States each year.

Patients typically first develop symptoms while awake, with the onset of hemorrhage often occurring after exertion from attendant increases in systemic blood pressure. Onset of a severe headache is typically abrupt, although this symptom may be minor or absent in up to 50% of patients. At presentation, patients are almost always hypertensive. The absence of hypertension in a patient with an acute intracranial event markedly decreases the probability of hypertensive intracerebral hemorrhage and suggests an alternate diagnosis.

Hypertensive hemorrhage occurs most commonly in deep cerebral structures, such as the putamen thalamus, and caudate. Hemorrhages occur less commonly in the frontal lobe, pons, and cerebellum. Initial signs may localize the likely site of hemorrhage, although rapid development of false localizing signs due to expanding hemorrhage with compression of the upper midbrain may occur.

Most cerebellar hemorrhages are associated with chronic hypertension. Less common causes include arteriovenous malformation, ruptured aneurysm, anticoagulation, blood dyscrasias, neoplasms, and trauma. The onset of acute cerebellar hemorrhage is usually dramatic, with severe headache, nausea, vomiting, appendicular and gait ataxia with variable cranial nerve abnormalities. However, patients with subacute cerebellar hemorrhage may present with nonspecific complaints, including headache, dizziness, and lethargy. Loss of consciousness at the onset is uncommon, although progression to coma occurs in 90% of patients within the first 24 hours.

Objective neurologic deficits in cerebellar hemorrhage may be subtle and consist of mild pupillary asymmetry, ipsilateral peripheral seventh nerve paresis, and ipsilateral nystagmus. Pupils are usually meiotic, remaining reactive even to coma. Although appendicular ataxia may not be present, a broad-based ataxic gait may be a valuable clue to the presence of intracranial pathology.

A patient suspected of having cerebellar hemorrhage should have an emergency CT head scan. Technetium brain scans are unreliable and are of little value in detecting pathology in the posterior fossa. MR scans are less sensitive than CT in detecting blood during the first 3 days. Lumbar puncture is contraindicated in patients with known or suspected cerebellar hemorrhage because of the risk of brain herniation. Neurosurgical consultation should be obtained promptly for patients with cerebellar hemorrhage. If the patient continues to deteriorate or if the hematoma is larger than 3 cm in size, emergency surgery is indicated. Smaller hematomas may be observed if the patient demonstrates no evidence of progression of hemorrhage or brainstem compression.

Initial management of the patient with hypertensive intracerebral hemorrhage requires urgent stabilization. Electrolyte and coagulation abnormalities should be corrected, and the patient should be fluid-restricted. The value of corticosteroids in this setting is debatable. The patient should be intubated with an endotracheal tube, as lethargy or coma increases the risk of aspiration or airway obstruction. Intubation should follow sedation and intravenous lidocaine to prevent stimulation that raises intracranial pressure causing recurrent hemorrhage. The degree of blood pressure control is controversial. Because most patients are hypertensive on presentation, blood pressure should probably be controlled to a systolic value of 160 mm Hg with intravenous vasodilators such as nitroglycerin or nitroprusside with a beta-blocker.

The present patient was taken to the operating room, and a cerebellar hematoma was removed. Postoperatively, the patient demonstrated return of mental status to baseline but retained an ataxic gait.

Clinical Pearls

1. Most cerebellar hemorrhages are associated with chronic hypertension. A constant finding in cerebellar hemorrhage is difficulty standing or walking.

2. Patients with subacute cerebellar hemorrhage may present with vague, nonspecific symptoms and minimal neurologic deficits. The recognition of truncal and gait ataxia may be valuable clues to the presence of posterior fossa pathology when other signs are subtle or absent.

3. The clinical course in cerebellar hemorrhage is difficult to predict. A stable patient with minimal neurologic deficits may deteriorate abruptly to coma and death without warning.

4. In contrast to most patients with hypertensive basal ganglia hemorrhages, neurosurgical intervention with hypertensive cerebellar hemorrhages may minimize morbidity and prevent mortality.

REFERENCES

1. Heros RC: Cerebellar hemorrhage and infarction. Stroke 13:106–109, 1982.
2. Little JR, Tubman DE, Ethier R: Cerebellar hemorrhage in adults: Diagnosis by computerized tomography. J Neurosurg 48:575–579, 1978.
3. Ott KH, Kase CS, Ojemann RG, et al: Cerebellar hemorrhage: Diagnosis and treatment. Arch Neurol 31:160–167, 1974.

PATIENT 5

A 21-year-old man with headache, facial pain and nasal discharge

A 21-year-old man presented with a five-day history of headache, right facial pain, periorbital edema, and nasal discharge. He had a history of "sinusitis" and had recently been treated with oral ampicillin for sinusitis.

Physical Examination: Temperature 101.4°; pulse 100; respirations 22; blood pressure 130/84. Eyes: right periorbital edema. ENT: purulent right nasal discharge; percussion tenderness over the frontal sinuses. Neurologic: lethargic; neck supple; no focal findings.

Laboratory Findings: Hct 42%; WBC 21,500/μl 95 PMNs. Serum chemistries: normal. Chest radiograph: normal. Head CT scan: pansinusitis with air-fluid levels.

Hospital Course: The patient was treated with nafcillin and chloramphenicol. Bifrontal sinus trephination with right external ethmoidectomy and sphenoid cannulation was accomplished with drainage of purulent fluid. Gram stain showed numerous PMNs and gram-positive cocci in chains. Antibiotics were continued and the patient improved over the first 4 days following surgery. Over the subsequent 2 days, however, his headache worsened, he became more lethargic, and his temperature increased to 102.4° F. A contrast head CT scan was obtained (below).

What is the most likely cause for the patient's clinical deterioration?

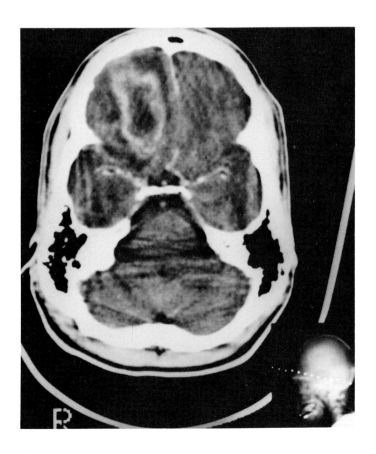

Diagnosis: Right frontal lobe brain abscess.

Discussion: Brain abscesses usually occur from direct extension of a parameningeal infection such as the sinus cavities, ear, or soft tissues around the face. The frontal and sphenoid sinuses are commonly implicated. A smaller percentage of brain abscesses are metastatic, with the source of infection being lungs (bronchiectasis, empyema, lung abscess) or heart (congenital right-to-left shunts). Less frequently, infection originates from a tooth abscess, infections of the skin or pelvic organs, or osteomyelitis. At times, the source of the abscess cannot be demonstrated.

Bacteria commonly associated with brain abscess include the anaerobic and microaerophilic streptococci. These organisms may occur alone or with diphtheroids and Bacteroides species. *Staphylococcus aureus* is frequently found in the brain abscess associated with penetrating head trauma, postcraniotomy, and bacteremia. The diagnosis can be made presumptively by contrasted CT scanning where the lesions often appear as ring-enhancing. When an initial CT scan is negative but suspicion remains, a radionucleotide brain scan or a repeat CT scan 48 to 72 hours later should be performed. Nuclear magnetic resonance head scanning also is a sensitive means of detecting brain abscess.

The clinical presentation of brain abscess varies from an indolent course with low-grade fever to acute toxicity simulating bacterial meningitis. Additional clinical features depend considerably on the anatomic location of the abscess. Frontal lobe infection may cause headache, impaired levels of consciousness, or focal and generalized seizures. In cerebellar abscesses, headache may be suboccipital and associated with nystagmus or cerebellar ataxia. The clinical course of brain abscess can be unpredictable, with symptoms evolving rapidly even in patients who appear stable. Brain abscesses may be multiple, particularly with a metastatic origin of infection, and have the least satisfactory outcome.

Urgent initiation of antibiotics and acquisition of culture specimens are the initial therapeutic approaches to brain abscess. Brain swelling usually necessitates delay of definitive surgical drainage of the abscess and may require brief courses of corticosteroids. Recently, CT-guided percutaneous needle aspiration of pus has obviated the need for craniotomy in many instances. Because of the fastidious nature of organisms causing brain abscess, isolation rates are often less than 50%. In patients with previous or concurrent antibiotic therapy for sinusitis or pneumonia, the isolation rate is significantly less. Patients require completion of at least a 4-week course of antibiotics, with longer treatment courses if the abscess cannot be excised.

Lumbar puncture is contraindicated in any patient suspected of having brain abscess because of the risk of herniation or intraventricular extension of the abscess. However, when lumbar puncture has been performed in patients with brain abscess, CSF usually is nondiagnostic. There may be a mild pleiocytosis or protein elevation, but organisms are seldom recovered.

The present patient had a CT-guided percutaneous needle aspiration of the right frontal brain abscess with removal of 10 ml of purulent fluid. Gram stain demonstrated PMNs and occasional gram-positive cocci in chains. He was treated with intravenous cefotaxime and metronidazole with a good result.

Clinical Pearls

1. Sinusitis and infections of the nasal cavity are a major cause of brain abscesses. Frontal and sphenoid sinusitis are most commonly implicated.

2. Maximal improvement in therapy of brain abscess occurs in patients treated with combined antimicrobial therapy and abscess drainage.

3. CT-guided needle aspiration of brain abscess can be effective for drainage and avoid the need for craniotomy.

REFERENCES
1. Chandrasekar PH, Kannangara DW, et al: Metronidazole therapy in brain abscess. Infect Surg, December: 927–930, 1983.
2. Garvey G: Current concepts of bacterial infections of the central nervous system: Bacterial meningitis and brain abscess. J Neurosurg 59:735–744, 1983.
3. Britt RH, Enzmann DR: Clinical stages of human brain abscesses on serial CT scans after contrast infusion: Computerized tomographic, neuropathological, and clinical correlations. J Neurosurg 59:972–989, 1983.

PATIENT 6

A 42-year-old man with progressive left-sided weakness, numbness, and ataxic gait

A 42-year-old man in previously good health was admitted with a 3-month history of progressive left-sided weakness, numbness, and gait ataxia.

Physical Examination: Temperature 98.6°; pulse 84; respirations 20; blood pressure 156/90. Neurologic: alert and oriented, pupils 2 mm equal and reactive; right sixth nerve palsy with intact facial strength; minimal left hemiparesis; decreased pin and light touch over the left side of the body excluding the face; mild ataxia of left upper extremity and a broad-based unsteady gait; DTR 3+ and symmetric; Babinski sign negative.

Laboratory Findings: Hct 42%; WBC 9,600/μl. Electrolytes, BUN and glucose: normal. Chest radiograph: normal. PPD: 18 mm induration. Heat CT with contrast: below. Lumbar puncture: opening pressure 160 mm H_2O, protein 73 mg/dl, glucose 52 g/dl, 4 WBC/μl (2 PMNs, 2 mononuclears), RBC 5/μl. Gram stain, India ink, and AFB stains: negative.

What diagnostic procedure would you recommend for this patient?

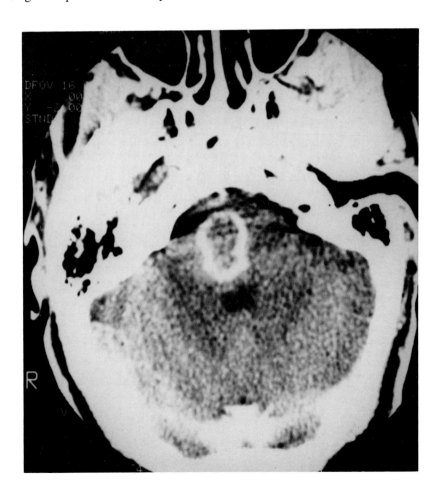

Diagnosis: Brainstem tuberculoma diagnosed at craniotomy.

Discussion: Intracranial tuberculomas are rarely encountered in the United States. The incidence in developed countries is approximately 0.15% of all intracranial space-occupying lesions; however, an incidence approaching 30% has been reported in developing countries. Tuberculoma may occur in any part of the brain but most commonly develops in the posterior fossa, especially in children. A past history of tuberculosis or evidence of tuberculosis outside of the CNS is found in only 30 to 50% of patients.

Signs and symptoms of intracranial tuberculoma are primarily related to local compression of adjacent cerebral structures from mass effect with attendant focal neurologic dysfunction, including cranial nerve and focal motor deficits. Nonlocalizing symptoms include headaches, seizures, confusion, and meningismus. Evidence of raised intracranial pressure presents an urgent situation requiring rapid diagnosis and therapy. Some patients may have systemic symptoms, such as fever, night sweats, and weight loss in the setting of a pulmonary infiltrate compatible with tuberculosis. Interestingly, onset of symptoms from a tuberculoma during the course of treatment or months to years after therapy for pulmonary tuberculosis is a reported scenario in developing countries.

Lumbar puncture demonstrates CSF with increased protein and minimal pleiocytosis if the lesion is contiguous to the meninges. Head CT scan frequently demonstrates a ring-enhancing lesion with central hypodensity. Without contrast, the lesion may be isodense and, thus, difficult to detect. The differential diagnosis based on the head CT includes primary brain tumor, metastatic carcinoma, lymphoma, abscess, parasitic cyst, and cerebral sarcoidosis.

Medical therapy of intracranial tuberculoma consists of a two- or three-drug regimen for 9 months. Treatment may be supplemented with corticosteroids if there is significant edema associated with the intracranial tuberculoma. Neurosurgical exploration may be indicated if the etiology of the space-occupying lesion is uncertain or if there is failure of medical therapy. Failure to diagnose intracranial tuberculoma may be associated with a fatal outcome. Successful therapy is usually associated with progressive shrinkage of the lesion, but paradoxical expansion of intracranial tuberculoma during treatment, while other manifestations of disease are improving, has been reported.

The patient underwent a suboccipital craniotomy with exploration of the posterior fossa and biopsy of the brainstem lesion. The tissue was negative for neoplasm but stained positive for AFB. The biopsy subsequently grew *Mycobacterium tuberculosis.* The patient was treated with rifampin, INH, and pyrazinamide. Over the following months, he demonstrated slow improvement of the left hemiparesis and ataxia. The right sixth nerve paresis persisted. Serial head CT scans over the following year showed progressive decrease in the size of the lesion.

Clinical Pearls

1. A history of tuberculosis or evidence of tuberculosis outside the CNS is often absent in patients with intracranial tuberculoma.

2. Although a presumptive diagnosis of intracranial tuberculoma can be made in the appropriate clinical setting, there are no conclusive diagnostic features that clearly differentiate intracranial tuberculoma from other lesions, such as malignancy.

3. Small- to medium-sized intracranial tuberculomas (< 2 cm in diameter) may respond to medical therapy alone. Larger lesions may require neurosurgical intervention for resolution.

REFERENCES
1. Chambers ST, Hendrickse WA, Record C, et al: Paradoxical expansion of intracranial tuberculomas during chemotherapy. Lancet 2:181–184, 1984.
2. Hilderbrand TB, Agnoli AL: Differential diagnosis and therapy of intracerebral tuberculomas. J Neurol 228:201–208, 1982.
3. Teoh R, Humphries MJ, O'Mahony G: Symptomatic intracranial tuberculoma developing during treatment of tuberculosis: A report of 10 patients and review of the literature. Q J Med 63:449–460, 1987.

CHAPTER 9

Ethics

Thomas A. Raffin, M.D.

PATIENT 1

A 68-year-old woman with the adult respiratory distress syndrome and ventilator dependency for 6 weeks

A 68-year-old woman underwent her second coronary artery bypass graft surgery. Following surgery she became septic and developed the adult respiratory distress syndrome with subsequent renal failure. She had been ventilator-dependent for 6 weeks and had required continued vasopressor support and frequent hemodialysis. Her mental status had progressively deteriorated, and the neurologist believed she had suffered numerous small cerebral infarcts. The cardiac surgeons asked for a consultation to determine what new therapies might be helpful.

Physical Examination: Temperature 100.2°; minute ventilation 16 L; peak inspiratory pressure 64 cm H_2O. Critically ill appearing woman. Chest: diffuse rales. Extremities: pedal edema; acrocyanosis of fingers and toes. Neurologic: responds only to painful stimuli.

Laboratory Findings: Hct 28%; WBC 14,600/μl, 82% PMNs; BUN 78 mg/dl, creatinine 7.2 mg/dl. ABG (FiO$_2$ 0.7): pH 7.43, PCO$_2$ 47 mm Hg, PO$_2$ 64 mm Hg. Chest radiograph: severe bilateral alveolar-interstitial infiltrates.

What is your assessment of the patient's clinical status and what recommendations should be made?

Diagnosis: Critically ill patient on long-term mechanical ventilation with essentially no chance to regain a reasonable quality of life.

Discussion: After careful examination of the patient and discussion with the family, the consultant realized that this patient had essentially no chance to regain a reasonable quality of life. Therefore, the task was to communicate this dismal prognosis to the cardiac surgeons and to determine whether they desired the consultant to assist in discussing possible plans with the family. Because the present patient was comatose and legally incompetent, she was unable to participate in discussions regarding these issues.

To gain insight into the ethical issues involved in the situation, one must be familiar with four fundamental ethical principles: beneficence, non-maleficence, autonomy, and justice. Beneficence, to "do good," dictates that the health care team attempt everything possible to preserve life. This principle underscores a commitment to the sanctity of life. Nonmaleficence directs health care personnel to do no harm (*primum non nocere*) and to alleviate suffering. Autonomy signifies that the patient is in charge. A legally competent adult who is not trying to commit suicide is the sole determiner of his or her own body. Thus, it is incumbent upon the physician or health care team to allow the patient to determine what should be done. If the patient is legally incompetent, then a legal surrogate must be identified. The fourth ethical principle, justice, entails fair allocation of medical resources. Derived from these four ethical principles, three key practical guidelines can assist in the decision as to whether or not to withhold or withdraw basic or advanced life support. First, it is necessary to identify who has decision-making authority. On the basis of the ethical principle of autonomy, the patient is always the primary authority. If the patient is legally incompetent, a legal surrogate must be found. If there is no family or loved ones, an interdisciplinary committee must be formed to serve as a legal surrogate or a state law that might dictate a different approach should be followed. The second practical guideline is to establish effective and sensitive communication with patients and families. The third practical guideline is to determine early in the course of a critical illness the patient's beliefs regarding quality of life issues and his or her wishes for extensive support and efforts to prolong life.

After the consultant decided that the present patient had essentially no chance of regaining a reasonable quality of life, he discussed the appropriateness of continued support with the referring cardiovascular surgeons. The surgeons requested that the consultant act as a facilitator in discussions with the family concerning withdrawal of advanced life support. The consultant explained the patient's prognosis and unlikely probability for recovery. Three days later, the family decided to withdraw advanced life support and the patient died.

Clinical Pearls

1. Ethical decision-making requires an understanding of four general ethical principles: beneficence, nonmaleficence, autonomy, and justice.

2. Three key practical guidelines are commonly used in ethical decision making: (1) to identify who is the source of authority; (2) to establish effective and sensitive communication with patients and families; and (3) to determine at an early stage what the individual believes about quality of life issues and what the patient's desires are for decision making.

REFERENCES
1. Ruark JE, Raffin TA, and the Stanford University Medical Center Committee on Ethics: Initiating and withdrawing life support: Principles and practices in adult medicine. N Engl J Med 318:25–30, 1988.
2. Luce JM, Raffin TA: Withholding and withdrawal of life support from critically ill patients. Chest 94:621–625, 1988.
3. Raffin TA: ICU survival in patients with systemic illness. Am Rev Respir Dis, in press.

PATIENT 2

A 44-year-old woman in a chronic persistent vegetative state for 9 months following a motor vehicle accident

A 44-year-old woman was in coma for 9 months following a motor vehicle accident. She was being fed by a nasogastric tube and did not respond to command or deep pain. Two neurology consultants agreed that she met the definition of being in a chronic persistent vegetative state. Her husband and family believed that she had essentially no chance to regain a reasonable quality of life and that her nasogastric tube feedings and other basic life support should be withdrawn.

Physical Examination: Vital signs normal. Neurologic: coma, no response to verbal commands or painful stimuli.

Laboratory Findings: Routine blood tests normal. Chest radiograph: normal.

Should basic life support be withdrawn?

Diagnosis: Chronic persistent vegetative state.

Discussion: The present patient is in a chronic vegetative state and is dependent on basic life support for survival. Withdrawal of life support will result in death. The goal of the physician and health care team is to determine what the patient would have wanted.

The principle of the need to identify the substituted judgment of the patient was established in the Karen Ann Quinlan case, which was adjudicated in 1976. In situations such as these, Living Wills are extremely helpful. In the absence of a Living Will, the family and loved ones can help to identify what the patient thought about quality of life issues before a serious illness. Their input can assist in determining whether or not the patient would have wanted to remain on nasogastric tube feeding if there were essentially no chance for regaining a reasonable quality of life.

The withdrawal of basic life support, such as hydration or nutrition by nasogastric feeding tubes or intravenous lines, is controversial at present. Of interest, approximately 15 states have supported the withdrawal of basic life support from patients in a chronic persistent vegetative state. In 1986, Massachusetts in the case of Brophy v. New England Sinai Hospital supported the withdrawal of nutrition and hydration from a fireman who was in a chronic persistent vegetative state. The Massachusetts court took this position because the evidence revealed the patient would never regain cognitive behavior, the ability to communicate, or the capability to interact purposefully with his environment. Most state courts that have addressed the withdrawal of nutrition and hydration from incompetent patients in chronic persistent vegetative states have treated it in the same way as withdrawal of advanced life support. There is no fundamental ethical difference, and thus far in 15 states there is clearly no legal difference.

Whenever discussing the withdrawal of basic or advanced life support, it is important for the physician or health care team member to discuss with the family or loved ones whether or not they feel any guilt. In most situations, families and loved ones experience guilt about the death of someone they love, and it is important to discuss these issues before the person has died. Some of the most damaging psychological trauma that occurs to families and loved ones following the death of a relative can be due to their own misgivings or guilt about some insignificant action they took in the past.

Clinical Pearls

1. Fifteen states have supported the withdrawal of basic life support from patients in a chronic persistent vegetative state. However, it is important that individual physicians and health care teams be familiar with their own state laws.

2. There is little ethical difference between the withdrawal of basic or advanced life support.

3. When considering withdrawal of basic or advanced life support from legally incompetent patients, the goal is to identify the patient's "substituted judgment." To do so, it is vital to communicate effectively with families and loved ones in order to understand what the patient would have wanted. By so doing, the ethical and legal principle of autonomy is upheld.

REFERENCES

1. Presidents Commission for the Study of Ethical Problems in Medicine and Biomedical and Behavioral Research: Deciding to Forego Life-Sustaining Treatment. Washington, D.C., U.S. Government Printing Office, 1983.
2. Brophy v. New England Sinai Hospital NESH, 497 N.E. 2d 626, Mass. 1986.
3. Ruark JE, Raffin TA, and the Stanford University Medical Center Committee on Ethics: Initiating and withdrawing life support: Principles and practices in adult medicine. N Engl J Med 318:25–30, 1988.

PATIENT 3

A 58-year-old man with severe COPD and respiratory failure who no longer wants aggressive treatment

A 58-year-old man with severe COPD has had severe dyspnea at rest for 2 years. He has been on multiple medications and continuous oxygen therapy. He has been admitted to the intensive care unit eight times in the preceding 12 months and has been on mechanical ventilation 4 times. He believes, as does his wife and family, that his quality of life is poor and he no longer wants aggressive medical treatment. He is in the emergency room and asks for your assistance.

Physical Examination: Pulse 148; respirations 52. Thin, extremely ill man in severe respiratory distress; markedly decreased breath sounds with a few rales and wheezes. Chest: decreased breath sounds.

Laboratory Findings: Hct 48%; WBC 11,000/μl. ABG (FiO$_2$ 0.30): pH: 7.26, PCO$_2$ 72 mm Hg, PO$_2$ 47 mm Hg. Chest radiograph (below): hyperinflation and changes compatible with severe COPD.

Should aggressive therapy be given to this patient?

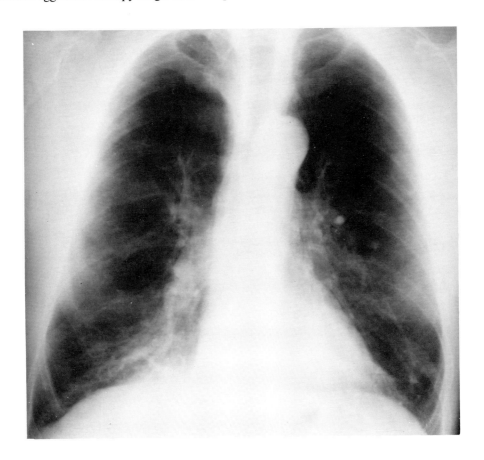

Diagnosis: Severe end-stage COPD in patient with respiratory failure.

Discussion: The present patient had end-stage COPD and no longer wanted to be admitted to an intensive care unit and placed on advanced life support. He was asking to be admitted to the hospital and to have his physician and health care team alleviate his suffering. This does not mean that the physician and health care team will help the patient to die. What it does mean is that they will provide pain-relieving medication if the patient is in significant discomfort from severe dyspnea.

In the same way we care for patients with terminal cancer or other terminal diseases, we often must care for patients with terminal COPD who do not want to die on a mechanical ventilator. Our goals as physicians are to restore health and to relieve suffering. It is crucial in a situation such as this to make sure that the patient, family, and loved ones have a clear understanding of the medical plan. In other words, if the patient has a cardiopulmonary arrest, the patient will not be resuscitated.

Furthermore, if the patient is being treated with morphine for severe discomfort from dyspnea, then the patient, family, and loved ones should know that morphine will probably hasten death, but that it is being given only to relieve suffering and will not be given in quantities specifically and purposefully to promote the patient's death. Morphine should be administered for pain to a patient with terminal COPD who no longer wants aggressive care in the same way it is delivered to patients with terminal cancer who no longer want aggressive care.

In this situation, it is important to write a "Do Not Resuscitate" order in the chart once the patient has given informed consent. It is always important to establish the code status of patients as early as possible. "Do Not Resuscitate" orders should be written and clearly noted in inpatient and outpatient records. It is a good idea to have a special sticker on the outside of charts to enable physicians to be aware of code status in emergencies.

If there is any difficulty in communication between the physician or health care team member and the patient, family or loved ones, then a facilitator should be called in. A facilitator is a person with special communication skills, such as a chaplain, priest, rabbi, social worker, or psychotherapist. Even though the physician may have good communication with the patient, family, or loved ones, a facilitator can be of tremendous value because he or she has the skill and the time to communicate effectively with all involved. Usually, physicians and other members of the health care team are under tremendous stress and have too little time to achieve the quality of communication that all would desire.

A "Do Not Resuscitate" order was written in the chart of the present patient, and he was not intubated. He received dyspnea-relieving medications and died 36 hours after admission.

Clinical Pearls

1. If the patient no longer wishes to receive aggressive care for terminal COPD or other diseases, it is entirely appropriate to use morphine to relieve suffering. The goal is not to hasten death but to relieve suffering.

2. It is important to establish as early as possible the "code" status of patients. "Do Not Resuscitate" orders should be written in inpatient and outpatient records. Unfortunately, timely determinations in many practice settings are the exception rather than the rule.

3. If there is any difficulty with communication, a facilitator should be called.

REFERENCES
1. Hyers TM, Briggs DD, Hudson LD, et al: Withholding and withdrawing mechanical ventilation. Am Rev Respir Dis 134:1327–1330, 1986.
2. Lo B, Saika G, Strull W, et al: Do-not-resuscitate decisions—A prospective study at three teaching hospitals. Ann Intern Med 145:1115–1117, 1985.
3. Bedell SE, Pelle D, Meher PL, et al: Do-not-resuscitate orders for critically ill patients in the hospital: How are they used and what is their impact? JAMA 256:233–237, 1986.

PATIENT 4

A 28-year-old man with fever, dyspnea, and hypoxemic respiratory failure from *Pneumocystis carinii* pneumonia

A 28-year-old man presented with a 5-month history of fatigue, cough, and increasing dyspnea on exertion. The patient gave a history of being in a high-risk group for AIDS.

Physical Examination: Temperature 101.1°; respirations 44. Thin, chronically ill appearing male with severe respiratory distress. ENT: thrush. Chest: bilateral rales.

Laboratory Findings: WBC 6,200/μl, 15% lymphocytes. ABG (100% O_2 face mask): pH 7.36, PCO_2 49 mm Hg, PO_2 53 mm Hg. Induced sputum: *Pneumocystis carinii.* Chest radiograph (below): diffuse bilateral infiltrates.

Because the patient had a poor prognosis for surviving intubation and mechanical ventilation, the health care team considered writing a "Do Not Resuscitate" order.

What issues should be considered when contemplating a "Do Not Resuscitate" order?

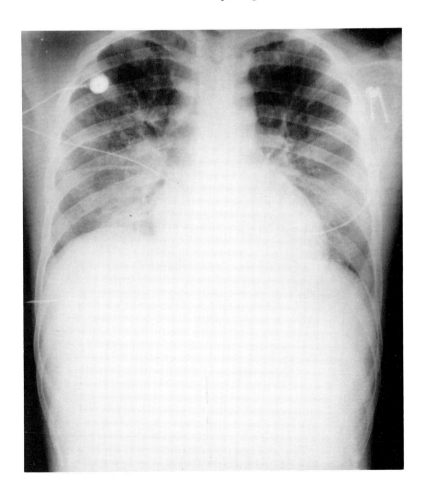

Diagnosis: AIDS with *Pneumocystis carinii* pneumonia and respiratory failure.

Discussion: The present patient had AIDS and respiratory failure from *Pneumocystis carinii* pneumonia. The severity of his hypoxic respiratory failure indicated that he would require intubation and mechanical ventilation for survival. Of paramount importance is the understanding that only this young man can make this decision. If he was legally incompetent, then the decision would be made by his legal surrogate, such as family or loved ones.

Physicians are increasingly being called upon to help make difficult decisions about intensive care for patients with AIDS. In most previous published studies, patients with AIDS who are in respiratory failure have a poor prognosis, with a mortality from 85 to 100%. In the past 2 years, however, several new studies have indicated improved outcomes. Recent data from San Francisco indicate that the mortality rate for AIDS patients in respiratory failure who require mechanical ventilation is closer to 55 to 70%. It is not yet clear whether this increased survival is due to changes in patient selection or improved treatment.

Physicians and health care team members must optimize truth-telling in order to facilitate optimal decision making. Since communication is difficult and emotionally wrenching in these situations, it is important to create an environment that optimizes communication. Physicians and health care providers should be sensitive to the fact that stress often impairs the judgment of patients and families. Patients and families should be encouraged to ask questions and express feelings. Not only does this help to decrease their intimidation, but it also provides the physician and health care team members an opportunity to verify whether they have been clearly understood.

It is extremely useful for patients to have filled out Living Wills. Forty states have passed Living Will legislation. Some states refer to them as Living Wills, whereas others use the names Natural Death Act Directive or Durable Power of Attorney for Health Care. In a Living Will a person can state that, if there is no chance to regain a reasonable quality of life, life support be either withheld or withdrawn. This is of great assistance to families and loved ones, because in most situations patients have not expressed their ideas about quality of life to the people closest to them.

Most individuals who are asked whether or not they would support a "Do Not Resuscitate" order being written decide against it. They would like a chance to see if advanced life support could provide an increased chance of survival with a reasonable quality of life. It is recommended that when patients refuse to accept a "Do Not Resuscitate" order, the health care provider ask a second question: Does the patient wish advanced life support to be stopped after 72 hours if it looks as though there is essentially no chance to regain a reasonable quality of life? Most patients would support withdrawing life support if this second question is asked. Physicians and health care providers should be prepared to ask seriously ill patients both questions.

The present patient decided after difficult deliberation to undergo intubation and mechanical ventilation. He died 2 weeks later.

Clinical Pearls

1. Over the past 5 years, AIDS patients who are in respiratory failure and require mechanical ventilation have had mortality rates ranging from 85 to 100%. Recently, several groups have reported lower mortality rates ranging from 55 to 70%. Patients with AIDS must be made aware of these changing statistics.

2. It is helpful for patients to have Living Wills before they become critically ill. Forty states have passed Living Will legislation. The great majority of patients, including health care providers, do not have Living Wills.

3. Physicians and other health care providers should talk with seriously ill patients about whether or not they wish to have a "Do Not Resuscitate" order. If the patient requests full CPR, a second question should be asked: Would the patient want advanced life support withdrawn after 72 hours if, in the judgment of the physicians and health care team, the patient has, in essence, no chance to regain a reasonable quality of life?

REFERENCES

1. Gilfix M, Raffin TA: Withholding and withdrawing extraordinary life support: Optimizing rights and limiting liability. West J Med 141:387–394, 1984.
2. Raffin TA: Value of the living will. Chest 90:444–446, 1986.
3. Steinbrook R, Lo B, Moulton J, et al: Preferences of homosexual men with AIDS for life sustaining treatment. N Engl J Med 314:457–460, 1986.
4. Wachter RM, Luce JM, Lo B, et al: Life-sustaining treatment for patients with the acquired immunodeficiency syndrome. Chest 95:647–652, 1989.

INDEX

Page numbers of complete chapters are in **boldface** type.